治癌实录

续新

吴　锦　吴宇光　王　俊◎著

中国科学技术出版社

·北京·

图书在版编目（CIP）数据

治癌实录续新 / 吴锦，吴宇光，王俊著 . — 北京：中国科学技术出版社，2024.5

ISBN 978-7-5236-0476-2

Ⅰ . ①治… Ⅱ . ①吴… ②吴… ③王… Ⅲ . ①肿瘤—中西医结合—诊疗 Ⅳ . ① R73

中国国家版本馆 CIP 数据核字 (2024) 第 040488 号

策划编辑	韩　翔　于　雷
责任编辑	于　雷
文字编辑	卢兴苗
装帧设计	佳木水轩
责任印制	李晓霖

出　　版	中国科学技术出版社
发　　行	中国科学技术出版社有限公司发行部
地　　址	北京市海淀区中关村南大街 16 号
邮　　编	100081
发行电话	010-62173865
传　　真	010-62179148
网　　址	http://www.cspbooks.com.cn

开　　本	710mm×1000mm　1/16
字　　数	198 千字
印　　张	24.25
版　　次	2024 年 5 月第 1 版
印　　次	2024 年 5 月第 1 次印刷
印　　刷	北京盛通印刷股份有限公司
书　　号	ISBN 978-7-5236-0476-2/R·3181
定　　价	68.00 元

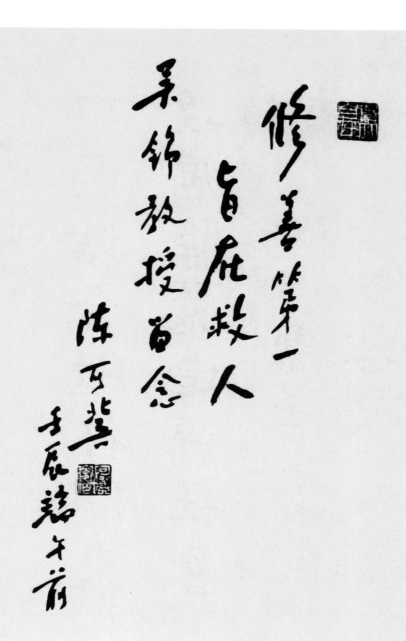

修善篤第一
旨在救人

采锦教授留念

陈可冀
壬辰禧午前

中国科学院院士、中国中医科学院陈可冀教授题词

為吳錦教授題詞

中西結合繼往開來
攻癌降魔造福社會

鄭耀宗 教授

中国科学院院士、香港大学前校长郑耀宗教授题词

為吳錦教授題詞

中西結合
造福人羣

周肇平 教授

香港中西医结合医学会创会会长、香港大学医学院前院长周肇平教授题词

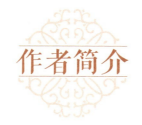

作者简介

　　吴　锦　我国首位获得中西医结合医学博士学位的教授。曾任国家卫生部临床药理基地主任、中国中医科学院研究员、香港大学中医药学院创院教授、香港中文大学中医学院客座教授等。长期带领团队进行中西医结合的深入研究，运用天然有效的生命修复方法，在各类癌症和疑难病症的治疗方面取得了重大成就。

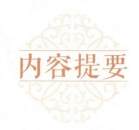

内容提要

　　恶性肿瘤死亡率在我国疾病谱中居首位，且高于世界平均水平。世界卫生组织提出，1/3 的癌症完全可以预防，1/3 的癌症可以通过早期发现得到根治，1/3 的癌症可以运用现有的医疗措施延长生命、减轻痛苦、提高生活质量。早期发现、早期诊断、早期治疗是预防癌症的关键。

　　本书作者为资深中西医结合治疗肿瘤学专家，她将自己从事中西医抗癌工作的亲身经历与智慧融入书中，用深入浅出、通俗易懂的语言向读者分享了自己治疗癌症的经验与心得。全书共两部分，第一部分作者用临证过程中 51 位患者的真实病案，简要描述了中医药治疗癌症的经过及用药；第二部分是较为详细地介绍了作者根据长期经验总结的日常养生和康复方法。

　　本书语言通俗易懂，病案真实可信，适合广大中医临床工作者、癌症患者及家属、中医药爱好者阅读参考。

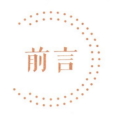

前言

　　癌症是全球最严重的疾病，根据国际最新癌症流行病学数据，大约每天新增 5300 个癌症患者。男性终生患癌率为 40.2%，女性为 38.5%。癌症发病年龄降低，发病率升高是总的趋势。随着全球人口增长和预期寿命增加，癌症逐渐成为常见病和多发病。

　　最新报道指出，全球癌症发病率仍呈迅速上升趋势。世界卫生组织（简称世卫组织）公布的最新数据表明，每年有 1000 多万人死于癌症，有 1930 多万新发癌症病例。我国每年癌症死亡人数达 300 万，居高不下，尤其是在我国香港，癌症已是头号杀手，短短 20 年间新症增幅高达 60%。

　　人人都想拥有健康的身体，但往往事与愿违。虽然医学在不断进步，癌症的发病率和死亡率却年年攀升。当前现代医学治疗癌症，主要是化疗、放疗、手术和靶向、免疫等抗癌药物。然而，治疗未必理想和有效，患者往往竭力忍受治疗带来的痛苦，却仍然避免不了癌症复发、转移，最终失去生命，这样的案例数不胜数。前来诊治的大多都是晚期，常规治疗无效的患者。尽管如此，生命修复中医药治疗仍然取得了良好的治疗效果。其疗效的关键在于不能因循守旧，治癌理论和临床治疗必须有发展和创新。

　　本书在已出版的治癌实录系列丛书基础上，通过真实病案介绍了晚期癌症患者采用中医药生命修复疗法，达到生命之树常青的效果。书中介绍的所有病案都是真实的，仅是我们多年来治疗患者中的少数代表。有些患者愿意公开自己的照片，以鼓励更多的患者；有些患者不愿公开照片，则对照片面部进行了遮挡处理。

书中列出了不同癌症的主要治疗原则和常用中药，治疗所用药物全部都是天然中药，没有化学合成药，也没有毒性强烈的药物。因为我们根本就没有考虑过使用强烈杀伤的方式去治疗癌症。中医药生命修复疗法治疗癌症方面的效果确切，目前我们总结了大量晚期癌症的病例，并进行了医学统计学处理。结果显示，治疗效果明确，且显著优于当前国际所见和各地报道。

书中的 51 个真实病案，一些是经治疗后长期健康生活的病例；另一些是在本书出版时，虽治疗时间不长，但已有康复趋势的病例。这些足以证实中医药生命修复疗法在抗癌治疗的不同阶段均有明确疗效。

本书介绍的养生和康复方法，是除了药物治疗外，可以长期锻炼且有利于健康的方法。随着社会的发展，不断有新的有损健康或易导致疾病的各种因素出现，我们更应遵循自然规律时代行之有效的健身方法和日常生活方式，将防癌、抗癌作为重要的关注点，为维护公众及个人健康而共同努力。

希望患者朋友可以抛开担忧和压力，树立信心，鼓起勇气，把握时机，科学治疗，一定能够与癌抗争，并战胜癌症。中医药学博大精深，源远流长，我们希望能够继续发扬光大，以便为患者、为社会贡献微薄之力。

吴　锦

liferepairjmt@gmail.com

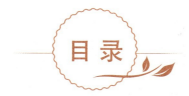

目 录

为癌症患者却病延年

晚期肺癌康复 25 年

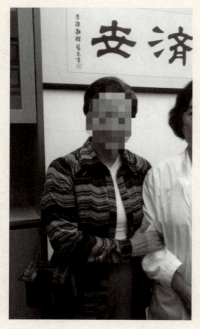

❶ 李太太于 2024 年 2 月前来诊治时合影留念

李太太曾于 20 世纪 90 年代患气管炎、肺气肿等慢性病，常有咳嗽、胸闷、痰多等症状，起初以为不是大病，但几个月都不见好转，遂再次去医院检查，经医院检查后确诊是患上肺癌第 Ⅲ 期，按照医师的建议是尽快做手术。李太太于 1999 年确诊后立即动手术，切除了肺部的 2 个肿瘤，手术后病理报告证实为肺腺癌。后又经过 1 年多的休养，感觉身体有些气力了，心想从此便可以放心了。没想到才刚过 2 年，于 2002 年年初又开始出现咳嗽、气短、胸闷等症状，经检查发现是肿瘤复发，双肺发现了 4 个肿瘤病灶。李太太到处找专家会诊，但都认为病情极其严重，且因双肺都有肿瘤，不适宜再次手术，并无确实有效的治疗方法。在这种束手无策的情况下，只好选择前来求助于我。

当时她身体状态很差，精神压力也很大，瘦弱不堪，胸闷、气短、呼吸困难，每次呼气之后，都需要大口换气，并不能正常自如的呼吸。经过我们认真细致的辨证分析及治疗，半年多后，她的 4 个肿瘤病灶全部消失。从患肿瘤至今，已经过去了 25 年，李太太一直持劳家务，健康快乐地生活着，并且每年都会检查身体，状况亦正常良好。晚期肺癌是当今常见，且是死亡率最高的恶性肿瘤之一。李太太虽经手术切除肿瘤，仍不能避免复发。因她年龄较大，手术后，长期有劳损虚弱的表现，加上肿瘤复发，生长速度快，有虚实夹杂的复杂情况，治疗中应当攻补兼施，祛邪与扶正并重，终使患者恢复健康。

如今 86 岁的李太太，完全称得上是健康高寿了。她从未做过化疗、放疗及靶向、免疫等治疗，仅靠生命修复的传统中医药治疗恢复健康。

治疗原则

益气固本，软坚化瘀，消瘤。

常用中药

1. 黄芪、人参、西洋参、龙葵、山慈菇、石见穿、土鳖虫、生大黄、杏仁等。
2. 同时服用消瘤丸。

影像学、病理学检查报告及诊疗记录

1. 2002 年 6 月检查报告显示，肺癌手术后，肺部发现 4 个新的肿瘤病灶，分别位于右肺下叶、左肺底部、右肺底部、左肺上叶。

2. 2002 年 12 月检查报告显示治疗效果很好，双肺、纵隔、肺门、胸膜、胸壁和骨等部位均无肿瘤复发。

3. 2015 年 11 月检查报告显示双肺病灶钙化和形成瘢痕，无肿瘤复发。

4. 2018 年 4 月检查报告显示无肿瘤复发迹象。

5. 2022 年 10 月 25 日 CT 检查报告显示，肺部有钙化结节、无肿瘤复发。

附：患者检查报告

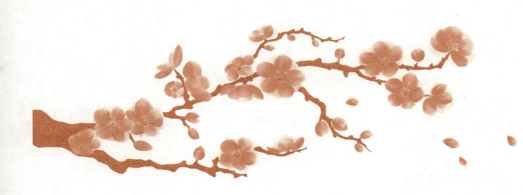

■ ■ ■■■■ HOSPITAL
· **SCANNING DEPARTMENT**
(CT, MR, NM, Mammography, U/S, Bone Densitometry)
■■ ■

Tel.: ■■■■ ■■ ■■■■■

REPORT FOR MRI/CT/NM SCANNING EXAMINATION

OUR REF. :	■■ ■ ■	**EXAM. DATE :**	**Tue, 18 Jun, 2002**
NAME :	Tse■■ ■		
ID No. :	■		
AGE / SEX:	64 F	**HOSPITAL :**	OUT-PATIENT
DATE :	Tue, 18 Jun, 2002		
EXAM. :	CT of Thorax		
CONTRAST MEDIUM :	Iopamiro 370	**REF. DR. :**	■ ■■■ ■

Time Report Leaves Department Delivery
Tue, 18 Jun, 2002   PM DHL

CLINICAL HISTORY:

Bronchioalveolar cell carcinoma for follow-up. Small meningioma in brain, definite, not a metastasis also for follow-up.

RADIOLOGICAL REPORT:

5 mm collimation high resolution axial helical scans have been performed with and without contrast injection. One set of non-contrast images from the previous examination on 1 December, 2001 is also printed for comparison. A minute 2 mm nodule is shown in the anterior aspect of the right lower lung field is again shown (page 4, image 39). This lesion was present in previous examination also image 39. Previous opinion was said it is benign and this is a correct diagnosis. In the meantime the lesion has not increase in size at all.

There are total of four new lesions identifiable. One is located in the antero-medial aspect of the right lower lung about 2.5 cm above the level of the 2 mm lesion and shown in image 34. Its size is 26 x 19 mm along the transaxial plane. It is immediately subpleural in location and close to midline. Prior to contrast injection, density measurement ranging from 5 to 20. After contrast injection, there is enhancement ranging from 15 units to 40 units. A second lesion is shown in the shape of a fan and it is quite small in size measuring no more than 2 cm in diameter and is located in the posterior portion of the left lung base (image 47). It did not exist in previous examination. A third lesion is noted in the posterior right lung base. It is quite hazy in character and poorly defined in the boundaries. 1 mm images show the same characteristics. It may well be an area of pneumonitis and so is the second lesion. A fourth lesion is shown which is of the same hazy character and located in the postero-medial aspect of the left upper lung.

Post-contrast scan shows no sign of any mediastinal or hilar lymphadenopathy. Regional bones show no metastatic disease.

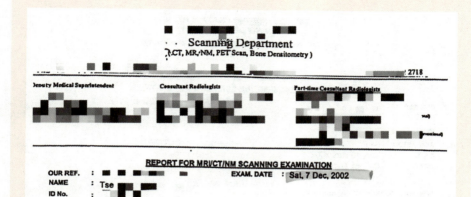

Scanning Department
(CT, MR, NM, PET Scan, Bone Densitometry)

2718

Deputy Medical Superintendent   Consultant Radiologists   Part-time Consultant Radiologists

REPORT FOR MRI/CT/NM SCANNING EXAMINATION

OUR REF.   :
NAME   : Tse
ID No.   :
AGE / SEX   : 64 F
DATE   : Mon, 9 Dec, 2002
EXAM.   : CT of Thorax

EXAM. DATE   : Sat, 7 Dec, 2002

HOSPITAL   : OUT-PATIENT

REF. DR.   :

Time Report Leaves Department
Mon, 9 Dec, 2002   AM DHL

CONTRAST MEDIUM : Iopamiro 370

CLINICAL HISTORY:

Bronchio-alveolar cell tumour, treated, for sequential follow-up.

RADIOLOGISAL REPORT:

Helical scan has been performed with high resolution technique. Left upper lung field shows linear densities representing scars both in the peripheral lung and in the perihilar region. Comparison with previous examination indicates that all the shadows existing in the lungs were previously presented including the small nodule in the anterior aspect of the right lung base (image 44) which has not been enlarging at all with the passage of time. Post-contrast scan demonstrates that the different major areas of the mediastinum are also normal without enlarged lymph node while the regional bones including the thoracic spine show no sign of plastic or lytic lesion.

OPINION :

This post-treatment follow-up study is quite satisfactory. Last examination was done exactly 3 months ago in 7th Sept. 2002. No change is observed and there is no sign of any recurrence of tumour in the lungs, mediastinum, hilum, pleural space, regional bones or chest wall.

NO. OF FILMS: 9 14" x 17"

SIGNED:

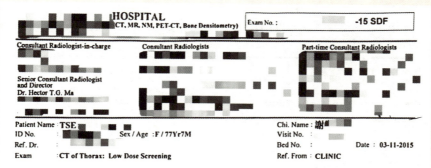

HOSPITAL
(CT, MR, NM, PET-CT, Bone Densitometry)   Exam No. :   ▪ -15 SDF

Consultant Radiologist-in-charge	Consultant Radiologists	Part-time Consultant Radiologists

Senior Consultant Radiologist
and Director
Dr. Hector T.G. Ma

Patient Name : **TSE** ▪ ▪   Chi. Name : 謝▪▪
ID No.   :   Sex / Age : F / 77Yr7M   Visit No. :
Ref. Dr.   :   Bed No. :   Date : 03-11-2015
Exam   : CT of Thorax: Low Dose Screening   Ref. From : CLINIC

Clinical Information / History:

Remote history of alveolar cell carcinoma of lung (left side as I remember). Treated in Sloan Kettering Cancer Center in New York and cured. For routine follow-up.

Radiological Report:

Left hilum is elevated which is related to previous surgical procedure. Localised pleural thickening is found along mediastinal aspect of left pleural space. Excessive pericardial fat pad is shown in the left sided cardiophrenic angle. Lungs are clear with no sign of any recurrence of lung neoplasm. Minimal scarring is shown in different locations of left lung. Several small calcific nodules are found in different areas of the right and left lungs. Hilum and mediastinum as well as axilla and supraclavicular regions are normal.

OPINION:

Scarring and calcification sites are found in different areas of both lungs but there is no suggestion of recurrence of lung malignancy identified.

NO. OF FILMS 7   14" x 17"   (DDMM) (HHMM)   REPORT & FILMS SENT OUT :
NO. OF COLOR PRINTS   NO. OF CDR 1   'WET' FILMS SENT   03-11-2015
Remark : 1 old film   RETURNED

Report No. : ▪ ▪   Authorized and Reported
                                                          on 03-11-2015 @ 16:56 by

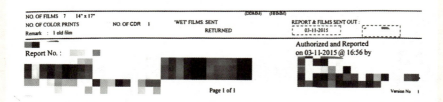

Page 1 of 1   Version No 1

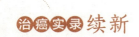

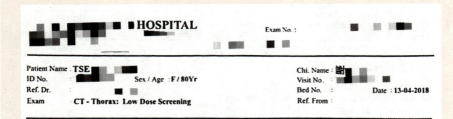

HOSPITAL   Exam No. :

Patient Name : TSE	Chi. Name : 謝
ID No. : Sex / Age : F / 80Yr	Visit No. :
Ref. Dr. :	Bed No. : Date : 13-04-2018
Exam : CT - Thorax: Low Dose Screening	Ref. From :

IMAGING REPORT:

Clinical Information:

Remote history of alveolar cell carcinoma of lung (left side) treated in Sloan Kettering Cancer Center in New York. For long term follow-up.

Imaging Technique:

Non-contrast axial helical scan of the thorax with low dose technique was performed.

Imaging Findings:

Linear five calcified fibrotic scars are noted in the anterior aspect of the left apex. Tiny calcified granuloma is also shown in the posteromedial aspect of the right mid lung. Another non-calcified nodule is also shown in the medial aspect of the right mid lung. Major airway shows rather extensive wall calcifications and spotty calcifications are also found in the aortic arch. No other abnormal shadow is noted in both lung fields and the appearance of the lungs is about the same as in previous examination performed in November 2015.

Opinion:

No active disease is shown in the lungs. History of alveolar cell carcinoma treated back in the remote past is noted. There is no sign of malignant recurrence. Tiny non-calcified and calcified but non-active tuberculomas are shown in the lungs. No active disease of any kind is noted at this point in time.

No. of image prints : 4   No. of DVD : 1

Remark :

Report No. :

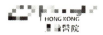

Patient ID:	Case No:
	Patient Type: OutPatient ()
Name: TSE	Referrer: Dr
	Sherwin
Sex: F DOB:	Exam Date: 25.10.2022
Accession No:	

Radiological Examination Report

IMPRESSION:

Reference made with previous CT dated 24-Sep-2021 at ▒▒▒ hospital.

1. Evidence of left upper lobectomy and wedge resection. No definite gross focal mass lesion detected over the surgical sites to suggest local recurrence. Compensatory hyperinflation of the rest of the left lung is noted.

2. Atelectasis is noted in the right middle and lower lobes.   Bilateral dependent basal atelectases noted.

3. A small left lower lobe lung cyst measuring 0.9cm is seen, which is similar.

4. A ground-glass opacity measuring 1.1x0.7cm is seen in the right upper lobe of the lung showing no significant interval change.

5. Calcified granulomas measuring 0.5cm are seen in the medial right upper lobe and posterior right upper lobe.   A calcified nodule measuring 0.6x0.5cm is similarly seen in the right middle lobe of the lung.

6. Nodularity seen in the right adrenal, which is similar.

7. A left renal cyst measuring 6.6cm is seen.   A tiny non-obstructive right renal stone measuring 0.2cm with CT number of 150HU is noted.

8. Coarse benign calcifications in both breasts measuring up to 0.2cm.

Dr
Consultant Radiologist
MBBS (HK), FRCR, FHKCR, FHKAM (Radiology)

Approved Date: 26.10.2022 08:39

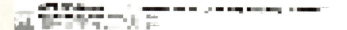

病案 2

重症肌无力和乳腺癌康复 20 年

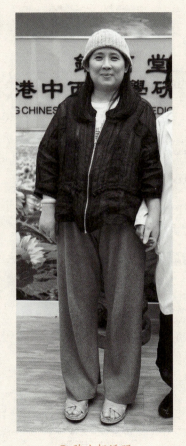

❶ 陈小姐近照

2004 年，陈小姐得了严重的疾病，开始的时候她只是感觉双腿疼痛，随后开始无力走路并且逐渐加重，到医院就诊却一直检查不出原因，只能一直不停地看病和吃药。但是全身和双腿的无力状况越来越严重，甚至到后来完全不能行走。2008 年，她不仅完全不能走路，需要坐在轮椅上，同时还出现了眼睑下垂、不能吃东西、嘴巴张不开、吞咽困难、双手无力抬起等严重症状，并伴有全身抽筋、疼痛、呼吸困难，经医院检查确诊为重症肌无力。此后，她不停地前往医院进行各种治疗。2009 年，她在医院接受住院治疗长达数月还是没有任何好转，医生亦不讳言，告知重症肌无力是由于神经传导异常引起的，因此没有好的治疗方法，只能靠打针、用药来维持非常短时间的作用，除此之外，没有更好的治疗方法。

2011 年，陈小姐坐着轮椅找到我们，希望采用中医药生命修复疗法治疗。她当时的身体非常虚弱，气喘、严重呼吸困难、眼睑下垂，坐在轮椅上亦没有一点力气，不仅不能够站起来，不能抬起双腿，而且双手无力症状非常严重，连一张纸都拿不起来，属于完全瘫痪的状态。在这样严重的情况下，她的生命随时面临危险，只能求助于生命修复的中医药治疗。于是我们给她精心治疗，全身调理，并根据她的具体情况，进行五脏六腑，十二条经络的调补，经过一段时间治疗，她逐渐感觉身体有一点力气了，可以慢慢地吃一点流质固体的食物，也可以慢慢地抬起双手去做一些简单的动作。随后她可以慢慢地自己写字、洗脸、刷牙，双腿也可以活动一点了，例如短暂的抬腿，慢慢地站立和行走一段距离，一步一步地慢慢恢复。

到 2013 年，陈小姐可以自行站立和行走，身体状况完全恢复了，没有人看得出她曾经是一个瘫痪的、坐在轮椅上完全不能动的严重患者。陈小姐千恩万谢、高高兴兴地离开了。大约过了 1 年，陈小姐又来找我们。她这次来全程是自己走进来的，与正常人行走没有任何区别。她非常感激地说出回来的原因，第一是来看望我们并表示感谢，第二是她又面临一个严重的问题，经过检查发现患了乳腺癌。原本她是准备采取手术切除肿瘤的方法，但是因为她曾经有重症肌无力的病史，医院方面非常担心，因重症肌无力的病史可能会在手术过程中导致生命危险，所以没有人敢给她打麻醉动手术，医生亦明确说明不能够为她动手术。

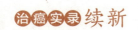

陈小姐思前想后，只好又来找我们寻求帮助。她乳腺的肿块非常明确且明显，经过检查及分析，我们尽快为其配以中药及相关治疗。经过1年多的治疗，她乳房内的肿块消失，乳腺也完全恢复正常了。后来她未再去医院做更多的检查，因为她自觉目前身体非常健康正常且高兴快乐。

重症肌无力是一种由神经-肌肉接头处传递功能障碍所引起的自身免疫性疾病，全身骨骼肌均可受累，表现为无力，不能活动。在当今，医学高度发达的情况下，仍然是疑难大病，无法治愈，再加上乳腺癌，更是雪上加霜，严重威胁到她的生命。在经过生命修复治疗之后，这两个疑难大病都治好了，真是皆大欢喜。

 治疗原则

健脾益肾，疏肝散结。

常用中药

1. 人参、黄芪、肉苁蓉、锁阳、柴胡、山慈菇、贝母、蜂房、当归、白芍等。
2. 同时服用消瘤丸。

影像学、病理学检查报告及诊疗记录

1. 2015 年 9 月 9 日和 9 月 24 日磁共振造影等检查报告证实乳腺癌，另一侧乳腺亦考虑为癌变。

2. 2015 年 8 月 10 日病理学检查报告证实为浸润性乳腺癌。

附：患者检查报告

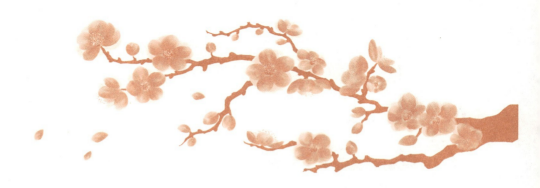

時間:2015/10/14 15:34:32

■ 醫院
■ Hospital

電子病歷

影像報告
乳房磁振造影-有/無造影劑報告

病歷號：■ ■   姓名：陳   出生日期：1967/11/15   第1頁

醫院代碼：■   帳號：■   身分證號：■   性別：女
科別：乳房醫學中心   醫師：■
檢查日期：2015/09/09   報告日期：2015/09/14   照會單號：■
報告編號：

檢查項目
MRI With/Without Contrast--Breast
疾病診斷
174.9 (ICD-9-CM_Breast cancer, female)

影像發現
Hx: biopsy proven left breast cancer, left lower breast. LMP 8/15.
Breast MRI with axial STIR, axial T1WI, axial TSE T2WI (SPAIR), axial DWI, pre-contrast and post-contrast 3D dynamic FS FLASH shows:
1. There are scattered fibroglandular densities (breast composition b) with moderate background parenchymal enhancement
2. an irregular, heterogeneous enhanced mass about 1.4cm at left deep lower central breast, compatible wtih biopsy proven breast cancer
3. there are asymmetrical clumped non-mass enhancement at left central to lower central breast, with susp appearance. Suggest tissue sampling.
* mammography showed left 12 o'clock calcifications, suggest also further correlate with left magnification views.

應斷
1). known left breast malignancy (mass at left lower central breast), suggest appropriate management
2). other is susp finding (BI-RADS 4A), left central to lower central region, suggest tissue sampling.
3). mammography showed calcifications at left upper central breast, suggest left magnification views.

確認醫師：■
--以下空白--

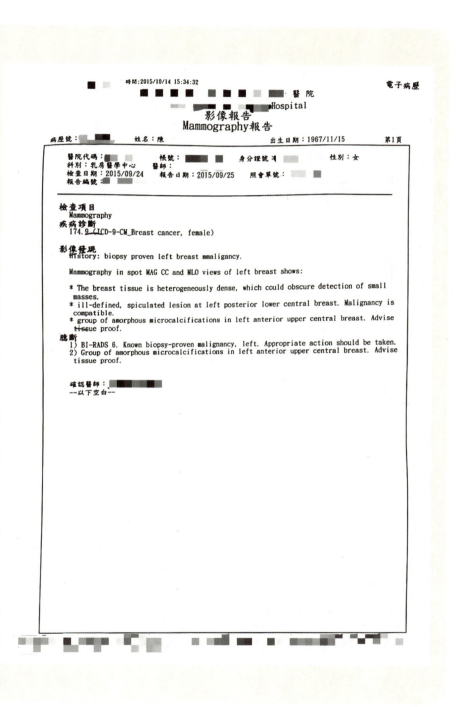

時間:2015/10/14 15:34:32 ■ ■ ■ ■ ■ 醫院　　　　　電子病歷
■ ■Hospital

影像報告
Mammography報告

病歷號：■ ■　　姓名：陳　　　　出生日期：1967/11/15　　第1頁

醫院代碼：■　　　帳號：■ ■ ■　身分證號:■　　　性別：女
科別：乳房醫學中心　醫師：
檢查日期：2015/09/24　報告日期：2015/09/25　照會單號：■ ■
報告編號：■ ■

檢查項目
Mammography

疾病診斷
174.9 (ICD-9-CM_Breast cancer, female)

影像發現
History: biopsy proven left breast mmaligancy.

Mammography in spot MAG CC and MLO views of left breast shows:

* The breast tissue is heterogeneously dense, which could obscure detection of small masses.
* ill-defined, spiculated lesion at left posterior lower central breast. Malignancy is compatible.
* group of amorphous microcalcifications in left anterior upper central breast. Advise tissue proof.

臆斷
1) BI-RADS 6. Known biopsy-proven malignancy, left. Appropriate action should be taken.
2) Group of amorphous microcalcifications in left anterior upper central breast. Advise tissue proof.

確認醫師：■ ■ ■
--以下空白--

015

時間:2015/10/14 15:33:58

電子病歷

■■■■■ 醫院
Hospital

病理部 病理組織檢查報告

MALIGNANCY

病歷號:■■■■	姓名:陳■■	出生日期:1967/11/15	第 1/1 頁
外科病理號碼:■■■■ ■		收件日期:2015/08/06	
檢體:b	科別:■■(總院)	初次報告日期:2015/08/10	
性別:女	年齡:047/09	身分證字號:■■■	

組織由來:

臨床診斷:

病理組織學診斷:

Breast, left, stated as 5.5 o'clock and 1 cm from nipple, core biopsy, invasive carcinoma of no special type

The specimen submitted consists of 5 tissue stripes measuring up tc 1.5 x 0.2 x 0.1 cm in size, fixed in formalin.

Grossly, they are yellow and soft.

All for section.   Jar 0

Microscopically, it shows infiltration of nests and focally linear cords of polygonal tumor cells in the stroma. In situ lesion is also seen. Immunohistochemically, tumor cells are positive for E-cadherin, ER(>90%) and PR(>90%). An invasive carcinoma of no special type is considered.

Ref: nil

負責醫師:■■■■■■   確認者:■■■■■■■■■■

此認此報告為惡性

西元2014年3月25日病歷委員會修正通過電子病歷版本

文件編號 ■■■■■ 版次 ■

■■■■■■■■■■■■ ■ ■■ (病歷複製本釋出專用紙)

凶险小细胞肺癌康复记

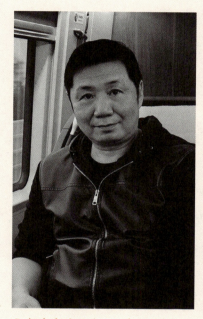

杨先生近照（2024年1月）

杨先生患有多种慢性病，如高血压、甲状腺功能亢进症、脂肪肝、肝功能障碍等。但他认为这都是些常见病、慢性病，并无大碍。当时55岁的他事业有成，孩子亦已长大无须操心，太太很能干，持家有道，让他感到生活无忧无虑，因此想要筹备一个大型的旅游计划，到处游山玩水。但是从2017年年初开始，他偶尔会有胸闷气短的感觉，起初认为问题不大，因为他既不抽烟也不喝酒，应该没有什么需要担心的。随着咳嗽越来越频繁，家人还是劝他尽快到医院做检查。初步检查的结果真是出乎意料，报告显示肺部有个很大的阴影，医院要求他尽快住院做进一步检查。住院以后，医生为其抽取肺部活组织，并进行病理检查，报告显示为小细胞肺癌，这个结果让全家人都感到非常震惊，措手不及。肺癌有很多种类型，而小细胞肺癌是其中恶性程度最高的一种，具有进展快、转移早、易复发等特点。这时杨先生全家人都笼罩在非常悲伤的情绪之中。当时经过 CT 检查，发现肺部的肿块非常大，有 8cm 左右，同时肿块已经侵犯了周围组织，支气管和肺的血管已经被肿瘤包围并堵塞了。医生建议尽快动手术以及做化疗、放疗治疗。但是他在咨询过后，认为这些治疗的效果都难以评价，长期疗效不明确，并无完全治愈的方法。

经朋友介绍，他前来要求我们给予中医药治疗。当时杨先生胸闷气短、咳嗽频繁，并且常伴有咯血的状况，在为他进行辨证分析和治疗的过程中，都配合得很好，不仅按时吃药，而且按照要求做一些全身调理，例如教他能够恢复整体免疫功能的站桩锻炼。在学习呼吸锻炼的时候，他的状况已非常虚弱，即使是站在地上练习，几分钟也坚持不下来，做 1～2 分钟就没有力气了。不过，他一直以毅力坚持，每天都练习，慢慢地能够坚持的时间也越来越长。这样治疗了数月之后，他深感症状缓解，胸部不再发闷，并且胸闷气短的感觉也消失了。随后他到医院进行复诊，医生为他再做检查，报告显示他体内的肿瘤已经消失了。2017 年 12 月再次行 CT 检查，报告同样显示其肿瘤已经消失，并且特别注明了支气管开口通畅。因为他以前的检查报告上说明，支气管是被完全堵塞了的。杨先生又去医院里找原来的主诊医生复诊，医生对这样的结果感到非常吃惊，更直言说这是不可能的，杨先生也由此深深明白生命修复中医药的效果确实很好。肿瘤消失之后，杨先生又按照医生的意见做了一些放射性的预防性治疗，同时坚持继续服用中药，现在的他已经非常健康了。然而，由于放疗的损伤，他的肝脏受到影响，引起转氨酶增高，但是这些状况都在进一步的调理中逐步恢复了。

小细胞肺癌是肺癌中恶性程度最高的类型，并且很容易发生扩散、浸润、转移。癌细胞的生长速度及复发率都较其他类型肺癌为高，所以是非常难于治疗的。最近再次见到杨先生，发现他身体非常好，完全看不出来曾经得过这样严重的疾病。他说已经7年了，朋友们都为他感到高兴，其实他在患病后，因为有很多放心不下的事情，所以早早安排好了后事，没想到现在完全康复，能够健康地生活和工作了。

治疗原则

解毒化瘀，攻邪消瘤。

常用中药

1. 重楼、蜂房、僵蚕、海浮石、八月炸、浙贝母、鱼脑石、半夏、鱼腥草、山慈菇等。
2. 同时服用消瘤丸。

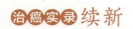

影像学、病理学检查报告及诊疗记录

1. 2017年2月23日CT检查报告证实，右下肺中心型肺癌，肿瘤大小达8.1cm×6.0cm。右肺下叶支气管闭塞，肺门及纵隔淋巴转移，淋巴结大小达4.9cm×3.2cm。

2. 2017年3月3日出院报告证实，小细胞肺癌伴多处淋巴结转移（广泛期），并患有多种疾病如高血压病、甲状腺功能亢进症、脂肪肝、肝囊肿等。

3. 2017年12月14日CT检查报告证实，肺癌8.1cm的肿瘤已消失，仅有少许慢性炎症。

附：患者检查报告

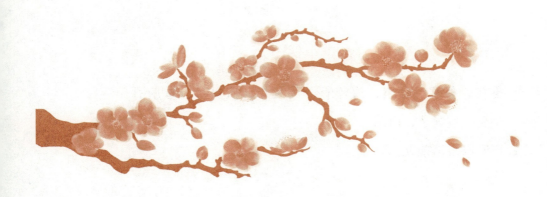

■■■■■■■■ ■医院

CT 检 查 报 告 单

门诊号：	姓名：杨	姓名拼音：YANG	性别：男	年龄：56
科别： 呼吸科二病区		影像号：	检查时间：2017-02-20 17:27	

检查项目

胸部CT平扫+增强（新）

临床诊断

右下肺门阴影伴纵隔淋巴结肿大待查：肺癌合并纵隔淋巴结转移可能

影像描述

肺窗：双肺透过度正常，右肺下叶肺门见大小约为8.1cm×6.0cm的不规则软组织肿块，右肺下叶支气管闭塞，平扫CT值为42HU，增强扫描病灶CT值最高为63HU，强化尚均匀；病变包绕右侧下肺静脉，与右心房关系密切。气管、支气管通畅，未见狭窄。叶间裂无增厚及移位。

纵隔窗：胸廓对称，胸廓骨质结构及软组织未见异常；右肺门及纵隔气管隆突下见增大淋巴结，大小约为4.9cm×3.2cm。血管结构清晰，心脏形态未见增大。肝内见多发低密度灶。

影像诊断及建议

右下肺中心型肺癌，并右肺门及隆突下淋巴结转移。

肝内多发低密度灶，囊肿可能，建议结合腹部检查。

报告医生：	审核医生：	报告时间：2017-02-23 14:55	

■■■■■■■ ■■ 医 院

出 院 介 绍 信

杨■（门诊号■■■ ■ 住院号■■■），于2017年2月13日入我院至2017年3月3日
出院，在我院住院计18天。

最后诊断：1. 右下肺小细胞癌伴右肺门、隆凸下淋巴结转移（广泛期）；2. 左锁
骨上窝多发低回声结节、双颈部淋巴结肿大伴代谢轻度增高待查；3. 右下肺阻塞性肺
炎；4. 高血压病；5. 甲状腺功能亢进症；6. 脂肪肝、肝囊肿可能、肝功能不全。

出院（转院）时病员状况：患者一般情况可，仍诉咳嗽，伴轻度恶心。查体：神志
清，精神好。双肺呼吸音粗，未闻及干湿性啰音。心律齐，腹软，无压痛，双下肢无水
肿。

需休息天数及其他建议：1. 注意休息、避免着凉；2. 出院带药：甲巯咪唑片10mg
口服 2/日（每4周复查甲状腺功能，根据甲功结果调整用药）；硝苯地平控释片30mg 口
服 1/日（监测血压，根据血压水平调整用药，心内科随诊）；富马酸比索洛尔片5mg 口
服 1/日；双环醇片50mg 口服 3/日；乙酰半胱氨酸胶囊0.2g 口服 3/日；威麦宁胶囊
2.4g 口服 3/日；盐酸昂丹司琼片 4mg 口服 2/日；3. 定期复查血常规、肝肾功能，如
出现白细胞下降，肝功能损伤可给予升白、保肝治疗；4. 2017年3月23日返院行下周
期"依托泊苷+顺铂"方案化疗；5. 定期呼吸科、肿瘤科、内分泌科随诊，不适随诊。

科主任：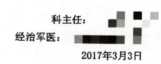

经治军医：

2017年3月3日

■■■■ ■■ ■ ■ 医院

CT诊断报告单

病人姓名:杨■	性别:男	年龄:55 岁	床号:	住院号:
病人编号:■■	科别:肝胆外科	检查日期:2017.12.14	检查号:■■	

检查设备: CT64_GE

检查项目: 胸部CT平扫+气管重建

检查方式:
轴位平扫

影像表现:

双侧肺纹理清晰,右肺下叶肺门周围可见片状异常密度影,各大支气管及分支开口通畅,右侧胸膜增厚;纵隔及双肺门区未见肿大的淋巴结影。

印象:

右肺下叶肺门周围片状异常密度影,考虑感染可能,建议治疗后复查;右侧胸膜增厚

(原肺癌 8.5×6cm)

报告医师:■ 报告日期: 2017.12.14

审核医师:■ 审核日期: 2017.12.14

*本报告谨供临床医师参考,不作为法律依据!

病案4

晚期恶性间皮瘤康复 15 年

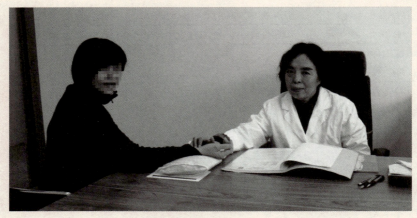

🎧 季小姐于 2023 年 2 月前来诊治时合影留念

20 岁正是人生的青春年华，但是季小姐在相当一段时间内都被疼痛缠身。她经常感到腹痛、胸痛、腰痛，以及消化不良。随后发现腹部越来越胀、越来越大，于是到医院检查，发现有腹水，经进一步的检查后，发现腹腔里面有大量的肿瘤，这种情况让季小姐以及她的父母都非常吃惊并深受打击。2010 年 3 月，她于澳大利亚的医院动手术，打开腹腔以后所见到的肿瘤严重程度，让医生们都感到吃惊，因为肿瘤已经弥漫性的大量转移到腹腔里的所有脏器。肿瘤有大有小，医生真是不知道如何下手才好，最后只能决定做一些选择性切除。当时医生考虑把部分腹腔相关器官切除，但因不能同时切除大量的器官，最后只选择切除了十二指肠、胆囊、脾脏和部分肝脏，这只能是一种姑息性的、短期的治疗。其实当时她的盆腔脏器和卵巢也都布满了肿瘤，但是考虑到季小姐是个年轻的女孩子，所以只切除了一侧而保留了另一侧的卵巢，同时切除了肿瘤侵犯的部分直肠。负责手术的医生以及其他的医生，都对患者的父母说得很清楚："这种弥漫性恶性间皮瘤，是恶性肿瘤中预后最坏的肿瘤之一，对她来说，只能是短期生存，没有长期希望。"经过这样大型的手术之后，季小姐一直在慢慢恢复中。但她也顾不得大型手术带来的严重创伤和身体反应，在手术后不到1个月，就赶紧开始了化疗。即使在化疗期间，出现呕吐、脱发、不能进食，她都坚持下来了，就是盼望身体能早日恢复健康。在第4次化疗以后，经检查发现她的癌症指数越来越高，正常值在35以下的癌抗原CA125，竟然达到了300多。手术后的第5个月，经检查发现手术切除的部位和腹腔里，又增加了大量肿瘤，发生了很多新的转移灶。在这种严峻的情况下，季小姐和她的父母只能把希望寄托在中医药生命修复疗法上。弥漫性恶性间皮瘤从医学文献上讲，即使仅发生在胸膜或腹膜，也都是一种致死性肿瘤，一般中位生存期是4～12个月。更不用说腹腔和盆腔脏器已经全部受到侵犯。季小姐只好停止化疗，前来接受中医药生命修复疗法治疗。

当时她腹痛严重，身体非常虚弱，在逐步调理之下，她的身体也在一步一步地恢复中。经过生命修复的治疗，在手术后

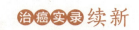

第7个月，经过检查，发现全腹腔和盆腔的肿瘤在大量复发之后，已经有了明显地减少和控制。接着又治疗了一段时间，大部分肿瘤已经消失。大家再接再厉，努力治疗，季小姐亦非常积极配合。很快地，季小姐就恢复了健康，在随后多次的检查中都没有发现肿瘤的复发和转移。直到现在，已经过去15年了，季小姐再没有为疾病的纠缠而烦恼，在疾病得到控制之后第7年，她结婚了，建立了幸福的家庭，现在的她生活美满、幸福健康。

祛邪攻毒，扶正抗癌。

常用中药

1. 桃仁、红花、薏苡仁、鳖甲、田七、三棱、莪术、牡蛎、大黄、海藻、昆布等。
2. 同时服用散结丸。

026

影像学、病理学检查报告及诊疗记录

1. 2010 年 3 月 31 日手术后病理检查报告证实为恶性间皮细胞瘤，卵巢、脾脏、胆囊、阑尾等脏器均有肿瘤病灶。

2. 2010 年 8 月 16 日手术后，化疗后 5 个月的检查报告，显示肿瘤增多，恶化，活性增强，在膈下、腹腔、脾曲、盲肠、结肠、盆腔、髂部等都有大量肿瘤病灶。癌抗原 CA125 也明显增高。

3. 2010 年 10 月 28 日检查报告显示，大量肿瘤病灶消失。

附：患者检查报告

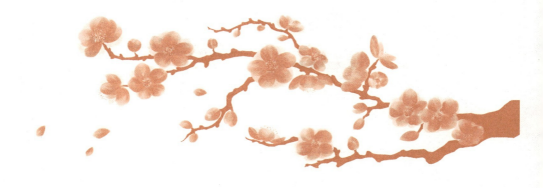

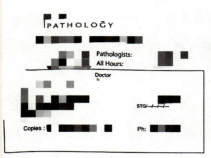
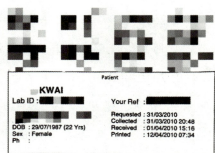

PATHOLOGY

Pathologists:
All Hours:

Doctor

STG/–/–/–/–

Copies :   Ph :

Patient

KWAI

Lab ID :

Your Ref :

DOB : 29/07/1987 (22 Yrs)
Sex : Female
Ph :

Requested : 31/03/2010
Collected : 31/03/2010 20:48
Received : 01/04/2010 15:16
Printed : 12/04/2010 07:34

Phoned to:
Date/Time: 31.03.10

MICROSCOPIC:

1. Paraffin sections confirm the frozen section report of lymph node with no evidence of metastatic neoplasm.

2. Sections show multiple deposits of epithelioid malignant tumour in lymph nodes within tissue loosely adherent to the ovary and to the spleen, and there are tumour deposits on the serosal surfaces of the ovary and the gallbladder. Smaller tumour deposits are present on the serosal surface of the appendix. The serosal surfaces also show fibrinous adhesions and there is subserosal oedema and congestion with mild neutrophil infiltration.

The tumour deposits are composed of epithelioid cells with abundant eosinophilic cytoplasm in a tubulo-papillary pattern, many of the cells exhibiting a deciduoid appearance. Occasional tumour cells show intracytoplasmic lumina containing mucicarmine and alcian blue-positive mucin. The nuclear features of the tumour are relatively bland and the mitotic rate is low. Focally, multinucleated giant cells are present within the tumour and there is a patchy lympho-plasmacytic infiltrate. Immunoperoxidase stains for calretinin and HBME1 show only focal staining of rare cells within the tumour. Stains for pancytokeratin and CA125 are positive within the tumour cells, whilst stains for CK5/6, CK7, CK20, Ber-EP4, BG8, WT-1, TTF-1, CEA, CD117, CD34 and MOC31 are negative. The immunohistochemical staining pattern is somewhat anomalous for malignant mesothelioma. However, in view of the review report of this patient's original diagnostic tumour biopsy (SEALS 10H01141, 10K0330843), in which strong positive staining for CAM 5.2, WT-1 and EMA were noted as well as focal staining with calretinin and D240, and the histological appearances in this specimen, the findings are considered consistent with malignant mesothelioma of tubulo-papillary epithelioid subtype. The relative failure of the tumour cells to stain with calretinin and HBME1 and the now negative staining with CK5/6 and WT-1 may represent an effect of chemotherapy on the tumour.

No intrinsic abnormality is identified in the hemicolectomy specimen and the mesenteric lymph nodes are negative for malignancy. The gallbladder mucosa shows autolysis, but no significant intrinsic abnormality is seen. Sections of the splenic and ovarian parenchyma also show no significant abnormality.

DIAGNOSIS:

1. **MESENTERIC LYMPH NODE**   -   **NO EVIDENCE OF MALIGNANCY**

2. **PERITONECTOMY, RIGHT HEMICOLECTOMY,GALLBLADDER, APPENDIX, OVARY WITH FALLOPIAN TUBE AND SPLEEN**   -   **MULTIPLE PERITONEAL AND LYMPH NODAL DEPOSITS OF MALIGNANT TUMOUR, FAVOUR MALIGNANT MESOTHELIOMA, TUBULO-PAPILLARY EPITHELIOID TYPE**

Reported by

NATA ●RCE
NATA Accreditation No.

Page 2 of 2

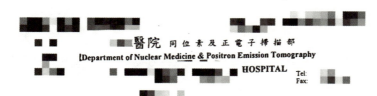

醫院 同位素及正電子掃描部
[Department of Nuclear Medicine & Positron Emission Tomography]
HOSPITAL
Tel:
Fax:

Functional parameters of these lesions are tabulated below:

Kwai	Current Study Date (16/8/10)				Prior Study Date(22/1/10)				
	in mm				in mm				
Site	LD	PD	SUVmax	TLG	LD	PD	SUVmax	TLG	TLG% change
R subphrenic lesion	28.0	13.9	6.1	9.6	13.8	8.3	3.9	2.2	328.7%
L groin node	23.8	13.0	10.4	10.9	12.5	11.3	5.8	2.9	278.2%
Peritoneal mass of splenic flexure	Not active				54.5	35.7	10.0	103.6	-100.0%
Lesion at or adjacent to caecum	Not active				18.0	12.4	7.3	6.7	-100.0%
Bilateral POD mass	Not active				44.0	22.7	12.2	103.9	-100.0%
L external iliac node	Not active				15.6	10.0	5.1	4.2	-100.0%
New Lesion:									
Peritoneal focus beneath segment III	18.4	13.3	4.1	4.1					
Rt anterior pelvic cavity	13.4	8.2	1.5	0.5					
Sigmoid colon	32.6	23.9	3.1	15.1					
Transverse colon	22.3	10.8	2.8	5.8					
Rt nasopharynx	29.8	20.6	5.4	18.0					

Note: LD=longest diameter; PD=diameter perpendicular to LD; TLG=total lesion glycolysis (vol x SUVmean)

Impression:

1. Post surgical resection of prior active peritoneal lesions in the splenic flexure, adjacent to caecum, descending colon, bilateral POD and the left external iliac node.
2. Worsening of active foci over right anterior subphrenic and left groin regions. Patchy activities around the capsular surface of liver, along the colon and bilateral anterior pelvic cavitiy are suggestive of active peritoneal disease. These may account for elevated CA 125 level.
3. Incidental findings of swollen right nasopharynx with increased ^{18}FDG activity. Correlation with nasopharyngoscopy and EBV DNA titre may be helpful to differentiate benign entity like focal nasopharyngitis from malignant pathology, or as clinically indicated.
4. No other ^{18}FDG-avid lesion in the remaining body survey.

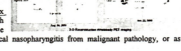

Thank you very much, ███ for your referral.

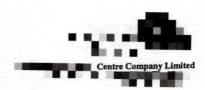

Centre Company Limited

KWAI ▓▓▓▓ Pre and Post Contrast CT scan of Thorax, Abdomen and Pelvis continued 28-10-2010

The spleen is not enlarged. The pancreas and adrenals are unremarkable.

Both kidneys are of normal size and appearance with normal enhancement pattern. There are no calculi, cysts, masses or hydronephrosis. The para renal fat and fascia are not thickened.

The bladder and the rectum are normally defined. The pelvic sidewalls are intact. The uterus and right adnexa are normal. There is a newly developed 2.6 cm left ovarian cyst. No adnexal mass or hydroureter is found. The inguinal hernias are again noted and unchanged.

Nodes:
Compared with last study, following changes are observed at the nodal stations:
- Left SCF, 0.3-0.85 cm (0.5-1.1 cm before)
- Pericardial, 0.75-1.0 cm (0.6-0.9 cm before)
- Pre-aortic and para-aortic, 0.4-0.9 cm (0.65-1.35 cm before)
- Left internal iliac, disappeared (0.8 cm before)
- Left external iliac, resolved (0.7-1.6 cm before)

Subcutaneous tissues:
No abnormal subcutaneous mass is seen. The breasts are symmetrical and normally defined.

Bones
The scanned skeleton in general is unremarkable. Normal bone density is noted.

Vasculatures:
There is no evidence of aneurysm or dissection in the abdominal and thoracic aorta. The common iliac arteries are also unremarkable and normal calibre

COMMENT:
1. Status treated malignant mesothelioma of the peritoneum.
2. The previously seen omental thickening had all resolved. Since patient did not receive treatment, they are more likely to be due to post operative inflammation.
3. The pelvic lymph nodes had also disappeared. The anterior mediastinal nodes seen in the last CT were actually thymus.
4. The residual nodes at the retroperitoneal and the left SCF are smaller.
5. The pericardial nodes are stable.
6. No distant metastases are noted in the lungs, liver, adrenals or bone.
7. The mildly dilated small bowel loops in the mid abdomen are unchanged.
8. Newly developed simple left ovarian cyst.

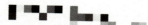

晚期恶性黑色素瘤已渡 17 年

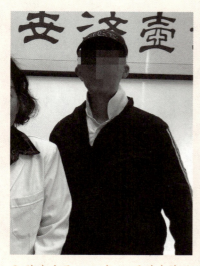

🎤 陈先生于 2023 年 10 月前来诊治时合影留念

陈先生在 17 年前经检查发现颈部有肿瘤病灶，于 2007 年做了颈部的肿瘤切除手术，经化验检查，确诊为恶性黑色素瘤。手术后本以为问题解决了，没想到仅 3 个月，就发生了腮腺、耳部及多处淋巴的转移。他又于 2008 年做了腮腺等部位的手术，清除淋巴结。但自此以后他经常有咳嗽、痰多等症状，到医院检查后发现，双肺都有多发的结节，中间及上腹部也有多处淋巴结节。于是陈先生前来接受中医药生命修复疗法的治疗，经过几年中医药的治疗之后，病情逐渐稳定。他以为可以松口气了，于是便忙于工作，2～3 年没有再服用中药和前来复诊。不料在 2018 年年初，他的左足趾发生溃疡，急忙到医院做检查，得知为肿瘤转移，于是做了局部清理。医院也直言他的病情非常严重，因原发部位在头部，而后到足部转移，说明全身都有肿瘤细胞的存在和蔓延。之后陈先生便开始认真服用我们的中药，再次检查时已无肿瘤复发。在此期间曾有足部另一处发生溃疡，他表示与以前的癌症溃疡情况一样，但经过中药调理并加中药外敷后，溃疡逐渐愈合，并没有再次进行手术。

2020年年初，经全身检查显示，他的身体已恢复了正常。时至今日，陈先生患恶性黑色素瘤已经17年了，治愈后一直按时检查身体，未发生复发或转移的情况，就又重新投入他忙碌的工作之中。恶性黑色素瘤是黑色素细胞来源的恶性程度非常高的肿瘤。其病因有多种说法，尚未完全清楚。关于这种癌症的分期，如已发生远处转移，则属于最晚期的恶性肿瘤，预后非常差。经医院早年就告知化疗和放疗等治疗并无良好的效果，所以他一直没有接受化疗和放疗等。在长达17年的生活中，也曾因中断治疗而导致肿瘤远处转移。但经积极治疗之后恢复正常，说明生命修复的中医药治疗有确切的治疗效果。

治疗原则

排毒化浊，祛邪抗癌。

常用中药

1. 丹参、虎杖、土茯苓、生大黄、薏苡仁、猫爪草、猕猴梨根、牡丹皮、半枝莲、野菊花等。
2. 同时服用攻毒散。

影像学、病理学检查报告及诊疗记录

1. 2019 年 6 月 19 日病理活检报告，证实足部为远处转移而来的恶性黑色素瘤。

2. 2020 年 4 月 16 日检查报告，证明 2007 年 7 月曾行耳部恶性黑色素瘤切除，并证实无肿瘤复发转移。

3. 2021 年 8 月 27 日 CT 检查报告，证实全身包括脑、胸、肺、腹、盆腔等均无肿瘤复发和转移。

附：患者检查报告

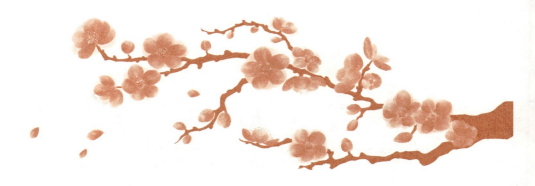

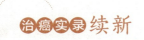

Histopathology Report

Name:	CHAN ███ 陳█	Laboratory No.:	██
Sex/Age:	M / 59Y	Hospital:	OFFICE
HKID/PP No.:	████	Consulting Doctor:	█ ████
Patient No.:	█		
Ward/Room:		Date Received:	19 June 2019
		Other Lab. No. :	████

SPECIMEN
Left toe (5th) skin lesion.

CLINICAL SUMMARY
Biopsy of left 5th toe skin lesion.

MACROSCOPIC EXAMINATION
Specimen labeled "Left 5th toe skin lesion". Received in formalin is a greyish congested skin ellipse measuring 5 x 2 mm across and 2 mm thick. All submitted in one block after bisection along long axis. (SW/hl)

MICROSCOPIC DESCRIPTION
The skin lesion shows ulcerated surface, comprising tumour nests and isolated cells with necrosis and extending to base. The lesional cells are epithelioid, with vesicular large nucleus, prominent nucleolus and brisk mitosis. Immunohistochemistry shows that the lesional cells are positive for S-100 protein and melan-A, while negative for epithelial marker AE1/3. Features are those of malignant melanoma.

DIAGNOSIS
Left 5th toe skin, biopsy
–   Malignant melanoma.

(End of report)

Report Date:	21 June 2019	Print Date:	21 June 2019	Page: 1 of 1

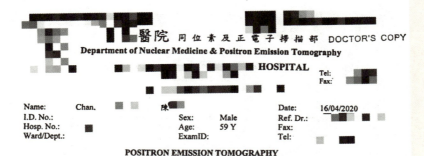

醫院 同位素及正電子掃描部 DOCTOR'S COPY
Department of Nuclear Medicine & Positron Emission Tomography

HOSPITAL

Tel:
Fax:

Name:	Chan,	陳		Date:	16/04/2020
I.D. No.:			Sex: Male	Ref. Dr.:	
Hosp. No.:			Age: 59 Y	Fax:	
Ward/Dept.:			ExamID:	Tel:	

POSITRON EMISSION TOMOGRAPHY
(¹⁸F-FDG ONCOLOGY)

History:

A 59 year-old gentleman has history of melanoma of left ear with excision in 7/2007. Left post-auricular lymph node metastasis with neck dissection in 2008, no adjuvant chemoradiotherapy necessarily. However, he complained of left big toe nail bed pigmented lesion, biopsy confirmed melanoma. PET here in 02/2018 showed a mildly hypermetabolic lesion in the left big toe nail bed, consistent with biopsy confirmed melanoma with surrounding inflammatory activity, and suspected left femoral nodal metastasis. He underwent left big toe amputation with left groin nodal dissection (sentinel node showed metastasis). No adjuvant therapy. Patient complained of left 5th toe ulcer. Biopsy confirmed melanoma involvement. PET here in 06/2019 showed activity at left 5th toe and left ear. He has amputation of left 5th toe and resection of left ear lesion, confirmed melanoma recurrence. No adjuvant therapy. PET here in 10/2019 showed no recurrence or metastasis. He is clinically well. Non-smoker. No TB. Known fatty liver and HBV carrier. PET for reassessment.

Radiopharmaceutical: 9.4 mCi F-18 Fluorodeoxyglucose (¹⁸FDG) injected intravenously.

Findings:

Limited whole body CT transmission and PET emission imaging began at 65 minutes after radiopharmaceutical administration (blood glucose 4.9 mmol/l), spanning a region from vertex to toe. 60 mg Spasmonal was given p.o. 15 min before ¹⁸FDG administration.

Liver tissue normal reference uptake has a SUVmax of 2.86.

Comparison is made with previous PET study performed here on 16/10/2019. Patient is status post left 1st and 5th toes amputation and left ear partial resection for melanoma.

In bilateral lower limbs, there is mildly improved mild activity at the left 5th toe amputation bed. Otherwise, there is no new focal abnormal metabolism in the left big toe amputation site. No new focal hypermetabolic cutaneous lesion is present in the rest of body survey. There is no new hypermetabolic lymphadenopathy in bilateral popliteal fossae or inguinal regions. There is more prominent activity at distal interphalangeal joint of right 5th toe. Previous mild soft tissue activity in the intercondylar fossa of left femur and right patella are further improved.

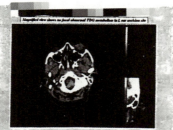

In the head and neck region, there is no new focal hypermetabolic pathology in the left ear excision site or left postauricular region. Previous bilateral submandibular lymph nodes are largely stable with low-grade activity. Bilateral jugular chains and supraclavicular fossae are clear. Nasopharynx and thyroid gland are unremarkable.

035

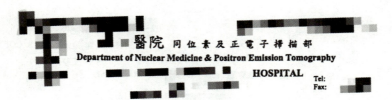

醫院 同位素及正電子掃描部

Department of Nuclear Medicine & Positron Emission Tomography

HOSPITAL

Tel:
Fax:

In thorax, prior small ground glass opacity at the anterior aspect of RML with low-grade activity has resolved. Normal parenchymal and pleural activity is seen in other lung segments. No new pleural or pericardial effusion is found and there is no new hypermetabolic lymphadenopathy in bilateral hila or mediastinum or axillae.

In the abdomen and pelvic region, previous focal activity at the superior aspect of the right testis is further improved. Left testis is unremarkable. There is normal size and metabolism of the liver, spleen, pancreas and bilateral adrenal glands. No new hyperdense gallstone. Kidney configuration is normal. Left urinary bladder diverticulum is noted. There is no focal hypermetabolic thickening in the stomach and bowel activities are mild and physiologic. Prostate gland is persistently enlarged but with no focal abnormal metabolism. Bladder diverticulum is noted. No new pelvic ascites is noted.

Skeletal survey shows no hypermetabolic focal marrow lesion in axial or proximal appendicular skeleton.

Functional parameters to compare these 2 studies are tabulated below:

CHAN,			16-Apr-2020				16-Oct-2019			
		in mm		F-18 FDG		in mm		*F-18 FDG*		TLG
Site		LD	PD	SUVmax	TLG	LD	PD	SUVmax	TLG	%change
Activity at Lt 5th toe amputation site		-	-	1.5	-	-	-	1.7	-	-
Focal uptake in distal interphalangeal joint of R 5th toe		-	-	2.5	-	-	-	1.8	-	-
Rt submandibular LN		6.0	5.0	3.1	0.2	6.0	4.9	3.6	0.2	0.0%
Lt submandibular LN		10.1	7.7	1.8	0.6	10.0	7.6	2.1	0.6	0.0%
Rt testis uptake		13.1	7.4	3.6	1.5	20.2	12.7	4.7	5.8	-74.1%

Note: LD=longest diameter; PD=diameter perpendicular to LD; TLG=total lesion glycolysis (vol x SUVmean)

Impression:

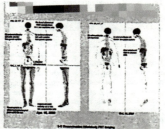

1. No metabolic evidence of local tumor recurrence at the left ear or left big toe. Prior mild activity at the left 5th toe amputation site is improved, suggestive of improving residual inflammation. It warrants follow-up monitoring for confirmation.
2. Bilateral submandibular nodes are stable with mild activity, suggestive of reactive adenitis. No evidence of interval nodal metastases.
3. Previous focal uptake at the superior right testis is further improved, favoring resolving inflammation.
4. There is more prominent activity at distal interphalangeal joint of right 5th toe, suggestive of degenerative arthritis. Previous activity in the intercondylar fossa of left femur and right patella is improved, confirmed improving stress related change or degeneration.
5. Prior GGO at the anterior RML with mild activity is resolved, confirmed inflammatory change.
6. No new suspicious focal pathology in the remaining body survey to suggest distant metastasis.

Thank you very much, ▮ ▮, for your referral.

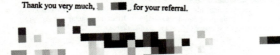

醫院

MEDICAL IMAGING DEPARTMENT

Patient's Name	: CHAN	**Unit Record No.**	:
Sex	: M	**Age**	: 60
Examination Date	: 27-AUG-2021	**Accession No.**	:

Ward / Class	: RADI	**Attending Doctor**	:

EXAMINATION / PROCEDURE REPORT

Clinical Information : melanoma.

CONTRAST MEDIUM: 85ml Iopamiro 300.

CT SCAN OF BRAIN, THORAX, ABDOMEN AND PELVIS (PLAIN AND CONTRAST)

FINDINGS:
Correlation with previous PET CT report dated 06 May 2021 was made.

CT Brain:

The ventricles are not dilated.
No focal lesion is detected in either cerebral hemispheres.
No abnormal enhancing lesion or enhancement is noted.
Gray-white differentiation is preserved.
No evidence of intracranial haemorrhage is seen.
No abnormal extra-axial fluid collection is seen.
The major venous sinuses are patent.

CT Thorax:
Bilateral apical pleural thickening and fibrotic changes are seen.
A 0.3 cm non-specific lung nodule is noted in the posterior segment of left lower lobe. No focal lung mass is seen. No focal consolidation or collapse is noted.
No evidence of bronchiectasis is seen.
No mediastinal or hilar lymphadenopathy is noted.   Small prevascular lymph node measuring 0.4 cm is seen.
No pleural effusion is present.
No gross destructive bony lesion is noted.
Previous left neck dissection is noted.

CT Abdomen and pelvis:

(Electronically Signed)

Approved on : 28-AUG-2021 11:51 PM
Page 1 of 2

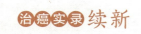

Hospital 醫院
MEDICAL IMAGING DEPARTMENT

Patient's Name	: CHAN	Unit Record No.	:
Sex	: M	Age	: 60
Examination Date	: 27-AUG-2021	Accession No.	:

Ward / Class	: RADI	Attending Doctor	:

EXAMINATION / PROCEDURE REPORT

Liver is normal in size and attenuation. A 0.7 cm hypodense non-enhancing lesion is seen in the posterior segment of the liver, favouring cyst. No focal hepatic mass lesion is noted. The biliary system is not dilated.
Portal vein is patent.

The gallbladder is unremarkable. No adrenal mass is noted. Spleen is not enlarged. Pancreas is unremarkable.

Bilateral kidneys are normal in sizes and smooth in contour. No hydronephrosis or renal stone is noted.

No ascites is noted. Small para-aortic lymph nodes measuring up to 0.4 cm are seen. A slightly enlarged left common iliac lymph node measuring 0.8 x 0.9 cm, left external iliac lymph node measuring 1.2 x 0.9 cm and left groin lymph nodes measuring 1.3 x 1.1 cm and 0.9 x 0.7 cm are seen.

The large bowel is not well distended for proper assessment. No evidence of intestinal obstruction is noted.

No pelvic mass lesion or intraabdominal collection is seen. Urinary bladder is not well distended. A urinary bladder diverticulum is noted on the left side of the urinary bladder.

No gross destructive bony lesion is seen.

IMPRESSION:
1. A 0.3 cm non-specific lung nodule is noted in the left lower lobe. Further followup study is suggested.
2. Slightly enlarged left common iliac, left external iliac and left groin lymph nodes are seen. Sizes are similar when compared to previous PET CT report dated 06 May 2021.
3. Small prevascular and para-aortic lymph nodes up to 0.4 cm are seen.
4. Small hypodense non-enhancing lesion in segment VII of liver is favouring cyst. No other focal hepatic mass lesion is seen.
5. No evidence of brain metastasis is detected.

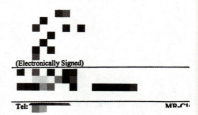

(Electronically Signed)

Approved on : 28-AUG-2021 11:51 PM
Page 2 of 2

Tel: MR-CT

晚期肠癌放弃化疗 15 年

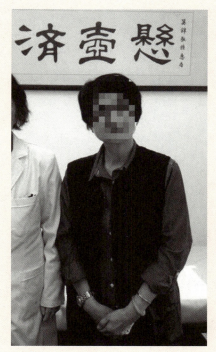

雷小姐于 2024 年 2 月前来诊治时合影留念

2009 年，雷小姐经常感到腹痛、排便困难，有时甚至排血便，于是到医院做检查。检查报告显示她的直肠上部有恶性肿瘤，并在肠周围、髂骨前、左髂部有大量的淋巴转移。她于 2010 年 8 月做了手术切除，手术后的病理检查报告诊断，证实为直肠与结肠腺癌，并伴有大量淋巴转移，仅切除的肿瘤周围，就有 19 个有癌转移的淋巴结，已属晚期。2011 年 3 月，PET 检查报告显示，髂部主动脉、腔静脉、腔静脉旁均有转移，需尽快化疗。但在做了 1 个疗程的化疗后，因不良反应很严重，雷小姐感觉无法坚持下去，但医院里的医生告诉她，1 次化疗还远远不够，一定要坚持继续化疗，否则会有生命危险。即使完成化疗，也不能保证不会复发和转移，因为已存在大量的淋巴转移。于是她前来生命修复治疗求助，她说化疗太辛苦，无法再坚持下去了。在医院的出院小结中，也有讲明她停止化疗，改用中药治疗。从此她一直用生命修复方法治疗，同时每年做检查，了解身体状况，如今15年过去了，肿瘤完全消失，一直没有复发。

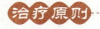

益气养阴，散结消瘤。

常用中药

1. 太子参、黄药子、生地黄、玉竹、石斛、玄参、川贝母、浙贝母、生大黄、全蝎等。
2. 同时服用散结丸。

影像学、病理学检查报告及诊疗记录

1. 2010年9月24日报告显示为肠腺癌，肠系膜有大量质硬肿大的转移淋巴结，病理报告证实，25个淋巴结中有19个已发生转移，属于晚期 $T_4 N_2$ 肠癌。

　　2. 2012 年 8 月 14 日 CT 检查报告证实于 2010 年 9 月手术。手术后 2011 年 3 月检查发现有大量转移病灶。因化疗副作用太大，1 个疗程后即停止化疗，而改用中药并持续中药治疗。以前检查到的盆腔、腹股沟、腹膜后转移淋巴结全部消失，没有见到肿瘤复发。

　　3. 2021 年 7 月 15 日肠镜检查显示肠道无任何肿瘤复发迹象。

附：患者检查报告

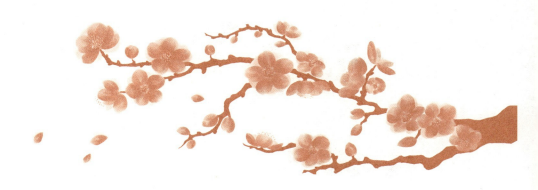

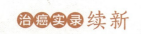

CENTRE 中心

Consultant

Hospital

24th Sep, 2010

Ref: Lui _____ F/56 i.d. _____

Dear Consultant,

I would like to refer this patient to you for adjuvant chemotherapy. Madam Lui presented to me with per rectal bleeding and passage of mucus. I performed colonoscopy examination on 11/9/2010 and found a tumour at upper rectum. Biopsy of tumour confirmed adenocarcinoma. PET-CT scan was performed which showed no evidence of distant spread. I and Dr. Chu Kin Wah performed laparoscopic anterior resection on 14/9/2010. The operation was smooth and she recovered uneventfully.

Intraoperatively the tumour was localized, there was no adjacent invasion and there was no peritoneal deposit. The colorectal anastomosis is at 7cm from the anal verge and just above the peritoneal reflection. Multiple hard and enlarged lymph nodes were palpable in the mesentery. The pathology examination reported T4N2 disease (19/25 lymph nodes). All resection margins were clear.

I enclose relevant reports for your reference. Please kindly offer your expert management on adjuvant chemotherapy. Thank you for taking care of this patient, if there is any enquiry please free feel to contact me, my pager number is 7388 5630.

Best Regards,

電話 Tel
傳真 Fax

網址 Website

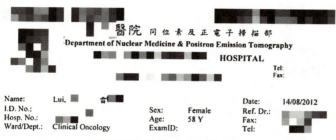

醫院 同位素及正電子掃描部
Department of Nuclear Medicine & Positron Emission Tomography

HOSPITAL

Tel:
Fax:

Name:	Lui,		Date:	14/08/2012
I.D. No.:		Sex: Female	Ref. Dr.:	
Hosp. No.:		Age: 58 Y	Fax:	
Ward/Dept.:	Clinical Oncology	ExamID:	Tel:	

POSITRON EMISSION TOMOGRAPHY
(^{18}F-FDG ONCOLOGY)

<u>History</u>:

A 58 year-old lady had laparoscopic resection of upper rectum in 09/2010, T3N2b disease, followed by chemotherapy and radiation therapy. PET here in 03/2011 showed mildly active nodes along right iliac vessel, aortocaval and paracaval regions. After 1 more cycle of chemotherapy, it was stopped due to side-effects. She switched to herbal medicine but later complained of right lower limb swelling. PET in 6/2011 showed improvement of myositis and nodes. She continued with herbal medicine, but sustained a recent minor trauma to her lower right chest wall. Hysterectomy for fibroid, cholecystectomy and appendectomy.

<u>Radiopharmaceutical</u>: 10.9 mCi F-18 Fluorodeoxyglucose (^{18}FDG) injected intravenously.

<u>Findings</u>:

Limited whole body CT transmission and PET emission imaging began at 84 minutes after radiopharmaceutical administration (blood glucose 5.4 mmol/l), spanning a region from base of skull to upper thigh. 60 mg Spasmonal was given p.o. 15 min before ^{18}FDG administration.

Liver tissue normal reference uptake has a SUVmax of 2.53.

The current examination is compared with prior study of 06/2011. The rectal anastomosis is marked by radiopaque sutures. It shows no metabolic evidence of local tumor recurrence. The anastomotic bowel loops show normal activities. The hypermetabolic lymph nodes previously observed in the right pelvic cavity, right groin and retroperitoneum have completely resolved. No evidence of hypermetabolic lymphadenopathy detected during this evaluation. There is still mildly increased gluteal muscle activity just adjacent to right hip joint, consistent with mild inflammatory activities, bilateral involving both sides. Physiologic bowel activities are noted in the ascending and transverse colon. There is no interval 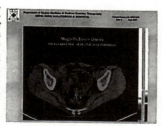 lymphadenopathy within the mesentery or omentum. The liver, adrenal glands, pancreas and spleen show normal size and metabolism. Kidney configuration is normal.

In the thorax, there remains normal parenchymal and pleural activity of bilateral lung segments. The tiny nodule in the inferolateral LUL is still ~2-3 mm, stable and without abnormal metabolism. No pleural or pericardial effusion. There is no lymphadenopathy in bilateral hila, mediastinum, supraclavicular fossae or jugular lymphatics.

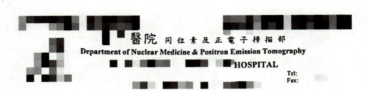

醫院 同位素及正電子掃描部
Department of Nuclear Medicine & Positron Emission Tomography
HOSPITAL

Tel:
Fax:

Skeletal survey shows no abnormal marrow metabolism. Specially, there is no abnormal activity involving the right lower chest cage to suggest the presence of metabolically active pathology.
Functional parameters to compare these 2 studies are tabulated below:

Lui,	Current Study Date 14.08.2012				Current Study Date 15.06.2011				SUVmax% change
	in mm				in mm				
Site	LD	PD	SUVmax	TLG	LD	PD	SUVmax	TLG	
Rt gluteal muscle	-	-	3.0	-	-	-	3.4	-	-12.1%

Note: LD=longest diameter; PD=diameter perpendicular to LD; TLG=total lesion glycolysis (vol x SUVmean)

Impression:

1. No PET/CT evidence of local recurrence or regional metastatic lymphadenopathy given patient's history of treatment for rectal malignancy.
2. All the previously detected hypermetabolic pelvic, groin and retroperitoneal nodes have metabolically and physically resolved.
3. Mild residual gluteal muscle activities adjacent to bilateral hips suggest mild myositis.
4. Stable 2-3 mm lung nodule in the LUL, likely benign.
5. No evidence of interval distant metastasis.

Thank you very much, ████ for your referral.

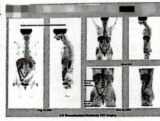

Colonoscopy Report

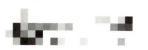

Patient Name: Lui	**Date of Procedure:** 15/7/2021
Patient No.:	**Doctor in Charge:**
ID No.: -	**Endoscopist:**
Gender: Female	**Mac by Anaesthetist:**
Date of Birth: -	
Age: 67 Y	

INDICATIONS: Per rectal bleeding 大便出血

PROCEDURE: Colonoscopy 腸鏡
Polypectomy at large intestine 結腸瘜肉切除術

SEDATION: Dormicum 4 mg, Pethidine 10 mg, Propofol Lipuro 1% 20 mg

EQUIPMENT: CF-HQ290L 2853058

SPECIMEN: Transverse colon polyp 橫結腸瘜肉

FINDING: Good bowel preparation
Scope to caecum
Ileocaecal valve and appendiceal orifice identified
3mm polyp at proximal transverse colon
The polyp was completely removed with biopsy forcep
Rest of colon and rectum showed normal vascular and
mucosal pattern
coloanastomosis at 7cm from anal verge, smooth outline
Mild haemorrhoids present

DIAGNOSIS: Colonic polyp 腸瘜肉
Haemorrhoid 痔瘡

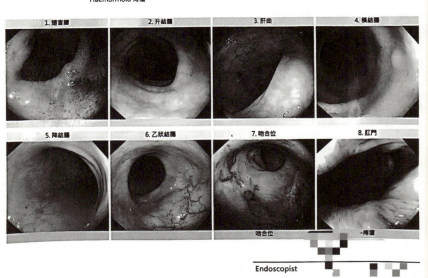

Endoscopist

045

病案7

晚期乳腺癌长寿之星

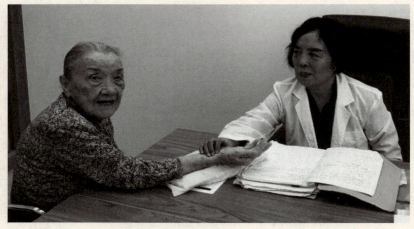

🎙 刘女士前来就诊时合影留念

　　如今人人谈癌色变，癌症给社会带来的危害性毋庸置疑。患了癌症后，虽经现代化的医学治疗，但英年早逝者也不胜枚举。然而，也有很多的癌症患者，经过正确的治疗能够很好地生存下来。本书所列举的病案都是很好的例子，也是我们用生命修复的中医药治疗的成千上万的患者中的一些代表。

　　为增强战胜癌症的信心，再举一位105岁的刘女士为例。刘女士自幼生活艰辛，父母早逝，她有3个弟弟妹妹，自己是老大。从16岁就挑起了一家生活的重担，不仅像母亲一样照顾弟弟妹妹，每天还要起早打理几亩田地，养活一家的生活。那时全家人吃了上顿没下顿，时常忍饥挨饿。一家人衣食住行的生活重任全由她一人担当。夜半时分，她也常在昏暗的油灯下缝补衣服，大半辈子都是这样受苦过来的。70多岁时，因为儿子在香港的生意做得越来越好，女儿也嫁了富裕人家，才过上了舒适的日子。刘女士在儿子家住，也时常去女儿家闲住几日，无忧无虑。但是世事难料，在刘女士近80岁时，准备好好享受老来福时，却查出患有乳腺癌并已有淋巴转移。

在儿子的安排下，她先在医院做了肿瘤切除手术，接下来就要进行化疗和放疗。刘女士住进了医院准备化疗和放疗时，看到同病房的患者在化疗期间都非常痛苦，有脱发、呕吐、不能进食的情况，也有人虽然经受住了这些痛苦，但依然因不能根治而离世。刘女士感到很害怕，但又知道与儿子女儿是无法商量的，他们一定会坚持要做这些治疗。思前想后，最终在半夜时分，自己擅自跑出医院，回到家里，以后无论谁来劝说，就是不去医院。就这样在家里不做治疗的日子过了不到1年，她胸部有些地方的皮肤开始发硬，成为一块一块的硬结。去医院检查的结果是乳腺癌皮下组织转移、淋巴转移，已经是晚期。刘女士还是不愿去化疗。但是当听说能够采用中医药生命修复疗法治疗时她很有兴趣，很快就前来进行治疗。那时她精神疲惫、瘦弱不堪、上肢水肿、胸部皮肤有溃烂。我们对她的治疗以通经破滞、养肝败毒为主。

经过约半年治疗，她的皮肤恢复正常，3 年后结节均消失，气色好转、食量恢复、体重增加。此后她间断的前来治疗，也一直坚持养生保健，她说现在虽然已 105 岁了，但并未感到老，甚至比年轻时精神还好。她是当之无愧的抗癌长寿之星。

治疗原则

通经破滞，养肝败毒。

常用中药

1. 当归、白芍、炮山甲、露蜂房、丹参、郁金、香附、鳖甲、王不留行、红参、当归、黄芪、刺五加等。
2. 同时服用化症丸。

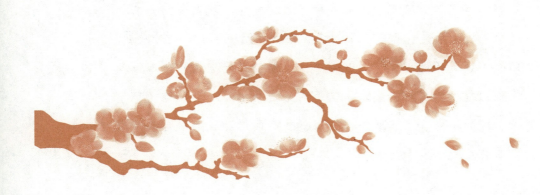

晚期鼻咽癌康复 18 年

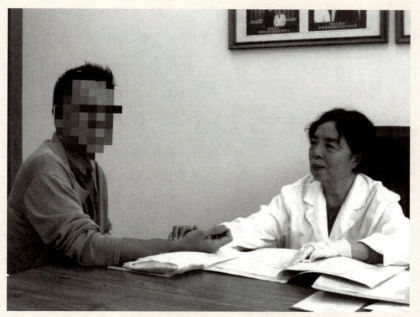

● 方先生于 2024 年 1 月前来就诊时合影留念

方先生 30 多岁，在一家公司当经理，每日忙忙碌碌。半年多来，他经常感到头痛、耳鸣、鼻塞、眼痛、视物模糊、眩晕等。起初以为是因为工作太忙、经常熬夜，过一阵子就会没事。但没多久，他的病情加重，视物模糊、耳鸣如潮、头痛剧烈，逼不得已去医院找医生，医生为他做了不少检查，其中包括活组织检查，确诊为鼻咽癌晚期。医生安排他做电疗，并告知他的病情已属晚期，有广泛的骨转移，各鼻窦、筛骨、蝶骨、颅骨和颈椎等，都有大范围的转移，而且肿瘤已侵犯视神经，即使做了电疗，肿瘤也会复发并继续转移，导致失明的概率也很大。

方先生深感压力，经过一番考虑，决定求助于生命修复治癌，一边电疗，一边前来服用中药。电疗之后，他一直坚持不懈地服用中药治疗。由于采用的中药以养阴清解、化痰祛邪为主，故有效地减缓了电疗的副作用，例如口干、失眠、耳鸣和不能进食等；更可喜的是，他体内严重的肿瘤转移全部消失。如今已过去了18年，肿瘤并没有复发和转移，当时医生说他或会在1~2年之后复发及转移，结果这个预言并未发生，他战胜了癌症。

随着医疗水平的提高，鼻咽癌的治疗水平较过去已有明显改善，虽然放疗对癌细胞有杀灭作用，但是此治疗的不良反应大、损伤大，对于晚期鼻咽癌治疗仍不尽人意。患者接受放疗以后，以中医药学的观点来说，一般认为有火热毒邪入侵，导致热毒过盛、化火灼津，患者有口干、咽喉干燥疼痛、吞咽困难等阴虚内热及严重的放射性损伤症状。更为重要的是，其他地方的转移病灶仍需大力治疗和控制，才能防止癌症卷土重来。在这种情况下，生命修复的中医药治疗进一步发挥了很好的养阴、攻毒、抗癌作用，使患者完全康复。方先生已经很多年没有前来诊治了。2022年3月我们电话回访时，他很高兴地说现在一切都好。

治疗原则

解毒攻邪，散结消瘤。

常用中药

1. 柴胡、黄芩、郁金、猕猴梨根、鱼脑石、鱼腥草、夏枯草、野菊花、桔梗、板蓝根等。
2. 同时服用消瘤丸。

影像学、病理学检查报告及诊疗记录

1. 2006 年 8 月检查报告证实鼻咽癌，并有广泛转移。
2. 2008 年 7 月检查报告证实肿瘤消失无复发。

附：患者检查报告

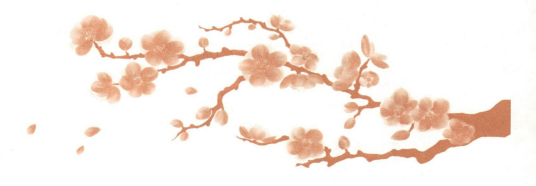

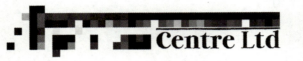

Centre Ltd

Specialists in Radiology

Exam. No.:	Name: Fung ████
Date of Exam. : 28th August, 2006	I/D. No.: ████
Referring Doctor: ████	Date of Birth: 08-12-1968

PLAIN & CONTRAST MRI SCAN OF THE BRAIN & NASOPHARYNX

Pre-contrast axial T1-weighted, proton density, T2-weighted, FLAIR/SPIR and Diffusion weighted images; sagittal T1-weighted images and coronal T2-weighted and T2*weighted images were obtained through the brain. Axial and coronal T1-weighted, T2-weighted and STIR images were obtained through the nasopharynx and axial T2-weighted images were obtained through the neck.

Post-contrast axial and coronal T1/MTC images were obtained through the brain; axial and coronal T1/SPIR images were obtained through the nasopharynx and axial T1 weighted images through the neck.

GIVEN CLINICAL DATA:- NPC confirmed by histology.

REPORT:-

A large irregular mass lesion is seen in the roof of the nasopharynx consistent with a mass lesion from nasopharyngeal carcinoma. It is seen involving the left fossa of Rosenmuller and obliterating the left eustachian tube opening. No significant infiltration into the right fossa of Rosenmuller is seen and no obliteration of the right eustachian tube opening is noted. The lesion is seen extending anteriorly into the posterior part of the left nasal cavity and also involving the inferior part of the left posterior ethmoidal and left sphenoidal sinuses. No involvement of the right nasal cavity and the rest of the paranasal sinuses is seen. No para-pharyngeal extension is noted and no involvement of the rest of the skull base and pterygoid bones is seen. The basal foramina appear normal and no intracranial extension of the lesion is noted. No posterior extension to involve the capitus longus muscles or inferior extension to the oropharynx is seen. No extension into the orbits is seen.

A few more prominent than usual left retropharyngeal lymph nodes are seen with the largest one measuring about 9 mm in the greatest diameter and this measurement is just within the normal limit.

A 1 cm lesion is seen in the inferior part of the right submandibular region and it has an internal area having very high signal intensity in the T2 weighted and STIR images and low signal intensity in the post-contrast images. The appearance is suggesting a partially cystic lesion. It appears to be within the inferior part of the right submandibular gland in the coronal images suggesting a lesion within the submandibular gland more suspicious of a submandibular mass like pleomorphic adenoma than a necrotic intra-submandibular gland lymph node.

No other suspicious lymph node or lymph node enlargement is seen in the rest of the cervical and supraclavicular regions.

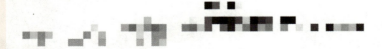

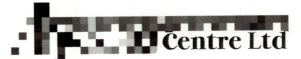

Specialists in Radiology

Centre Ltd

No abnormal marrow signals or marrow enhancement to suggest metastasis is seen in the cervical spine and the skull.

A small ill-defined area having medium to low signal intensity in the T1 weighted images is seen in the pre-pontine cistern. It is having signal intensity quite similar to that of CSF in the T2 weighted and STIR images. It is hyperintense in the FLAIR and Diffusion weighted images. It does not appear to be enhancing in the thin axial post-contrast images but is suspiciously enhancing in the thin coronal post-contrast images raising the suspicion of slight associated abnormal enhancement. No significant compression on the adjacent pons is seen and no significant displacement of the adjacent blood vessels is noted. Its MR appearance does not favor a dural metastasis, meningioma or neuroma and it appears a bit prominent to be due to flow artifact in this pre-pontine cistern. It raises the suspicion of an epidermoid cyst.

No other site of abnormal contrast enhancement is seen in the rest of the intracranial region and no evidence of dural metastasis or brain metastasis is seen.

There is no area of significant abnormal signal intensity noted in the brain. No suggestion of infarction, haemorrhage, chronic ischemic change, demyelinating disease, encephalomalacic changes or encephalomyelitis is noted in the brain.

The pituitary gland appears normal. The cavernous sinuses are unremarkable. The main cranial nerves are unremarkable. No chronic subdural effusion or hydrocephalus is seen. No lesion is seen in the cervicomedullary junction.

Retained secretion is seen in the posterior ethmoidal sinus. Further slight mucosal thickenings are seen scattered in the rest of the paranasal sinuses. No significant mucosal thickening is seen in the mastoid regions.

IMPRESSION:-

Nasopharyngeal carcinoma in the nasopharynx with left nasal cavity and early left posterior sphenoidal sinuses involvement.

The more prominent than usual lymph nodes in the left retropharyngeal region have sizes within the normal limits favouring reactionary changes than early metastasis though the latter cannot be excluded.

The lesion in the right submandibular gland is most suspicious of a submandibular mass like pleomorphic adenoma rather than cavitating metastatic lymph node though the latter cannot be excluded. Further aspiration biopsy for pathological confirmation would be helpful.

There is a suspicious signal area seen in the pre-pontine cistern as described above. It is most suspicious of an epidermoid cyst and further follow-up MR examination for progress is suggested for more information.

Thank you for your referral.

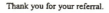

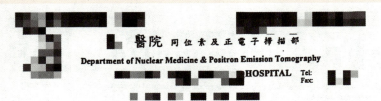

醫院 同位素及正電子掃描部

Department of Nuclear Medicine & Positron Emission Tomography

HOSPITAL Tel:
Fax:

<u>Impression</u>:

1. Negative PET scan showing no evidence of local tumor recurrence.
2. There is no evidence of lymph node or distant metastasis.

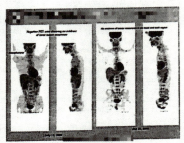

Thank you very much, ▮ ▮ for your referral.

为保胎儿拒绝化疗康复 18 年

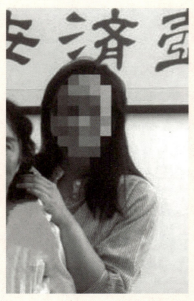

林女士2023年12月前来诊治时合影留念

林女士留学澳大利亚，1999年毕业后留在当地工作和生活，她和丈夫一直想要孩子，但多年来一直未能如愿。直到2006年，30岁的林女士终于有喜了，夫妻俩很是高兴，商量着为小宝宝准备衣物等必需品。然而，怀孕后不久，林女士便感到两侧乳房胀痛并有肿胀物，她以为是妊娠的正常反应。但为慎重起见，她还是去医院做了检查，结果发现两侧乳房各有1个肿块。医生称是良性的乳腺纤维瘤，要她尽早进行手术切除，以免影响日后哺乳。据医生所说，因为是良性肿瘤，手术切口很小，仅将肿瘤取出即可，并不需要做大面积切除，对乳腺组织也不会有损伤和影响。于是，林女士便做了双侧乳腺的小手术，将肿瘤取出，以为从此万事大吉。没想到几天后，医生又来电话，要她尽快再次手术，原来切除的2个肿瘤经过检验后，发现右侧为纤维瘤，而左侧为乳腺癌，同时已发生淋巴转移，需要尽快做较大面积的切除手术，同时将腋下等转移的淋巴组织一并切除。医生表示化验结果显示，肿瘤恶性程度很高，要求林女士先做流产，再进行手术和化疗。

林女士听后犹如晴天霹雳，她怎么也不敢相信自己得了癌症，更不敢相信要做流产除掉胎儿。她反复恳求医生，希望能够保住胎儿，但是医生的回答很坚决，流产是唯一的选择，否则连大人也保不住。林女士走投无路，只能联系香港的父母和亲朋，请他们帮忙打听有无其他办法。很快就获悉香港生命修复中医药治癌的事情，林女士当即决定马上前来香港，只要有一丝希望，她都要去尝试。

林女士于 2006 年 5 月初来香港求诊，当时已怀孕 19 周，由于长途奔波加上心情紧张、悲伤劳累，导致腹痛、胎动不安，其舌淡、脉弦细，有流产的迹象。抗癌中医药治疗与西医治疗大不相同，可尽量在医治肿瘤的同时避免流产。治疗 1 周后，林女士的腹痛次数减少，随后继续进行抗癌、保胎同时治疗，患者精神好转，心情也逐渐开朗，2006 年 9 月下旬，喜得麟儿。患者生产以后，乳腺会分泌大量乳汁，这对乳腺癌患者来说是非常严峻的考验，治疗稍有不妥，病情就会立刻加重并加快转移。但借助正确的抗癌中医药治疗方法，患者终于闯过了这道难关，母子平安。现在过去了 18 年，她的儿子也 18 岁了，全家生活愉快。林女士亦留在香港工作多年，她很注重儿子的成长，一有时间就带他去游玩和学习不同课程。林女士从未做过化疗和放疗，甚至连澳大利亚医生严格要求需要大面积切除恶性肿瘤，以及腋部转移淋巴结和周围组织，也完全没有接受，靠着抗癌中医药治疗，她战胜了癌症。

治疗原则

固肾安胎，解郁疏肝，散结攻毒。

常用中药

1. 菟丝子、桑寄生、阿胶、川续断、佛手、山核桃皮、贝母、白芍、蜂房、海藻、昆布等。
2. 同时服用消瘤丸。

影像学、病理学检查报告及诊疗记录

1. 2006 年 4 月 19 日澳大利亚的医生写信证实林小姐怀孕 17 周，并患乳腺癌，伴有淋巴转移，要尽快做化疗及放射治疗。

2. 2006 年 11 月 7 日（分娩后 2 个月）PET/CT 报告证实患者拒绝化疗，左乳腺和腋下无肿瘤复发，右侧乳腺、腋下、淋巴及头、颈、胸、腹、骨盆、骨骼等部位均没有肿瘤转移和复发。

3. 2008 年 4 月 12 日检查报告没有肿瘤复发。

附：患者检查报告

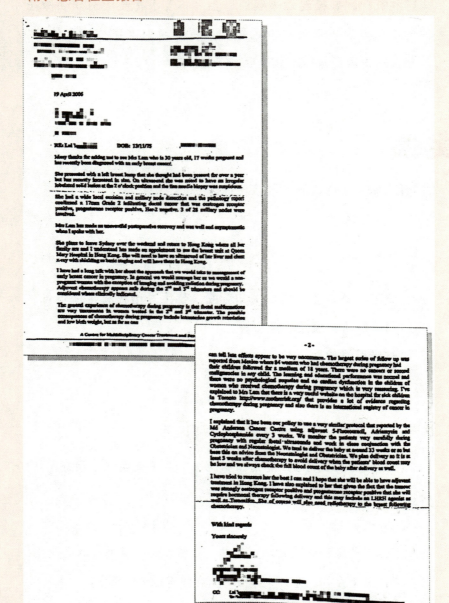

Hospital

Scanning Department
(CT, MR, NM, PET Scan, Bone Densitometry)

> **PET-CT** ▉▉▉▉
> **EXAM. DATE** 7 Nov, 2006

REPORT FOR MRI/CT/NM/PET SCANNING EXAMINATION

NAME Lam ▉▉ ▉▉

ID No. K47▉   **AGE** 30   **SEX** F

EXAM. PET-CT   of   **HOSPITAL** ▉▉▉▉▉▉▉▉▉▉
FDG - Whole Body Trunk

CLINICAL HISTORY:

T1N1 Ca breast with left lumpectomy and axillary dissection done in Apr 2006. Refused adjuvant chemo RT. PET-CT for progress.

Blood glucose level is 5.0 mmol/l.

RADIOLOGICAL REPORT:

RADIOPHARMACEUTICAL:

10.6 mCi F-18 deoxyglucose.

FINDINGS:

Whole body trunk PET scan was performed from the base of skull to the upper thighs. Serial tomographic images of the whole body trunk were presented in transaxial, coronal and sagittal projections. Plain CT of whole body trunk was performed for image fusion with PET scan.

No recurrent tumour is identified in the left breast and left axilla. The right breast, right axilla and internal mammary chain are not involved. No abnormal uptake is present in the mediastinum. No hypermetabolic nodule is present in the lungs. The head and neck and supraclavicular fossae are clear.

The liver shows uniform physiological activity. The spleen, adrenals, pancreas and other abdominal and pelvis visceral organs are unremarkable. Incidentally, mild focal uptake is present at the right iliac area, with SUV max. = 3.39. This is probably a reactive lymph node. Follow up assessment is recommended.

No focal lesion is present in the axial skeleton.

(The plain CT images are performed for anatomical correlation and localization of lesion seen on PET. This is not a complete diagnostic contrast CT study).

(SUV = Standardized Glucose Uptake Value.)

IMPRESSION :

FDG PET-CT scan demonstrates no evidence of recurrent tumour in the left breast and left axillae. The right breast, right axilla and internal mammary chain are unremarkable. No recurrent tumour is present in the head and neck, thorax, abdomen, pelvis and axial bony skeleton.

Thank you for your referral.

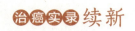

Hospital 醫院

MEDICAL IMAGING DEPARTMENT

Patient's Name	: LAM ▮▮▮	Unit Record No	: ▮▮▮
Sex	: Female	Age	: ▮▮
Examination Date	: 12/04/2008	Examination No	: ▮▮▮
Ward / Class	: ▮▮		

EXAMINATION / PROCEDURE REPORT

Examination : MM/Mammogram - Bilateral

BILATERAL MAMMOGRAM

The parenchymal density of both breasts is dense.

Architectural distortion in the upper outer quadrant of the left breast related to previous operation is detected.

No focal nodule, suspicious microcalcification, skin thickening or nipple retraction could be detected on both sides.

The axillary regions are unremarkable.

IMPRESSION

Architectural distortion in the upper outer quadrant of the left breast related to previous operation.

No mammographic evidence of malignancy.

Comparing with the previous study on 10.11.06, no significant interval change is detected.

Follow up mammogram and ultrasound is recommended.

<u>Statistical Information</u>

6-10% of malignancies are not identified by mammography. Negative mammogram findings should not delay ultrasound evaluation or biopsy of a clinically suspicious lesion.

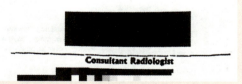

Consultant Radiologist

病案 10

选择生命修复避免大手术

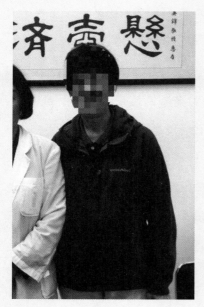

⊙ 郑女士于 2023 年 12 月前来诊治时合影留念

80 岁的郑女士，既往 20 年来一直有心慌、气短及胸闷的症状，早年诊断患有冠心病、高血压及高血脂，服用治疗心脏病和降压、降脂药物 10 多年了。慢性胃病、胃溃疡病史也有十几年。2020 年，自觉身体虚弱，胃痛、胸闷、气短，到医院再次进行身体检查，除了冠心病、高血压等慢性疾病加重，又患上了非常严重、恶性程度非常高的胃癌。经过专家会诊，医院和专家的意见都是让她先做心脏手术。除了冠心病之外，她的心脏还有严重的二尖瓣和三尖瓣反流，医院要求她先做心脏手术，这样才有条件进行下一步恶性肿瘤——胃癌的切除手术。随后经过检查又发现了肝血管瘤，也需要手术，这些疾病导致她的身体处于更加虚弱的状态。她的病情已非常严重，医生认为在这样的情况下，起码需要做 2～3 个手术。

郑女士认为自己已经 80 岁了，身体又非常瘦弱，很难承受这样的大手术，而且还不止要做 1 个，先要做心脏的，又要做胃癌的手术切除，还可能要做肝血管瘤的手术，郑女士实在没法承受动手术对她身体的打击。经过多方了解，她来到了我们这里寻求生命修复的治疗。郑小姐刚来的时候身体非常瘦弱，腹痛严重、心跳气短、精神状态非常差，经过我们对她的细心治疗，谨慎服用中药并且增加了针灸等治疗，她的身体慢慢强壮起来，上述的症状亦慢慢减轻甚至消失，不仅没有腹痛、腹胀等症状，她的心脏情况也有了很大的改善，已经没有气短、呼吸困难等情况。

经过 1 年左右的治疗，郑女士已经恢复了健康，为她检查的医院也认为现在没有必要再做心脏及其他手术。目前郑女士每天在家里帮助子女准备各种生活用品和食物，她的生活过得很充实，非常健康、愉快。

治疗原则

活血祛瘀养心，祛邪扶正攻毒。

常用中药

1. 桃仁、红花、瓜蒌、薤白、人参、三棱、莪术、丹参、当归、郁金、三七、土鳖虫、猕猴梨根、半枝莲等。
2. 同时服用消瘤丸、化瘀丸。

影像学、病理学检查报告及诊疗记录

1. 2021年4月20日检查报告显示郑女士有高血压、冠心病、二尖瓣及三尖瓣反流，医院提出应先做心脏手术，再做胃恶性肿瘤切除手术。

2. 2021年4月21日病理检查报告显示胃有分化程度很差的恶性肿瘤，为胃印戒细胞癌。

3. 2021年4月29日检查报告显示肝血管瘤，动静脉畸形。

附：患者检查报告

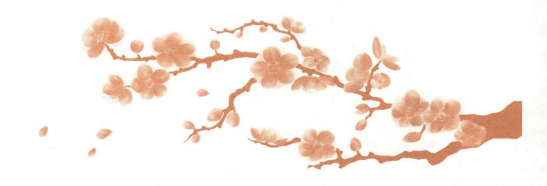

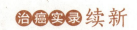

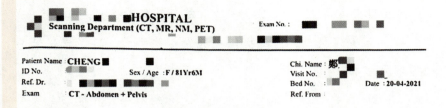

■HOSPITAL
Scanning Department (CT, MR, NM, PET)

Exam No. :

Patient Name : CHENG■ ■
Chi. Name : 鄭■
ID No. : ■
Sex / Age : F / 81Yr6M
Visit No. :
Ref. Dr. : ■
Bed No. : ■
Date : 20-04-2021
Exam : CT - Abdomen + Pelvis
Ref. From :

There is a thin wall left ovarian cyst. This may represent a residual physiological cyst. If there is clinical concern, follow-up ultrasound may be warranted.

There are bilateral renal cortical cysts with no suspicious features. The urinary bladder demonstrates a prominent wall which may be due to its lack of significant distension. Cystitis or neoplastic infiltration of the urinary bladder is not excluded and correlation with urinalysis / cystoscopy may be warranted.

There are signs of some dilated arteries and veins in the posterior subcapsular aspect of segment 7 of the liver. This is associated with a wedge-shaped area of contrast hyperenhancement during the arterial phase. The appearances are suggestive of an area of arteriovenous shunting and may be related to an arteriovenous malformation / atypical haemangioma. If there is clinical concern, follow-up imaging may be warranted. There are hepatic cysts with no suspicious features.

There is mild thickening of the gallbladder suggesting chronic cholecystitis with/without adenomyomatosis.

The pancreas is unremarkable. This is with the limitation that early pancreatitis may appear unremarkable on CT and correlation with serial amylase levels may be more sensitive.

The spleen, adrenal glands, small and large bowel and the stomach are unremarkable.

Limited scans through the lungs demonstrate minor dependent changes in the lung bases.

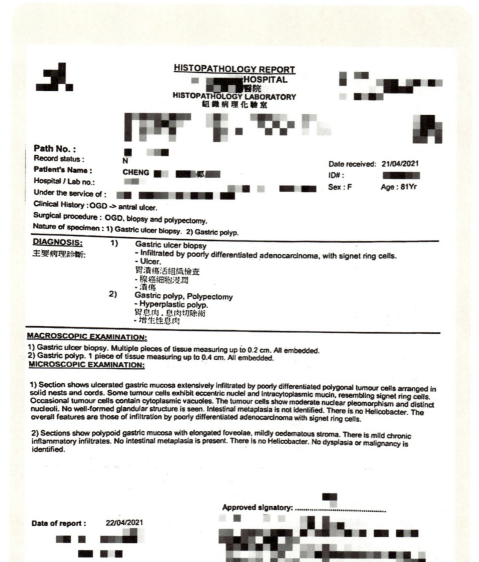

HISTOPATHOLOGY REPORT

█████ **HOSPITAL**
█████ 醫院
HISTOPATHOLOGY LABORATORY
組織病理化驗室

Path No. :
Record status :   N
Patient's Name :   CHENG █████ 怡█████   Date received: 21/04/2021
Hospital / Lab no.:   ID# :   █████
Under the service of :   Sex : F   Age : 81Yr
Clinical History : OGD -> antral ulcer.

Surgical procedure : OGD, biopsy and polypectomy.

Nature of specimen : 1) Gastric ulcer biopsy. 2) Gastric polyp.

DIAGNOSIS: 1)   Gastric ulcer biopsy
主要病理診斷: - Infiltrated by poorly differentiated adenocarcinoma, with signet ring cells.
                            - Ulcer.
                            胃潰瘍活組織檢查
                            - 腺癌細胞浸潤
                            - 潰瘍
                     2)   Gastric polyp, Polypectomy
                            - Hyperplastic polyp.
                            胃息肉，息肉切除術
                            - 增生性息肉

MACROSCOPIC EXAMINATION:
1) Gastric ulcer biopsy. Multiple pieces of tissue measuring up to 0.2 cm. All embedded.
2) Gastric polyp. 1 piece of tissue measuring up to 0.4 cm. All embedded.
MICROSCOPIC EXAMINATION:

1) Section shows ulcerated gastric mucosa extensively infiltrated by poorly differentiated polygonal tumour cells arranged in solid nests and cords. Some tumour cells exhibit eccentric nuclei and intracytoplasmic mucin, resembling signet ring cells. Occasional tumour cells contain cytoplasmic vacuoles. The tumour cells show moderate nuclear pleomorphism and distinct nucleoli. No well-formed glandular structure is seen. Intestinal metaplasia is not identified. There is no Helicobacter. The overall features are those of infiltration by poorly differentiated adenocarcinoma with signet ring cells.

2) Sections show polypoid gastric mucosa with elongated foveolae, mildly oedematous stroma. There is mild chronic inflammatory infiltrates. No intestinal metaplasia is present. There is no Helicobacter. No dysplasia or malignancy is identified.

Approved signatory: ....

Date of report :   22/04/2021

cw

22/04/2021 12:46:16   (Patient discharged before issue of this report.)   Page : 1 of 1

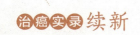

Medical Centre
■■醫務中心

Letter of Referral

Consultant
STH

29 April, 2021

Dear Dr.

CHENG ■■■ ■Female, DoB: 22/09/1939
Our ref.:

I learned that the above named lady has gastric ulcer which suspected to be malignant.

She has chronic hypertension, coronary artery disease (proven by CT scan), degenerative valvular disease and paroxysmal SVT and been FU in QEH. She also has consulted me intermittently in the past. She has no active cardiac symptom in her activities of daily living.

Clinical examination today found no ankle edema, clinic BP is on the high side though her fome BP are normal. There is no sign of heart failure. Bedside echocardiogram found good LV function, mild to moderate mitral and tricuspid regurgitation.

I believe her cardiac status is fit to have surgery in case she needs for resection of the malignancy. Aspirin can be stopped and I have added Vastarel MR 35mg bd which is a cardio-protective drug for potential ischaemia. There is no need for antibiotic cover for her valvular problem. Meticulous attention for fluid balance in the peri-operative period is required to prevent fluid overload.

Please feel free to contact me should you need further information. Thank you.

Best regards,

战胜晚期肺癌 20 年

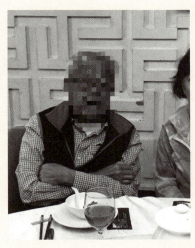

⌒ 潘先生于 2022 年 3 月前来合影留念

潘先生是位成功的企业家，于多地开设制衣公司，制造的男女服装品牌远销欧洲各国。近几年，他亦有向国内投资，发展酒店、旅游业等项目。潘先生是位大老板，公司里各个部门的职员众多，大家都认同老板是位工作认真、精明、精力充沛的人，对员工要求严格，一点小毛病也会被他发现，因此从不敢有过失，否则就担心会被"炒鱿鱼"。但是对于这位潘老板，有一件事是新来的年轻职员并不知道的，只有老员工才知道，原来这位老板患有肺癌，并发展到晚期，至今已有 20 多年。

2002 年年底，潘先生发现肺癌时已经 62 岁了。他立即到医院接受当时最先进的靶向治疗，但是服用靶向药物 3 个月后，肺部肿瘤不仅没有缩小，甚至还转移到胸膜上，令他的病情加重，肺部和胸膜都有癌肿，而且已属晚期。潘先生果断地放弃西医治疗，前来进行生命修复的中医药治疗。当时的他胸痛严重、呼吸短促、咳嗽频繁，他和家人都认为病情严重，不容乐

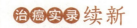

观。我们经过辨证分析后，决定采用益气养阴、排毒攻癌、软坚散结为治疗原则的中医药治疗。几个月后，他的病情明显好转，疼痛基本上已经消失，其他症状也明显改善。然而，他却因工作繁忙，加上缺乏耐心，对癌病也没有充分的认识，故停止治疗，不再吃中药。几个月后，他的病情再次加重，经常咳嗽甚至出现咯血症状，胸痛加背痛，急忙前来再次治疗，并表明这次不敢再随便停药了。就这样坚持了1年左右，患者检查发现双肺肿瘤已消失，并且没有出现新的转移病灶。而潘先生亦继续坚持治疗，数年后，改为间断服药，至今他仍努力工作，肿瘤也没有复发。

肺癌是发病率及死亡率很高的癌症，晚期肺癌更是凶险，同时肺癌也是我们治疗最多的癌症之一。这些成功治疗的案例，说明了晚期癌症都是可治的，不仅是化疗、靶向治疗、放疗等方法可用于治癌，还有天然的无毒、无副作用且更为有效的治疗方法。

扶正益阴，排毒攻癌，软坚散结。

常用中药

1. 北沙参、太子参、黄药子、生地黄、玉竹、石斛、玄参、
   川贝母、生大黄、全蝎等。
2. 同时服用散结丸。

影像学、病理学检查报告及诊疗记录

1. 2005 年 2 月 23 日 PET/CT 检查报告与 2004 年 6 月 17 日
检查比较，治疗反应良好，两肺未见有肿瘤病灶，胸部无肿大
淋巴。脑、颈、胸、骨盆均无转移病灶。

2. 治疗前肺及胸膜有恶性肿瘤。

3. 治疗后肺部 X 线片正常。

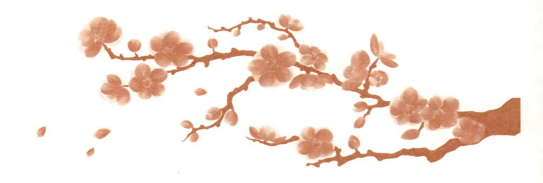

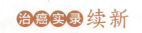

▬▬▬▬▬▬ Hospital

Scanning Department
(CT, MR, NM, PET Scan, Bone Densitometry)

▬▬▬▬▬▬▬▬▬▬▬ Tel:▬▬▬▬▬▬▬ Fax:▬▬▬▬▬

REPORT FOR MRI/CT/NM/PET SCANNING EXAMINATION

OUR REF. : ▬▬▬▬▬▬   **EXAM. DATE** : Wed, 23 Feb, 2005
NAME : Pun ▬▬▬▬▬
ID No. : E29▬▬▬

There is no abnormal hypermetabolic lesion in the head and neck and supraclavicular fossae. Bilateral axillae are normal.

The liver shows uniform physiological activity. Bilateral adrenals are normal. No significant positive finding is present in the abdomen and pelvis.

There is no focal lesion in the axial bony skeleton.

(The plain CT images are performed for anatomical correlation and localization of lesion seen on PET. This is not a complete diagnostic contrast CT study).

IMPRESSION :

Good clinical response when compared with the pretreatment study in 17 June 2004. No residual active tumor nodule is present in both lungs. No residual hypermetabolic lymph node is present in the thorax. No evidence of metastasis is noted in the brain, head and neck, thorax, abdomen and pelvis.

SIGNED: ▬▬▬▬▬▬▬▬

DR REPORT ▬▬▬▬▬▬

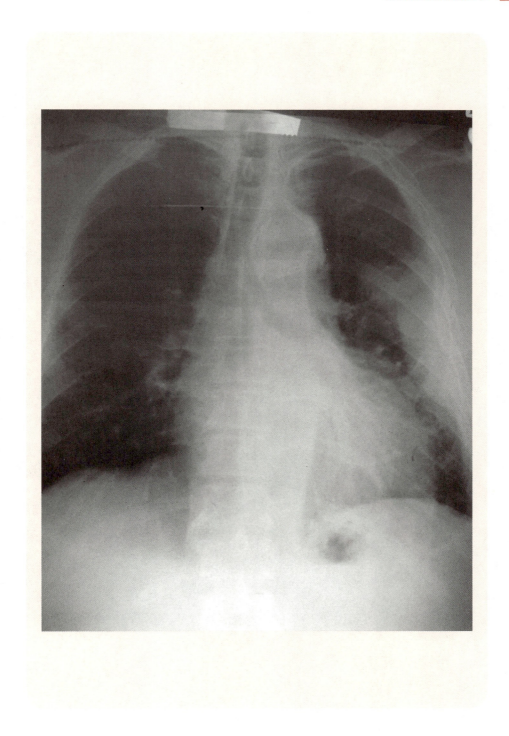

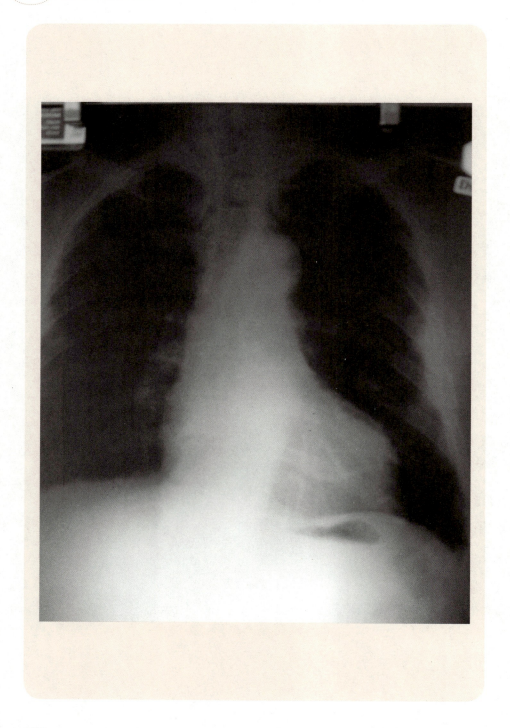

病案 **12**

晚期肺癌全身转移脑转移康复

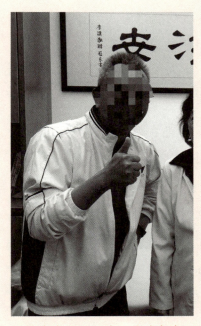

● 何先生于 2022 年 4 月前来诊治时合影留念

2016 年，何先生常常感到劳累、气喘不适，同年 5 月在颈部，锁骨上方发现肿大的淋巴结，于是到医院检查。经取材颈部肿大的结节并做病理检查，确定是来源于肺的分化程度很差，即恶性程度很高的，非小细胞肺癌的转移灶，医院尽快安排他做了 6 个疗程的化疗，随后他就在不停地治疗之中。放疗后，又做了 4 个疗程的化疗，但检查却发现癌指数异常升高，2018 年 5 月 PET 检查显示脑部及双肺发现转移；2018 年 8 月做脑放疗；2018 年 10 月脑转移灶加重，遂再做 6 个周期的免疫治疗；2019 年 7 月在做免疫治疗多次以后，发生治疗药物的耐药、抗药，继而又转为化疗加靶向治疗。期间发生严重的皮肤过敏反应，有红肿、脱皮状况，癌指数继续增高。2019 年年底及 2020 年继续化疗、靶向治疗；2020 年 7 月检查发现脑转移灶，肺部、肺门肿瘤均增大。于 2020 年 8 月做开颅手术取出 1 个脑转移肿瘤，然后继续放疗至 2020 年 10 月，但又发生了硬脑膜转移及面部肌肉的转移，再做放疗。2021 年 6 月又发现新的多发脑肿瘤、脑膜、肌肉、骨骼等转移，由于腰椎的癌肿转移压迫神经造成严重的腰痛、腿痛，日夜剧烈疼痛；遂于 2021 年 6 月 10 日再做腰部椎板切除手术，并再做脑部转移肿瘤及面部肌肉转移瘤的切除。但医生明确说明了位于脑部深层的肿瘤无法切除。手术后经检查发现严重脑水肿，肿瘤增大，且伴有严重尿潴留，更为严重的是在腰椎管腔内及腰部骨髓中有多发转移灶，导致双下肢瘫痪，完全不能活动。前列腺亦有病变需进一步检查，并有股骨转移。

经过以上长期严峻和危险的各种治疗之后，患者于再次手术后的 1 周多，即 2021 年 6 月 21 日前来就诊。当时的他非常虚弱，讲话困难近乎失语。需要坐在轮椅上由家人推着，双下肢完全瘫痪无知觉且不能动，在轮椅上还有一个大尿袋，小便无知觉完全依靠导尿，腿和足部水肿，疼痛严重。何先生患晚期肺癌已生命垂危，全身有大量转移病灶。脑部有多发转移，导致语言不清，思维混乱，不能书写。虽然做过 2 次脑部手术了，但医生说深部的脑肿瘤因危险性很大均没有手术切除，加上脊椎的肿瘤发展转移，并造成严重疼痛和瘫痪。我们决定除中药外，为他增加针灸等经络治疗。经过悉心的诊治，患者逐渐好转，于 2 周之后，腿部可逐渐轻微活动，稍稍有点感觉；于 3 周以后，可以稍短时间站立；1 个月左右，他已经可以扶持铁架行走几步，及后逐渐增多步行的次数。然而，这段日子内，他的颈部又再度出现大的肿块，以及尚有腰、腿部转移灶的严重疼痛，但经过悉心的治理后都逐渐得到缓解，之后由需要扶拐杖行走，到不再使用拐杖也能行走，身体多处的疼痛亦已消失。更可喜的是，思维和讲话都恢复正常，书写及语言表达能力也全部恢复。

在此期间，虽完全没有西医治疗，但私人医院里也多次催促他去做检查，以便再做化疗、放疗、免疫治疗等。我们的意见是不想让他在短时间内反复多次地接受放射线检查，故此何先生也多次拖延检查时间，最后医院再三催促，于2021年10月28日去做了检查，结果显示他的颅骨及脑内转移灶全部消失，就连面部肌肉肿瘤、椎管内多发肿瘤、肺部及肺门肿瘤、多发骨转移灶也一并消失，总共18个转移病灶全部消失了。医院亦表示何先生已不需要化疗、靶向及免疫等治疗了，何先生和家人都很开心。

我们建议他要继续巩固治疗一段日子，但他自认为已经没事了，还一心想着早日去上海谈生意。何先生在这样严重的病情下康复，说明了中医药生命修复疗法治癌效果明确，也说明了癌症不一定是绝症，即使是晚期癌症，只要使用了正确的治疗方法，也是能够康复的。这对于晚期癌症发生多处转移的患者，不是放弃，不是无药可医，而是对进一步的治疗和研究，提供了新的方向和方法。

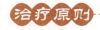

治疗原则

扶正祛邪，攻毒消瘤。

常用中药

1. 龙葵、山慈菇、玄参、白芍、鳖甲、丹参、石见穿、制附子、肉桂、生大黄、玄明粉、土鳖虫、全蝎等。
2. 同时服用消瘤丸、散结丸。

影像学、病理学检查报告及诊疗记录

1. 2020 年 7 月 25 日脑部 MRI 扫描显示肺部癌肿脑转移，准备做手术。

2. 2021 年 1 月 12 日脑 MRI 扫描显示左脑手术后，左颞叶和枕叶又有多发硬脑膜转移。

3. 2021 年 3 月 24 日面部骨 CT 显示左颞部肿瘤增大。

4. 2021 年 6 月 11 日腰椎 MRI 扫描显示大量腰椎转移、骨转移、膀胱扩张、双侧肾积水。

5. 2021 年 6 月 18 日脑 MRI 扫描显示脑部转移病灶增大及增多，脑水肿、颈部大量淋巴转移。

6. 2021 年 10 月 28 日 PET/CT 报告显示肺原发病灶消失，而且脑、骨、腰椎等全身 18 个癌转移灶全部消失。

附：患者检查报告

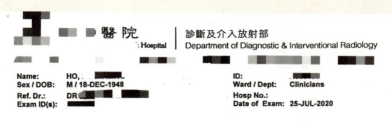

醫 院　診斷及介入放射部
: Hospital　Department of Diagnostic & Interventional Radiology

Name: HO, ▮▮▮▮▮L	**ID:**	▮▮▮▮▮
Sex / DOB: M / 18-DEC-1948	**Ward / Dept:**	Clinicians
Ref. Dr.: DR▮▮▮▮	**Hosp No.:**	
Exam ID(s): ▮▮▮▮	**Date of Exam:**	25-JUL-2020

MRI SCAN OF BRAIN WITH AND WITHOUT CONTRAST

<u>Clinical data:</u>
Ca lung. Brain metastasis in left temporal lobe, planned for surgery.

<u>Technique:</u>

Pre-contrast:
Axial T1 T2W SWI DWI & ADC map
Coronal FLAIR

Post-contrast (Gadolinium):
Axial T1 weighted
Coronal T1 weighted
Sagittal T1 weighted

<u>Findings:</u>
Previous MR scan dated July 3, 2020 is used for comparison.

A focal mass lesion is detected at the anterior left temporal lobe. It is T1-hypo, T2-hyperintense with avid heterogeneous contrast enhancement. Dark foci on SWI are present. The heterogeneous enhancing focus measures 2.2cm x 2.1cm x 2.6cm (Vs 2.7cm x 2.2cm x 2.8cm). Interval decreased perilesional white matter oedema is present at the left temporal lobe, left insula and left trigone. Interval decreased associated mass effect is found. Interval less compression of the left lateral ventricle with less sulcal effacement is seen. No midline shift is noted.

A few small hyperintense foci are found at bilateral periventricular white matters, especially around both occipital horns. No associated mass effect or perifocal white matter edema is seen. No abnormal contrast enhancement or restricted diffusion is noted. They are similar to the last MR scan.

No focal enhancing mass is demonstrated in the rest of brain, brainstem and cerebellum.
No intracerebral haematoma is seen.
No acute infarct on DWI and ADC map is evident.
Bilateral cavernous sinuses are unremarkable.
Basal cistern and suprasellar cistern are clear.

Ventricles and cerebral sulci are not dilated. No hydrocephalus is detected.
No extra-axial fluid collection or haematoma is evident.

Bilateral cerebellopontine cisterns are clear. Bilateral VII-VIII nerve complexes are preserved. No abnormal focal enhancing mass is found.
No abnormal leptomeningeal or pachymeningeal enhancement is noted.
Corpus callosum and the pituitary gland are normal.
Paranasal sinuses and mastoid aircells are clear.

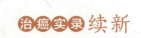

Exam(s) Ordered : MR
Exam No :
Completed Date : 12/01/2021 13:43

REPORT STATUS :
APPROVED

Main report only

MRI SCAN OF ▇▇▇ WITH AND WITHOUT CONTRAST

Clinical data:
Ca lung with brain secondary. Previous RT and brain resection. Reassessment.

Technique:
Pre-contrast: Post-contrast (Gadolinium):
Axial T1, T2, SWI, DWI & ADC map Axial T1
Coronal FLAIR Coronal T1
Sagittal T1

Findings:
Comparison is made with previous MRI dated 15 September 2020.

Evidence of previous left temporal craniotomy is noted. Focal enhancement about 1.7 x 1.1 cm in left anterior temporalis muscle is seen, ? post-operative change (series 9 image 4).

Interval decrease in size of the previously noted T1 hypointense and T2 hyperintense cystic lesion in the lateral aspect of left anterior temporal lobe is seen. It measures 1.4 x 2.1 x 0.8 cm versus 1.6 x 2.4 x 1.6 cm previously (craniocaudal x anteroposterior x transverse diameter). Thin rim enhancement is similar. Findings are suggestive of post-operative change.

Interval increase in vasogenic edema in the left anterior temporal lobe is seen. Interval development of multiple lobulated enhancing lesions up to 0.8 cm in thickness in the left middle cranial fossa around the left temporal lobe. Similar dural lesion about 1.3 x 1.2 x 0.9 cm in the lateral aspect of left anterior occipital lobe is noted. Findings are suggestive of dural metastases. Cavernous sinuses and Meckel's cave are grossly intact.

There are a few small non-enhancing T2 hyperintense foci in the periventricular white matter of bilateral cerebral hemispheres, especially around bilateral occipital horns, suggestive of nonspecific white matter change.

No other abnormal signal intensity or mass lesion in the brain is seen.

No abnormal enhancement or leptomeningeal thickening is demonstrated.

No evidence of intracerebral hemorrhage is noted.

Continued findings:
No evidence of restricted diffusion to suggest acute infarct is present.

Cerebral sulci and cisterns are not widened.
Grey white matter differentiation is within normal limit.
Ventricles are prominent in size similar to previous MRI.
No mid-line shift is seen.
No extra-axial collection is noted.

Impression:
1. Evidence of previous left temporal craniotomy. Focal enhancement about 1.7 x 1.1 cm in left anterior temporalis muscle, ? post-operative change. Suggest follow-up scan for progress.

2. Interval decrease in size of the previously noted cystic lesion in the left anterior temporal lobe. Thin rim enhancement is similar. Findings are suggestive of post-operative change.

3. Interval development of multiple enhancing lesions around the left temporal lobe and anterior left occipital lobe, suggestive of dural metastases. Interval increase in vasogenic edema in the left anterior temporal lobe.

4. No leptomeningeal thickening or enhancement is seen.

5. No intracranial hemorrhage is seen.

6. No acute cerebral infarct is noted.

7. Ventricles are prominent in size similar to previous MRI. No obvious hydrocephalus is seen.

19/1/2021

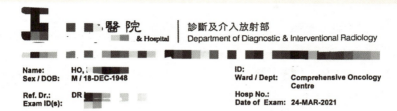

Name: HO,
Sex / DOB: M / 18-DEC-1948
ID:
Ward / Dept: Comprehensive Oncology Centre

Ref. Dr.: DR
Exam ID(s):
Hosp No.:
Date of Exam: 24-MAR-2021

CT SCAN OF FACIAL BONES WITH AND WITHOUT CONTRAST

Clinical data:

Ca lung with brain secondary. Right buccal mucosal mass ? nature.

Technique:
5 mm thick slice obtained at 5 mm intervals through the facial bones with and without contrast (Iopamiro).

Findings:

Comparison with previous MRI studies dated Feb 6, 2021 and Mar 3, 2021.

Previously noted ill-defined enhancing soft tissue mass at left temporal region shows interval increase in size. It lies at the anterior aspect of left temporalis and masseter muscles. It abuts onto the lateral wall of the left maxillary sinus and left maxillary bone. It now measures 2.5 x 1.8 x 3 cm (W x AP x H). It shows heterogeneous contrast enhancement, and contains no calcification. Its margin is irregular. No definite bony erosion is noted at the adjacent maxillary wall or maxillary bone. The left buccal wall appears slightly thickened.

Bilateral masticator muscles are unremarkable.

No enlarged upper jugular or submental lymph node is seen.

Bilateral submandibular glands are unremarkable.

Bilateral parotid glands are unremarkable.

Small retention cyst at right maxillary sinus. Other paranasal sinuses and mastoid cells are clear.

No gross mass is seen at the nasopharynx.

Page 1 of 2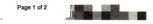

醫院 | 診斷及介入放射部
Hospital | Department of Diagnostic & Interventional Radiology

Name: HO,	**ID:**
Sex / DOB: M / 18-DEC-1948	**Ward / Dept:** Comprehensive Oncology Centre
Ref. Dr.: DR	**Hosp No.:**
Exam ID(s):	**Date of Exam:** 24-MAR-2021

<u>Impression:</u>

1. Previously noted ill-defined heterogeneous enhancing soft tissue mass at left temporal region, at the anterior aspect of temporalis and masseter muscles shows interval increase in size, compared with serial MRI studies. Recurrent tumour cannot be excluded. Suggest further correlation with tissue diagnosis.

2. Small retention cyst at right maxillary sinus.

Dr.
Department of Diagnostic & Interventional Radiology
MBBS(HK) FRCR FHKCR PDIP Epidemiology &
Biostatistics(CUHK)
MPH(CUHK) MMed (DR), NUS
FHKAM(Radiology)

Typed By :

Approved Date-Time:
25-MAR-2021 12:27 PM

Report read by :_____ Date_____ Time_____
Doctor's Signature   dd/mm/yy

 2 of 2

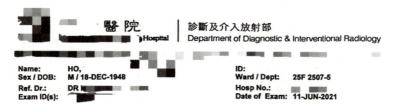

醫 院 | 診斷及介入放射部
Hospital | Department of Diagnostic & Interventional Radiology

Name:	HO,	ID:	
Sex / DOB:	M / 18-DEC-1948	Ward / Dept:	25F 2507-5
Ref. Dr.:	DR	Hosp No.:	
Exam ID(s):		Date of Exam:	11-JUN-2021

MRI SCAN OF LUMBAR SPINE WITH AND WITHOUT CONTRAST

Clinical data:

Ca lung. C/O L pelvic pain ? bone secondary.

Technique:

Pre-contrast:
Sagittal T1, T2, STIR, T1 fat saturation
Axial T2 weighted

Post-contrast (Gadolinium):
Sagittal T1 fat saturation
Axial T1 fat saturation

Findings:

Alignment appears satisfactory.
No definite vertebral body collapse is seen.
No abnormal focal marrow signal is noted.
Conus medullaris terminates at T12/L1 level.

Multiple intraspinal enhancing foci are noted in the lumbar spinal canal. The prominent ones are noted at L2, L3-4, L4 and L4-5 levels +/- inferior tip of spinal canal. Size measures up to about 0.4 x 0.6 x 1.0 cm.

Decreased T2 signal intensity is noted involving multiple intervertebral discs, consistent with disc desiccation change.
L4-5 and L5-S1 disc spaces are decreased.
At L1-2 level, no significant disc protrusion is seen.
At L2-3 L3-4 and L5-S1 levels, mild posterior disc protrusions are seen. No substantial central spinal stenosis is seen at these levels.
At L4-5 level, moderate disc protrusion with associated facet joint degeneration and ligamentum flavum hypertrophy are seen. Narrowing of the spinal canal and crowding of the cauda equina are noted. The AP dimension of the spinal canal is reduced to about 0.4 cm. Compromise of bilateral L4-5 intervertebral neuroforamina is noted.

Incidental finding of abnormal marrow signal loss is noted at the T3, T4 and T5 vertebral bodies on localizer images; worrisome of osseous metastases.

Urinary bladder is grossly distended. Mild bilateral hydronephrosis are noted.

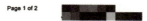
081

醫院 . Hospital | 診斷及介入放射部
Department of Diagnostic & Interventional Radiology

Name:	HO,	**ID:**	
Sex / DOB:	M / 18-DEC-1948	**Ward / Dept:**	25F 2507-5
Ref. Dr.:	DR	**Hosp No.:**	
Exam ID(s):		**Date of Exam:**	11-JUN-2021

Impression:

1. Multiple intraspinal enhancing foci in the lumbar spinal canal. The prominent ones are noted at L2, L3-4, L4 and L4-5 levels +/- inferior tip of spinal canal. Features are suspicious of metastatic lesions.

2. Spondylotic change of the lumbar spine. Features are most prominent at the L4-5 level, where spinal stenosis and crowding of the cauda equina are noted.

3. Incidental finding of abnormal marrow signal loss at the T3, T4 and T5 vertebral bodies; worrisome of osseous metastases.

4. Incidental finding of grossly distended urinary bladder and bilateral hydronephrosis.

Dr
Department of Diagnostic & Interventional Radiology
MBBS FRCR FHKCR FHKAM(Radiology)

Typed By :

Approved Date-Time:
11-JUN-2021 05:04 PM

Report read by :_____ Date _____ Time_____
                Doctor's Signature   dd/mm/yy

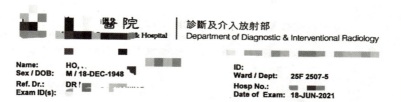

醫 院 │ 診斷及介入放射部
& Hospital │ Department of Diagnostic & Interventional Radiology

Name: HO, ..	**ID:**
Sex / DOB: M / 18-DEC-1948	**Ward / Dept:** 25F 2507-5
Ref. Dr.: DR	**Hosp No.:**
Exam ID(s):	**Date of Exam:** 18-JUN-2021

MRI SCAN OF BRAIN WITH AND WITHOUT CONTRAST

<u>Clinical data:</u>
CA lung. Brain metastasis.

<u>Technique:</u>

Pre-contrast:
Axial T1 T2 SWI DWI & ADC map
Coronal FLAIR

Post-contrast (Gadolinium):
Axial T1 weighted
Coronal T1 weighted
Sagittal T1 weighted

<u>Findings:</u>
Comparison is made with MR scan dated 1 Jun. 2021.

Evidence of left fronto-temporal craniotomy is noted.

Contrast enhanced tumoral thickening of the left temporalis muscle has increased in size, now measuring 1.3cm (previously, it measured 1.1cm) in maximal thickness. Extension into the underlying left frontal skull bone is noted.

Enhancing lesions are noted in the left temporal lobe with interval increase in size. The larger ones are listed as below:
1. Left anterior temporal, 2.0x3.1x3.1cm (previously, it measured 1.7x1.9x2.7cm)
2. Left posterior temporal, 0.90x1.5x2.0cm (previously, it measured 1x1.5x1.3cm).

Enhancing lesions are noted in the cerebellum with interval increase in size and number noted. The larger one is listed as below:

1. Left cerebellum, 1.1x0.66x1.0cm (previously, it measured 0.8x0.4x0.5cm).

The associated vasogenic edema has increased in size. Features are suggestive of progression of disease.

No obvious enhancing mass lesion is noted in the right cerebral hemisphere. No obvious leptomeningeal enhancement.

Ventricles are not dilated. No midline shift or extracerebral collection.

Page 1 of 2

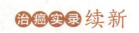

醫院   診斷及介入放射部
& Hospital   Department of Diagnostic & Interventional Radiology

Name:	HO, .	**ID:**	
Sex / DOB:	M / 18-DEC-1948	**Ward / Dept:**	25F 2507-5
Ref. Dr.:	DR	**Hosp No.:**	
Exam ID(s):		**Date of Exam:**	18-JUN-2021

<u>Findings:</u> (Cont'd)
T2 weighted hypointense signal in bilateral cerebral white matters appear similar. No restricted diffusion on DWI image to suggest acute ischaemia. Increased signal at the left mastoid air cell suggestive of mastoiditis.

Mucous retention cyst in right maxillary sinus has resolved.

Clustered enlarged left upper neck lymph nodes are seen. The biggest measures 0.97x0.99cm.

<u>Impression:</u>
Comparison is made with MR scan dated 1 Jun. 2021.

1. Evidence of left fronto-temporal craniotomy is noted.

2. Contrast enhanced tumoral thickening of the left temporalis muscle has increased in size, now measuring 1.3cm (previously, it measured 1.1cm) in maximal thickness. Extension into the underlying left frontal skull bone is noted.

3. Enhancing lesions are noted in the left temporal lobe with interval increase in size. Enhancing lesions are noted in the cerebellum with interval increase in size and number noted. The associated vasogenic edema has increased in size. Features are suggestive of progression of disease.

4. T2 weighted hypointense signal in bilateral cerebral white matters appear similar.

5. Increased signal at the left mastoid air cell suggestive of mastoiditis.

6. Mucous retention cyst in right maxillary sinus has resolved.

7. Clustered enlarged left upper neck lymph nodes are seen. The biggest measures 0.97x0.99cm.

Dr.
Department of Diagnostic & Interventional Radiology
MBBS(HK) FRCR(UK) FHKCR FHKAM(Radiology)

Typed By :

Approved Date-Time:
18-JUN-2021 05:58 PM

Report read by :_____   Date_____   Time_____
    Doctor's Signature   dd/mm/yy

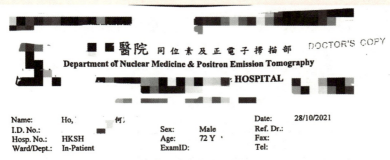

醫院 同位素及正電子掃描部
Department of Nuclear Medicine & Positron Emission Tomography

DOCTOR'S COPY

■ ■ HOSPITAL

Name:	Ho, 何			**Date:**	28/10/2021
I.D. No.:		**Sex:**	Male	**Ref. Dr.:**	
Hosp. No.:	HKSH	**Age:**	72 Y	**Fax:**	
Ward/Dept.:	In-Patient	**ExamID:**		**Tel:**	

POSITRON EMISSION TOMOGRAPHY
(^{18}F-FDG ONCOLOGY)

History:

A 72 year-old gentleman, spiculated nodule in 05/2016. PET in 2016 showed RML nodule and lymph nodes. Excisional biopsy of right supraclavicular node confirmed metastatic poorly differentiated non-small cell carcinoma of lung origin. He was given 6 cycles of Alimta and Taxol. PET in 10/2016 suggested improvement with residual right hilar nodes. Radiation therapy to right hilar nodes were given, then 4 cycles of chemotherapy. CEA rose to 4.9. PET in 05/2018 found active lesions in left temporal lobe and bilateral lungs. Radiation to brain then chemotherapy in ~08/2018. PET in 10/2018 found borderline worsening in RML nodule and right lower interlobar node. Given 6 cycles of Keytruda. PET in 03/2019 stable disease. PET here in 07/2019 on same treatment regimen worrisome of drug resistance. Treated with chemotargeted therapy, but stopped due to severe skin problem. CEA from 5.1 in 07/2019 to 8.7 in 11/2019. PET in 12/2019 showed stable RML lung tumor and right interlobar node. He had alimta. CEA at 6.6 in 07/2020. PET here in 07/2020 showed recurrent left temporal brain metastasis, worsening of RML lung tumor and left hilar node. Excision of left temporal lobe metastasis in 08/2020, then radiotherapy to RML in 10/2020. He developed dural metastasis, then Cyberknife to left temporal region. He noticed suspicious metastatic nodule anterior to the masseter muscle, treated with radiotherapy. PET here in 06/2021 showed progression with new nodal, brain, lleptomeningeal, muscle and bone metastases. He had lumbar laminectomy and excision of muscle and temporal lobectomy in 06/2021, followed by targeted therapy. Patient is asymptomatic. Known thyrotoxicosis treated medically in 1995. No TB.

Radiopharmaceutical: 9.8 mCi ^{18}F-FDG injected intravenously.

Findings:

Limited whole body CT transmission and PET emission imaging began at 60 minutes after radiopharmaceutical administration (blood glucose 6.3 mmol/l), spanning a region from base of skull to upper thigh. 60 mg Spasmonal was given p.o. before ^{18}F-FDG administration.

Liver tissue normal reference uptake has a SUVmax of 3.07.

Comparison is made with previous PET/CT study performed here on 11/06/2021. The spiculated primary lung tumor in lateral RML is metabolically resolved. Prior consolidation with atelectasis adjacent to the tumor bed in lateral segment of RML suggestive of post-irradiation change is improved. The pericystic GGO in posterior LUL has metabolically subsided. Previous patchy lung density in central and posterior aspect of RLL is largely stable. No new hypermetabolic nodule or mass is found in other lung segments. There is new small amount of right pleural effusion, without left pleural or pericardial effusion. Previous mildly hypermetabolic left hilar and right interlobar nodes are either stable or improved. No new hypermetabolic lymphadenopathy is present at rest of mediastinum or supraclavicular fossa. Previous bilateral

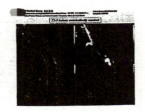

Ho

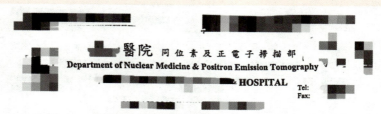

醫院 同位素及正電子掃描部
Department of Nuclear Medicine & Positron Emission Tomography
HOSPITAL
Tel:
Fax:

axillary lymph nodes remain metabolically resolved. Prior hypermetabolic lymph nodes at left submandibular, left retromandibular, left upper jugular level II and left intraparotid regions are all metabolically resolved. The right jugular chains are clear. Thyroid gland and nasopharynx are unremarkable.

Prior hypermetabolic soft tissue density in left infratemporal fossa just lateral to the left maxillary sinus, abutting the left temporalis muscle is metabolically resolved or excised. Prior hypermetabolic lesion in the lateral left temporal region operative bed, left parietal lobe (lateral periphery), left inferior temporal lobe as well as left cerebellum are no longer seen. Prior hypermetabolic lesion the left lateral frontal bone (associated with lytic change) and extending to adjacent left temporalis muscle has metabolically resolved.

In the abdomen, there is normal size and metabolism of the liver, spleen, pancreas and bilateral adrenal glands. No new hyperdense gallstone. No new focal hypermetabolic thickening is detected in the stomach and bowel activities are mild and physiologic. Kidney configuration is normal, without hydronephrosis or hydroureter. Distended urinary bladder has subsided. No new pelvic ascites is detected. There is no new hypermetabolic lymphadenopathy at retroperitoneum, mesentery or omentum.

Skeletal survey shows metabolic quiescence achieved in osseous lesions at the T3 body, T4 body, left T4 pedicle and transverse process, and T5 body. Prior small hypermetabolic foci in the spinal canal at T11, L4, L4/5 and S1 levels are all resolved. There is interval lumbar laminectomy with diffuse activity at the operative bed, suggestive of residual inflammatory and remodeling change. Diffusely increased muscle activity at bilateral temporalis muscle, prevertebral muscle at cervical region, bilateral temporalis muscles and left sartorius muscles suggestive of abnormal muscle strain are subsided. Stable faint activity at right proximal femur is non-specific.

Functional parameters to compare these 2 studies are tabulated below:

HO,	28-Oct-2021				11-Jun-2021				
	in mm		F-18 FDG		in mm		F-18 FDG		
Site	LD	PD	SUVmax	TLG	LD	PD	SUVmax	TLG	TLG %change
RML spiculated tumor	Resolved				8.8	7.1	2.3	0.3	-100.0%
Consolidation and atelectasis in RML	18.1	8.9	1.4						
LUL pericystic GGO	Resolved				8.0	5.7	1.2	0.1	-100.0%
Rt interlobar LN	10.8	7.8	2.7	1.0	11.1	8.0	3.4	1.3	-23.1%
L hilar node	11.2	9.4	3.4	1.4	15.8	12.0	3.2	2.7	-48.1%
L lateral frontal bone & adjacent L temporalis muscle	Resolved				40.2	22.7	15.4	83.1	-100.0%
L temporal region	Resolved				24.3	19.1	19.9	39.4	-100.0%
L infratemporal fossa	Resolved				21.3	13.0	6.0	9.7	-100.0%
L inferior temporal lobe	Resolved				14.4	10.4	9.4	4.9	-100.0%
Lesion at periphery of L parietal region	Resolved				8.7	7.2	9.9	1.7	-100.0%
L cerebellum	Resolved				9.8	7.3	8.3	1.3	-100.0%
L retromandibular node	Resolved				8.8	8.0	12.8	2.4	-100.0%
L submandibular node	Resolved				8.6	7.9	6.2	1.1	-100.0%
Small focus at R spinal canal at T11 level	Resolved				12.3	9.0	3.2	1.3	-100.0%
Small focus at anterior spinal canal at L4-5 level	Resolved				7.3	5.8	3.0	0.3	-100.0%
Small focus at L spinal canal at L4 level	Resolved				8.0	5.7	2.4	0.2	-100.0%
Small focus at R spinal canal at L4 level	Resolved				9.5	8.5	4.0	0.9	-100.0%
Small focus at spinal canal at S1 level	Resolved				6.9	6.2	2.4	0.3	-100.0%
T3	Resolved				10.4	8.1	4.6	1.0	-100.0%
T4	Resolved				32.9	25.4	10.5	58.0	-100.0%
T5	Resolved				27.0	13.0	9.3	16.0	-100.0%

Note: LD=longest diameter; PD=diameter perpendicular to LD; TLG=total lesion glycolysis (vol x SUVmean)

Ho,

醫院 同位素及正電子掃描部
Department of Nuclear Medicine & Positron Emission Tomography
& HOSPITAL

Tel:
Fax:

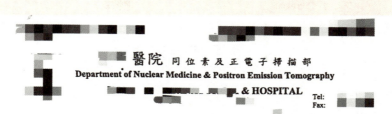

Impression:

1. The primary lung tumor in lateral RML is metabolically resolved. Post-radiation pneumonitis in the RML is improved.
2. The pericystic ground-glass opacity in posterior LUL is metabolically subsided with resolved solid component, suggestive of treated metachronous tumor.
3. The right interlobar and left hilar nodal metastases are either stable or mildly improved. Distal nodal metastases at left submandibular, left retromandibular, left upper jugular level II and left intraparotid regions are metabolically subsided.
4. Tumor deposit in left infratemporal fossa is resolved.
5. Tumor deposits at left frontal bone with extension to adjacent left temporalis muscle are also metabolically normalized.
6. Brain metastases in lateral left temporal region (around operative bed), left inferior temporal lobe, lateral left parietal lobe and left cerebellum are all met metabolically resolved.
7. Leptomeningeal metastases at spinal canal at T11, L4, L4/5 and S1 levels are metabolically subsided.
8. Bone metastases at T3, T4 and T5 are achieved metabolic quiescence.
9. No other suspicious focal pathology in the remaining body survey.
10. *In summary:* very good response to current treatment response.

Thank you very much, Dr.   , for your referral.

MSc(Epidemiology and Biostatistics)(CUHK)
Specialist in Nuclear Medicine, Department of Nuclear Medicine & P.E.T., HKSH

A835128 Ho, Koon Ming

病案13

肠癌肺转移康复

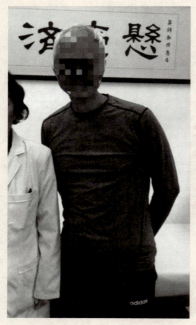

吴先生有一份稳定的工作，每天会锻炼身体，自觉身体很好，也有个幸福的家庭，儿女双全，感到非常满足。但是在2017年，他常感到肚子不舒服，甚至还有便血的情况，于是急忙到医院里去做身体检查。经过肠镜检查后，证实患有乙状结肠癌。

吴先生急忙抓紧治疗时机，在确诊是结肠癌之后的当月，也就是2017年7月份，行手术切除结肠的肿瘤及周围组织治

🔆 吴先生于2024年2月前来诊治时合影留念

疗。但是病理报告显示的结果不太乐观，他的肿瘤已经属于第Ⅲ期，并且有淋巴转移。经过病理学检查，他患的这种肿瘤是分化程度很差的肿瘤，也就是恶性程度很高的肿瘤，容易复发和转移，并且已经是第Ⅲ期了，也已经有淋巴转移。在接下来的1年中，吴先生一直在坚持做化疗，尽管化疗有严重的不良反应，令他感到非常痛苦，但他以顽强的意志一直坚持着。在

进行了 1 年多的化疗之后，他认为没事了，于是在 2018 年 7 月份又做了一次检查。检查显示，结果并没有那么乐观，在他的肺上发现了最少 4 个肿瘤结节。

经过朋友的介绍，吴先生急忙前来我们这里寻求进一步治疗。他当时精神压力很大、精神状态很差、全身疲乏无力，身心疲惫。他认为已经转移就很难治疗了，果断地结束了化疗，再加上化疗已经做了太长的时间，确实难以再继续下去。在往后的治疗过程中，他积极地服用中药，遵从医嘱，刮风下雨也从不间断来诊。这样治疗了 1 年，于 2019 年 10 月，他再次做检查，显示肺部的结节已经全部消失。

吴先生本来是不太相信中医药的，但是经过亲身经历，他现在非常相信中医药。在 2020 年的检查中，不仅肺部肿瘤结节全部消失，同时也检查了其他部位，肝脏、脾脏及其他器官都是正常的。吴先生非常高兴，对以后的生活和工作都充满了信心，更接受了公司的安排，担任总监负责更加重大的任务，他完全有信心能够胜任这个工作。

治疗原则

解毒化瘀，散结消瘤。

常用中药

1. 香附、郁金、槐角、皂刺、蜂房、白花蛇、薏苡仁、土茯苓等。
2. 同时服用消瘤丸。

影像学、病理学检查报告及诊疗记录

1. 2017 年 7 月 27 日 PET/CT 证实乙状结肠肿瘤，并有最少 4 个肺部肿瘤结节。

2. 2017 年 7 月 29 日手术后病理报告证实为低分化腺癌 PT_3N_1b，并有多个淋巴结转移，建议做舒缓辅助性化疗。

3. 2019 年 10 月 8 日 CT 报告证明腹腔、盆腔未见肿瘤。

4. 2020 年 10 月 21 日 CT 报告证实胸腔、腹腔、盆腔均未见有肿瘤，原肺部的多个结节肿瘤已不存在。

附：患者检查报告

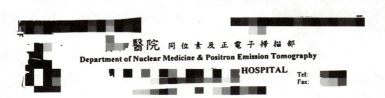

醫院 同位素及正電子掃描部
Department of Nuclear Medicine & Positron Emission Tomography
█████ HOSPITAL

Tel:
Fax:

Functional parameters of these lesions are tabulated as below:

NG, ████ ████	in mm		F-18 FDG Standard
Site	LD	PD	SUVmax
Lesion in sigmoid colon	31.6	26.7	8.1

Note: LD=longest diameter; PD=diameter perpendicular to LD

Impression:

1. A moderately hypermetabolic lesion of 32 mm LD x 27 mm PD and SUVmax 8.1 is identified in sigmoid colon. On transaxial view, it shows eccentric involvement. Diagnosis of malignant colonic pathology has to be considered first. Differential possibility includes tubulovillous adenoma. Correlation with recent histopathology result is recommended.

2. No enlarged or hypermetabolic node in the abdomen or pelvis.

3. Several (at least 4, up to 5 mm) non-^{18}FDG-avid pulmonary nodules in RUL (x 3) and lateral RML (x 1) are non-specific and can be due to granulomas. Nonetheless, follow-up study is recommended for serial monitoring.

4. No ^{18}FDG-avid lesion in the remaining body survey including the liver.

Thank you very much, Dr. ████ for your referral.

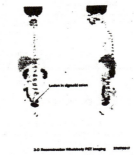

████

_____ ████ BChB, FHKCR, FHKAM (Radiology)
Specialist in Nuclear Medicine, Department of Nuclear Medicine & P.E.T., HKSH

E722366 Ng Chi Wa.doc

091

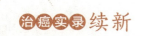

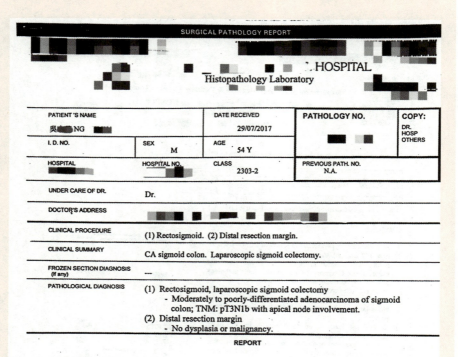

SURGICAL PATHOLOGY REPORT

. HOSPITAL

Histopathology Laboratory

PATIENT'S NAME 吳██NG ██		DATE RECEIVED 29/07/2017	PATHOLOGY NO. ██ ██	COPY: DR. HOSP OTHERS
I. D. NO.	SEX M	AGE 54 Y		
HOSPITAL ██	HOSPITAL NO. ██	CLASS 2303-2	PREVIOUS PATH. NO. N.A.	

UNDER CARE OF DR.	Dr.
DOCTOR'S ADDRESS	
CLINICAL PROCEDURE	(1) Rectosigmoid. (2) Distal resection margin.
CLINICAL SUMMARY	CA sigmoid colon. Laparoscopic sigmoid colectomy.
FROZEN SECTION DIAGNOSIS (If any)	---
PATHOLOGICAL DIAGNOSIS	(1) Rectosigmoid, laparoscopic sigmoid colectomy - Moderately to poorly-differentiated adenocarcinoma of sigmoid colon; TNM: pT3N1b with apical node involvement. (2) Distal resection margin - No dysplasia or malignancy.

REPORT

Macroscopic examination:

(1) Labelled "Rectosigmoid" is a previously-opened 13.5 cm. length of large bowel measuring 5 cm. in maximum circumference and with both resection margins measuring 5 cm. in circumference. There is a tan ulcerated tumour 3.6 cm. longitudinally by 4 cm. in lateral direction which occupies approximately 1/2 of the circumference of the bowel. It is situated 6 cm. and 4 cm. from the bowel resection margins. The tumour is 0.4 cm. in depth and has raised involuted edges. The cut surface shows tumour infiltrating through the muscle coat and into the adjacent fibrofatty tissue to a depth of 5 mm. It is well clear by 2 cm. from the underlying deep fibrofatty margin. Two apical lymph nodes 1.2 x 0.8 x 0.8 cm. and 1 x 0.7 x 0.7 cm, are present along with thirteen other pericolic lymph nodes the largest 0.7 cm. and which the smallest 0.2 cm. in diameter.

Blocks: (1A)&(1B) Nearest and further bowel resection margin, one piece in each; (1C) Full face of tumour, one piece; (1E) Tumour, 2 pieces with associated fibrofatty tissue; (1E) Random block, 2 pieces; (1F) Mesenteric resection margin and apical lymph nodes, 3 pieces; (1G) Pericolic lymph nodes, 13 pieces.

(2) Labelled "Distal resection margin" is a mucosal-covered rim of tissue 2.4 x 2 x 0.8 cm. Eight pieces with all tissue embedded excepted staple areas.

(CONTINUED ON NEXT PAGE)

Page 1 of 2

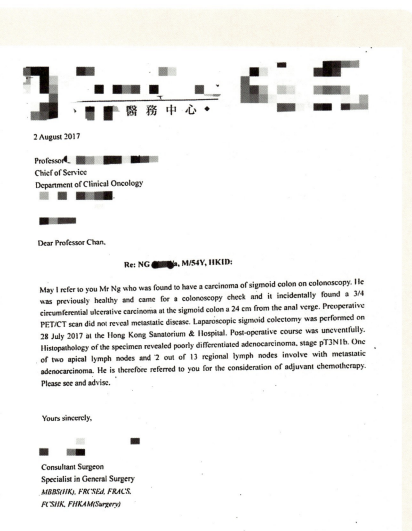

醫務中心 ◆

2 August 2017

Professor
Chief of Service
Department of Clinical Oncology

Dear Professor Chan,

Re: NG ___ a, M/54Y, HKID:

May I refer to you Mr Ng who was found to have a carcinoma of sigmoid colon on colonoscopy. He was previously healthy and came for a colonoscopy check and it incidentally found a 3/4 circumferential ulcerative carcinoma at the sigmoid colon a 24 cm from the anal verge. Preoperative PET/CT scan did not reveal metastatic disease. Laparoscopic sigmoid colectomy was performed on 28 July 2017 at the Hong Kong Sanatorium & Hospital. Post-operative course was uneventfully. Histopathology of the specimen revealed poorly differentiated adenocarcinoma, stage pT3N1b. One of two apical lymph nodes and 2 out of 13 regional lymph nodes involve with metastatic adenocarcinoma. He is therefore referred to you for the consideration of adjuvant chemotherapy. Please see and advise.

Yours sincerely,

Consultant Surgeon
Specialist in General Surgery
MBBS(HK), FRCSEd, FRACS,
FCSHK, FHKAM(Surgery)

醫院 Hospital 醫院 Hospital 影像及介入放射科 Department of Imaging and Interventional Radiology (DIIR) 檢驗報告 Examination Report	Case No.: HKID: Name: NG, (吳 Sex: **M** Age: **56y** DOB: **17-Oct-1962** Hosp / Spec / Ward: **PWH** / **ONC** / **CHF**	**R**
Accession no.:	Reg. Date: 08-Oct-2019 09:52	

DUPLICATE

Procedure: Abdomen +con., Pelvis+con.

Report:

CT ABDOMEN & PELVIS

Report:

Correlation is made with previous PET/CT dated 30.11.2018.

Colorectal anastomosis is again unremarkable with no suspicious thickening or mass detected.
Non-specific tiny hypoenhancing foci in both lobes of liver, probable tiny cysts.
No other suspicious focal hepatic lesion detected.
GB, CBD, pancreas, spleen, adrenals and kidneys (apart from cortical cysts) unremarkable.
Gastric and splenic varices are noted.
No ascites or lymphadenopathy.
Lung bases are clear.
No suspicious bone lesion.

COMMENT

1. Colorectal anastomosis is again unremarkable with no suspicious thickening or mass detected.
2. Non-specific tiny hypoenhancing foci in both lobes of liver, probable tiny cysts. No other suspicious focal hepatic lesion detected.

C
T

Report to : PWH/ONC/CHF Requested by	Reported by : DR. Oct-2019 11:11 Generated on : 08-Oct-2019 11:11 Reprinted by 04-Nov-2019 16:46

Page 1 of 1

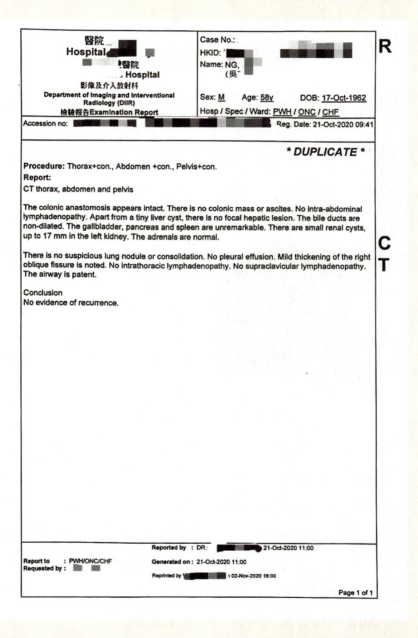

R

醫院
Hospital
醫院
Hospital
影像及介入放射科
Department of Imaging and Interventional
Radiology (DIIR)
檢驗報告 **Examination Report**

Case No.:
HKID:
Name: NG,
(吳

Sex: **M**   Age: **58y**   DOB: **17-Oct-1962**

Hosp / Spec / Ward: **PWH** / **ONC** / **CHF**

Accession no:

Reg. Date: 21-Oct-2020 09:41

C
T

* DUPLICATE *

Procedure: Thorax+con., Abdomen +con., Pelvis+con.

Report:

CT thorax, abdomen and pelvis

The colonic anastomosis appears intact. There is no colonic mass or ascites. No intra-abdominal lymphadenopathy. Apart from a tiny liver cyst, there is no focal hepatic lesion. The bile ducts are non-dilated. The gallbladder, pancreas and spleen are unremarkable. There are small renal cysts, up to 17 mm in the left kidney. The adrenals are normal.

There is no suspicious lung nodule or consolidation. No pleural effusion. Mild thickening of the right oblique fissure is noted. No intrathoracic lymphadenopathy. No supraclavicular lymphadenopathy. The airway is patent.

Conclusion
No evidence of recurrence.

Reported by : DR.   21-Oct-2020 11:00

Report to   : PWH/ONC/CHF

Requested by :

Generated on : 21-Oct-2020 11:00

Reprinted by   02-Nov-2020 16:00

Page 1 of 1

避免了第四次做手术

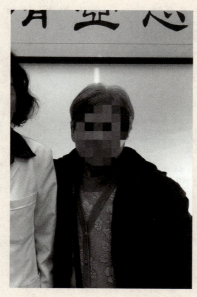

梁太太于2022年4月前来诊治时合影留念

梁太太患有糖尿病多年，骨关节炎、高血压病史也有多年，长期多病缠身，曾做过膝关节手术。2016年，她感到颈部不适，经超声波检查，发现甲状腺肿瘤，属多发性的甲状腺肿瘤。当时虽然并未明确显示是良性还是恶性，但由于肿瘤生长速度快，于是决定做手术。2017年4月，梁太太做了甲状腺全切除手术，手术后病理报告证实为恶性甲状腺乳头状癌。

随后在2017年7月开始进行放疗。2018年3月甲状腺癌复发并伴有淋巴转移和双肺结节，于是在2018年7月再次做手术切除复发的肿瘤和转移的淋巴结。手术后发现另一侧颈部出现转移的淋巴结。梁太太与家人经过慎重考虑，决定还是切干净为好，这样就不必再担心转移问题了。因此，2018年8月再次动手术切除转移的淋巴结，术后经检查确定为甲状腺转移性乳头状癌，于2018年10月及2019年10月都有增加放疗。

梁太太先后共进行了3次手术和3个不同阶段的放疗，原本全家都放下心头大石了，没想到，2020年9月4日检查时发现肿瘤再次复发，需要再次做手术，也就是进行第4次的手术。梁太太对此深受打击，精神崩溃，经多方打听以后，来到我们这里，选用了完全不同的中医药生命修复疗法。

当时的梁太太身体非常虚弱，颈部两侧都有多个可以摸到，且大小不同的坚硬肿块和结节。同时她还有严重头痛、呕吐、排尿困难、失眠、精神压力大，以及进食很少的状况。经过数月的治疗之后，她的颈部肿块和结节逐渐减少消失，身体状况开始改善，不适的症状也逐渐消失。由于她使用了中医药生命修复疗法，不仅避免了第4次手术，也避免了反复进行手术和放疗却无法控制癌症的生长和转移。

治疗原则

祛邪排毒，散结消瘤。

常用中药

1. 太子参、黄药子、生地黄、威灵仙、猕猴桃根、玄参、夏枯草、莪术、生大黄、全蝎、蜈蚣等。
2. 同时服用散结丸。

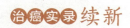

影像学、病理学检查报告及诊疗记录

1. 2018 年 3 月 1 日 CT 检查报告显示甲状腺癌全部切除后，又有肿瘤结节出现，双肺又有结节。

2. 2020 年 8 月 27 日报告显示手术后肿瘤再次复发。

3. 2020 年 9 月 4 日检查报告证实 2017 年 4 月 18 日行甲状腺全切手术，病理诊断为甲状腺乳头状癌 pT_3N_1。2018 年 3 月肿瘤复发再次手术，病理检查为转移性甲状腺癌。2020 年再次复发，考虑手术。

附：患者检查报告

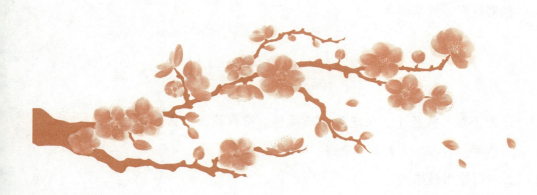

为癌症患者却病延年

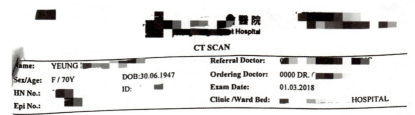

CT SCAN

Name: YEUNG	Referral Doctor:
Sex/Age: F / 70Y DOB:30.06.1947	Ordering Doctor: 0000 DR.
HN No.: ID:	Exam Date: 01.03.2018
Epi No.:	Clinic /Ward Bed: HOSPITAL

Exam: **CT THORAX (Plain)**

FINDINGS:

Known history of thyroid cancer with previous total thyroidectomy. There are a few soft tissue nodules over bilateral thyroid bed, measuring up to 1.2cm x 0.9cm on right side. Further assessment is helpful to exclude local or lymph node recurrence.

There are several soft tissue nodules in both lungs, measuring up to 0.3cm in posterior segment of right upper lobe, medial segment of right middle lobe and basal posterior segment of left lower lobe. They may represent post-inflammatory granulomas rather than pulmonary secondaries.

Fibrocalcific changes are found in apical segment of right upper lobe, with several calcified granulomas measuring up to 0.4cm, likely related to old infection. Follow up is helpful.

No "tree-in-bud" lesion or interlobular septal thickening. There is no pleural effusion or pneumothorax on both sides.

Major airways are patent. There is no definite bronchiectasis. There are several mediastinal lymph nodes, measuring up to 0.8cm in short axis distance, probably reactive in nature. A few calcified lymph nodes are found in right hilum.

Bilateral adrenal glands are not enlarged.

There are a few cysts in both lobes of liver, measuring up to 0.9cm in right lobe.

Mild irregularity over anterior end of right 7th rib, probably related to old injury.

IMPRESSION:

Known history of thyroid cancer with previous total thyroidectomy. A few soft tissue nodules over bilateral thyroid bed, up to 1.2cm x 0.9cm on right side. Further assessment is helpful to exclude local or lymph node recurrence.

DR.
CONSULTANT RADIOLOGIST
MBChB(CUHK), MMed(DR), NUS, M Med Sc(HK),
FRCR(UK), FHKCR, FHKAM(Radiology)
Authorized And Reported On 01.03.2018 18:18

Page 1 of 2

Typed By: 90334

P. 1

099

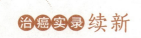

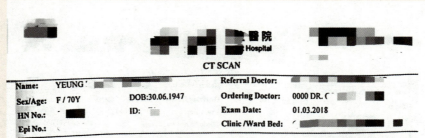

CT SCAN

Name:	YEUNG	**Referral Doctor:**	
Sex/Age:	F / 70Y	DOB:30.06.1947	**Ordering Doctor:**	0000 DR. C
HN No.:		ID:	**Exam Date:**	01.03.2018
Epi No.:			**Clinic /Ward Bed:**	

Several soft tissue nodules in both lungs, up to 0.3cm, may represent post-inflammatory granulomas rather than pulmonary secondaries.   Fibrocalcific changes in apical segment of right upper lobe, likely related to old infection.   Follow up is helpful.

Thank you for your referral.

DR.
CONSULTANT RADIOLOGIST
MBChB(CUHK), MMed(DR), NUS, M Med Sc(HK),
FRCR(UK), FHKCR, FHKAM(Radiology)
Authorized And Reported On 01.03.2018 18:18

▪ Hospital ▪醫院
MEDICAL IMAGING DEPARTMENT

Patient's Name	: YEUNG		Unit Record No.	:
Sex	: F		Age	: 73
Examination Date	: 27-AUG-2020		Accession No.	:
Ward / Class	:		Attending Doctor	:

EXAMINATION / PROCEDURE REPORT

The oesophagus appears unremarkable.

A hypermetabolic focus (SUVmax 5.3) is seen at the lower oesophagus, which could be due to physiological uptake.

ABDOMEN & PELVIS

Mild heterogeneous increased uptake is seen along the stomach, could be due to physiological uptake, though possibility of subtle tumour mass cannot be entirely excluded.

No abnormal bowel pattern, bowel wall thickening or bowel dilatation is seen. No increased uptake is seen along the bowel.

No abnormal tracer uptake is seen within the abdomen and pelvis.

Few tiny non-FDG avid liver cysts are seen. No other focal liver lesion or adrenal enlargement is seen.

The spleen, pancreas and both kidneys appear unremarkable except for non-FDG avid renal cyst.

No significant abdominal or pelvic lymphadenopathy is noted.

Small uterine fibroid is seen. No abnormal adnexal mass lesion is seen.

No ascites is noted.

SKELETON

Diffuse degeneration is seen along the spine. Lumbar spine scoliosis with convexity towards left side is seen.

No other abnormal tracer uptake is seen. No other significant focal bony abnormality is seen.

COMMENTS :

1. Status post thyroidectomy is noted. Evidence of left neck operation is also seen.
2. A hypermetabolic nodule (size=1 x 0.8 x 0.8cm, SUVmax 40.8) is seen along the left thyroid bed. Features are highly suspicious of tumour recurrence in the present clinical context.
3. A slightly prominent, hypermetabolic right lower neck posterior triangle lymph node (size=0.5 x 0.8cm, SUVmax 11.9) is seen. It is compatible with metastatic lymph node.

(Electronically Signed)
Dr.
Consultant in Radiology
MBBS(HK), FRCR, FHKCR, FHKAM(RADIOLOGY)

Approved on : 27-AUG-2020 03:22 PM
Page 2 of 3

Referral Letter
Hospital

To: Department of Surgery

Case no: [ ]
[Referral No.:]

04/09/2020

Dear Consultant In-charge,

Re: YEUNG, [   ] [   ]   Sex: F Age: 73y

Reason for referral: Thyroid cancer with neck relapse

Special consideration: For surgery

Reason for priority: Malignancy/ suspected malignancy

The above named patient has CA thyroid with Total thyroidectomy + level VI selective LN dissection done in your department 18/4/17
Pathology; papillary thyroid carcinoma
pT3N1a tumour, less than 0.1 mm from the peripheral margin.

RAI 80 mCi on 10.7.17

Neck recurrence in Mar 2018
Left mid cervical LN FNAC: metastatic papillary carcinoma

left 2-5b SND done on 18.7.2018 + right level VI LN dissection done on 10.8.2018
postop RAI 150 mCi 10.9.2018

3rd RAI 150 mCi given on 14.10.2019 for perssitent raised Tg

PETCT done on 27.8.2020 showed suspicolus of left thyroid bed recurrence wnt right lower neck level V LN met.
uptake in lower esophagus and stomach.

Please kindly see this patient for possibility of further excision of neck disease.
Please also kindly consider OGD assessment in view of PETCT findings.

Thank you very much.

Signature:
签名
Name in Block Letters:
姓名

ASSOCIATE CONSULTANT
Department of Clinical Oncology

請盡早到轉介之診所辦理預約的手續。此轉介信的有效期為發出日期的三個月內。
Please make appointment with the referred clinic as early as possible. This referral letter is valid for 3 months from the date of issue.

Printed on [   ] Printed by [   ]

Page 1 of 2

前列腺癌多发骨转移康复 15 年

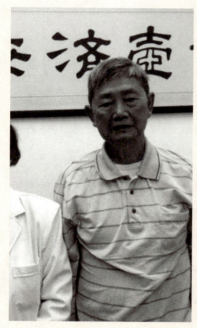

🔸 黄先生于 2024 年 2 月前来诊治时合影留念

2009 年时，黄先生经常发生排尿困难，尿急、尿频，且越来越严重，之后甚至出现了全身骨头疼痛的情况。由于疼痛逐渐加重，特别是晚上睡觉的时候，经常会被痛醒，有时就连呼吸也能感到疼痛，再加上腰痛令他不能弯腰，行走困难。于是他到医院去做检查，发现是前列腺癌，经过更进一步的检查显示，发现不仅是前列腺癌，还有多发性的骨转移，已经属于晚期癌症。当时医生说可以采取一些对症治疗的方案，但是没有根本的治疗方法，于是他急忙来到我们这里，求助于生命修复的抗癌治疗。

经过数月的治疗，他的疼痛逐渐减少直至消失，精神亦逐渐恢复了正常。因为治疗效果很好，所以黄先生放弃了所有的西医治疗，例如化疗、放疗、激素治疗等。他一直坚持按时吃药、按时治疗。2014 年，他再次检查时发现，多发性全身骨转移已经完全消失。黄先生深受鼓舞，继续认真治疗，身体恢复得也越来越好。2018 年做全身检查时，再次证明全身骨转移都已经消失。

2021 年，他去医院做例行检查时，当初的主诊医生见到他感到非常吃惊，因为当时患病的他已经是晚期癌症，于是便问他是做了什么？吃了什么东西？他告诉医生，是因为进行了生命修复的中药治疗。医院里的医生也不得不佩服地说："你真是幸运，活了这么久时间啊！"

前列腺癌是常见的男性恶性肿瘤，也是全球范围内主要的癌症杀手之一。前列腺癌发生多发性骨转移，已是癌症晚期，临床常见缓解疼痛、改善活动能力、防止病理性骨折等舒缓性治疗。而让骨转移全部消失者，尚属罕见。从发现癌症到现在已经过去 15 年，黄先生也已经 86 岁，现在的他仍感觉身体很好，没有什么不舒服，每天也会进行各种身体锻炼。

软坚散瘀，通滞攻毒。

常用中药

1. 龙葵、山慈菇、柴胡、白芍、鳖甲、丹参、路路通、猕猴梨根、菝葜、莪术、玄明粉、土鳖虫等。
2. 同时服用消瘤丸。

影像学、病理学检查报告及诊疗记录

1. 2010 年 8 月 3 日检查报告证实前列腺癌。

2. 2010 年 8 月 9 日检查报告确定在右髂骨、肋骨等处有骨转移。

3. 2014 年 6 月 25 日检查报告证实骨转移消失。

4. 2018 年 8 月 17 日检查报告再次证实骨转移消失。

附：患者检查报告

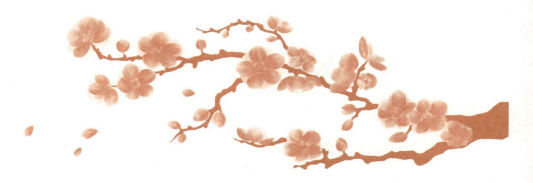

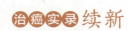

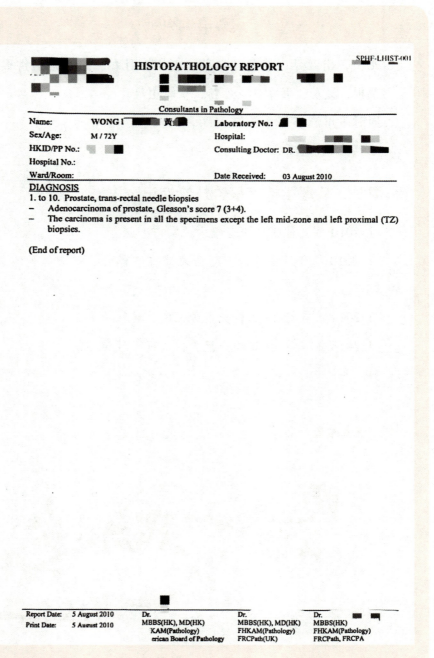

HISTOPATHOLOGY REPORT

SPHF-LHIST-001

Consultants in Pathology

Name:	WONG [黃	Laboratory No.:	
Sex/Age:	M / 72Y	Hospital:	
HKID/PP No.:		Consulting Doctor:	DR.
Hospital No.:			
Ward/Room:		Date Received:	03 August 2010

DIAGNOSIS

1. to 10. Prostate, trans-rectal needle biopsies

− Adenocarcinoma of prostate, Gleason's score 7 (3+4).

− The carcinoma is present in all the specimens except the left mid-zone and left proximal (TZ)
biopsies.

(End of report)

Report Date:	5 August 2010	Dr.	Dr.	Dr.
Print Date:	5 August 2010	MBBS(HK), MD(HK)	MBBS(HK), MD(HK)	MBBS(HK)
		KAM(Pathology)	FHKAM(Pathology)	FHKAM(Pathology)
		erican Board of Pathology	FRCPath(UK)	FRCPath, FRCPA

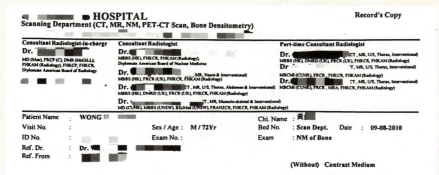

■ ■ ■ ■ HOSPITAL

Record's Copy

Scanning Department (CT, MR, NM, PET-CT Scan, Bone Densitometry)

Consultant Radiologist-in-charge	Consultant Radiologist	Part-time Consultant Radiologist

Dr. ■ ■
MD (Man), FRCP (C), DMR (McGILL),
FHKAM (Radiology), FHKCP, FHKCR,
Diplomate American Board of Radiology
■ ■ ■ ■

Dr. ■ ■ ■
MBBS (HK), FHKCR, FHKAM (Radiology),
Diplomate American Board of Nuclear Medicine

Dr. ■ ■ ■ MR, Neuro & Interventional
MBBS (HK), FRCR (UK), FHKCR, FHKAM (Radiology)

Dr. ■ ■ CT, MR, U/S, Thorax, Abdomen & Interventional
MBBS (HK), DMRD (UK), FRCR (UK), FHKCR, FHKAM (Radiology)

Dr. ■ T, MR, Musculo-skeletal & Interventional
MD (CUHK), MBBS (UNSW), BScMed (UNSW), FRANZCR, FHKCR, FHKAM (Radiology)

Dr. ■ ■ CT, MR, U/S, Thorax, Interventional
MBBS (HK), DMRD (UK), FRCR (UK), FHKCR, FHKAM (Radiology)

Dr ■ T, MR, U/S, Thorax, Interventional

Dr. ■ ■ CT, MR, U/S, Thorax, Interventional
MBChB (CUHK), FRCR , FHKCR, FHKAM (Radiology)

Dr. ■ ■ CT, MR, U/S, Thorax, Interventional
MBChB (CUHK), FRCR , MBA, FHKCR, FHKAM (Radiology)

Patient Name	: WONG ■	Chi. Name : 黃■	
Visit No.	:	Sex / Age : M / 72Yr	Bed No. : Scan Dept. Date : 09-08-2010
ID No.	:	Exam No. :	Exam : NM of Bone
Ref. Dr.	: Dr. W■ ■ ■		
Ref. From	: ■ ■ ■		(Without) Contrast Medium

Clinical Information / History:

Prostate biopsy confirmed Ca prostate. PSA = 92.

Radiological Report:

Whole body bone scan was performed after the intravenous injection of 25 mCi Tc-99m MDP.

FINDINGS :

Planar and SPECT images of the skeleton demonstrate intense abnormal uptake at the inferior aspect of the right ilium. This is most consistent with bone metastasis. No disease activity is demonstrated in other areas in the bony pelvis. Abnormal uptake is also demonstrated at L3 vertebral body. Again, this is most consistent with bone metastasis. No significant abnormality is demonstrated in other vertebra levels. Mild focal uptake is also demonstrated at the posterior aspect of the left 9th rib. This may represent subradiographic bone injury or early metastasis. The sternum, clavicles and scapulae are normal. No significant abnormality is present in the skull and extremities.

IMPRESSION :

Abnormal uptake is present at L3 and the right ilium. These are most consistent with bone metastases. Mild focal uptake at the 9th rib may represent subclinical rib injury or early metastasis.

Thank you for your referral.

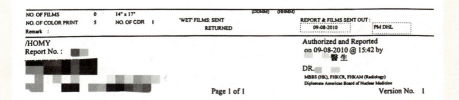

NO. OF FILMS	0	14" x 17"	(DDMM) (HHMM)	REPORT & FILMS SENT OUT :
NO. OF COLOR PRINT	5	NO. OF CDR 1	'WET FILMS: SENT	09-08-2010 PM DHL
Remark :			RETURNED	

/HOMY
Report No. : ■ ■

■ ■ ■ ■ ■ ■

Authorized and Reported
on 09-08-2010 @ 15:42 by
醫生

DR. ■
MBBS (HK), FHKCR, FHKAM (Radiology)
Diplomate American Board of Nuclear Medicine

Page 1 of 1   Version No. 1

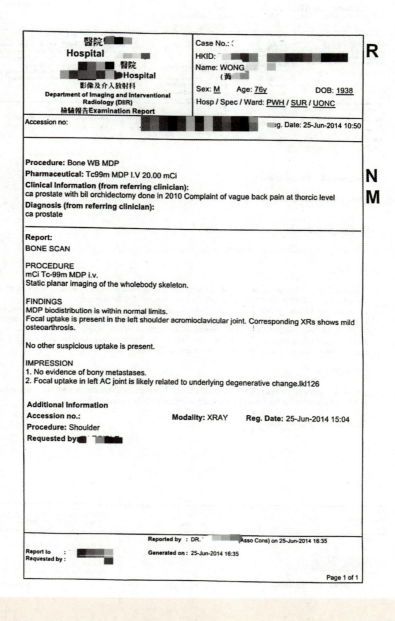

醫院
Hospital
醫院
Hospital
影像及介入放射科
Department of Imaging and Interventional Radiology (DIIR)
檢驗報告 Examination Report

R

Case No.:
HKID:
Name: WONG
（黃
Sex: M   Age: 76y   DOB: 1938
Hosp / Spec / Ward: PWH / SUR / UONC

Accession no:

g. Date: 25-Jun-2014 10:50

N
M

Procedure: Bone WB MDP
Pharmaceutical: Tc99m MDP I.V 20.00 mCi
Clinical Information (from referring clinician):
ca prostate with bil orchidectomy done in 2010 Complaint of vague back pain at thorcic level
Diagnosis (from referring clinician):
ca prostate

Report:
BONE SCAN

PROCEDURE
mCi Tc-99m MDP i.v.
Static planar imaging of the wholebody skeleton.

FINDINGS
MDP biodistribution is within normal limits.
Focal uptake is present in the left shoulder acromioclavicular joint. Corresponding XRs shows mild osteoarthrosis.

No other suspicious uptake is present.

IMPRESSION
1. No evidence of bony metastases.
2. Focal uptake in left AC joint is likely related to underlying degenerative change.lkl126

Additional Information
Accession no.:   **Modality: XRAY**   **Reg. Date: 25-Jun-2014 15:04**
Procedure: Shoulder
Requested by

Reported by : DR.   (Asso Cons) on 25-Jun-2014 16:35

Report to   :
Requested by :   Generated on : 25-Jun-2014 16:35

Page 1 of 1

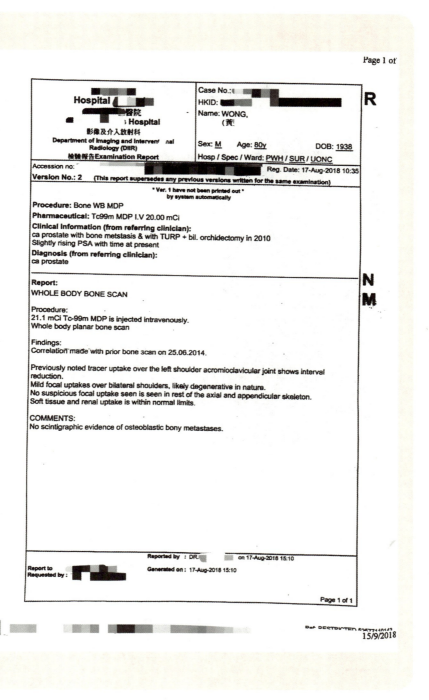

Hospital 醫院
Hospital

影像及介入放射科
Department of Imaging and Intervential nal
Radiology (DIIR)

檢驗報告 Examination Report

Case No.:
HKID:
Name: WONG,
(黃

Sex: **M**   Age: **80y**   DOB: **1938**

Hosp / Spec / Ward: **PWH** / **SUR** / **UONC**

R

Accession no:

Reg. Date: 17-Aug-2018 10:35

Version No.: 2   (This report supersedes any previous versions written for the same examination)

* Ver. 1 have not been printed out *
by system automatically

Procedure: Bone WB MDP

Pharmaceutical: Tc99m MDP I.V 20.00 mCi

Clinical Information (from referring clinician):
ca prostate with bone metstasis & with TURP + bil. orchidectomy in 2010
Slightly rising PSA with time at present

Diagnosis (from referring clinician):
ca prostate

N M

Report:
WHOLE BODY BONE SCAN

Procedure:
21.1 mCi Tc-99m MDP is injected intravenously.
Whole body planar bone scan

Findings:
Correlation made with prior bone scan on 25.06.2014.

Previously noted tracer uptake over the left shoulder acromioclavicular joint shows interval reduction.
Mild focal uptakes over bilateral shoulders, likely degenerative in nature.
No suspicious focal uptake seen is seen in rest of the axial and appendicular skeleton.
Soft tissue and renal uptake is within normal limits.

COMMENTS:
No scintigraphic evidence of osteoblastic bony metastases.

Reported by : DR.   on 17-Aug-2018 15:10

Report to
Requested by :   Generated on : 17-Aug-2018 15:10

Ref. RESTRICTED

15/9/2018

病案 16

晚期胰腺癌康复 14 年

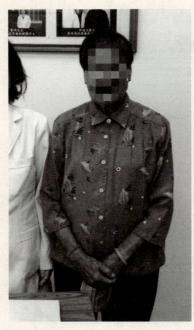

🔊 王太太于 2023 年 4 月前来诊治时合影留念

王太太今年 87 岁了，子孙满堂，个个都很孝顺，她的生活也过得非常快乐。谁都没想到，她在 14 年前就患了晚期胰腺癌，当时医院更是告知她的生命大概只有几个月的时间。2010 年，王太太因为黄疸、腹痛而做身体检查，报告显示明显胰腺癌。2010 年 10 月，她做了胰腺癌的手术，当时医生打开她的腹腔之后，发现肿瘤非常多，并且已经侵犯到胰腺周围神经，甚至侵犯到十二指肠位置。王太太做了手术以后，在恢复过程中得知，她的病情是非常严重的，同时还伴有心脏扩张，医生说手术也无法切除干净腹腔里的肿瘤，因为肿瘤的范围很大。

此后，王太太经常感到腹痛，但是到医院里去求助，医生却告诉她，已经尽了最大的努力，现在没有其他的办法了，唯一可以做的，就是服用吗啡止痛。因为她的疼痛非常严重，所以医生告诉她服用量可增大，只要能达到止痛的目的就可以。但是即使大剂量服用，她仍然感到痛楚，医生一再表明已经没有更好的治疗方法。在这种情况下，王太太只好求助于我们生命修复的治疗。

刚来的时候，她的身体非常瘦弱，而且腹痛严重，经常呕吐，不能进食。在她刚开始的治疗过程中，由于主要的症状是腹痛严重，所以除了服用中药，也加了针灸等方法来辅助治疗。这样过了1年多，她的腹痛慢慢地减轻了。随着疼痛的慢慢减轻，王太太一步步地减轻吗啡的剂量，她知道西医对这个病已没有更好的治疗方法，所以也没有再去医院检查。

此后，她就是按时的前来治疗并服用中药，就这样经过了2年的治疗，她的身体已经康复了，再也没有明显的疼痛，心脏的情况也在逐步好转。从患上晚期胰腺癌到现在，已经有14年的时间了，期间她没有再去医院，也从没有做过化疗、放疗等。只是按时吃中药，她的病也一直没有复发。胰腺癌是一个非常严重的疾病，且王太太的情况属于晚期，经过治疗之后，现在已完全恢复了健康。她腹腔的肿瘤经过手术之后，还有转移的病灶，当时的手术无法为她切除干净，但是经过生命修复的治疗后，最终还是恢复了健康，现在有时候还会前来调理。经过这么多年，她也深信生命修复治疗对肿瘤的治疗效果是毋庸置疑的。

治疗原则

解毒化瘀，散结消瘤。

常用中药

1. 柴胡、黄芩、半夏、厚朴、田七、延胡索、莪术、土鳖虫、山慈菇等。
2. 同时服用消瘤丸。

影像学、病理学检查报告及诊疗记录

1. 2010年11月10日手术后病理检测报告，证实为胰腺肿瘤紧贴手术切缘小于0.01cm。手术切缘有肿瘤浸润，有门静脉、十二指肠、周围神经等浸润。

2. 2020年9月21日检查报告显示癌指数均在正常范围，无复发迹象。

附：患者检查报告

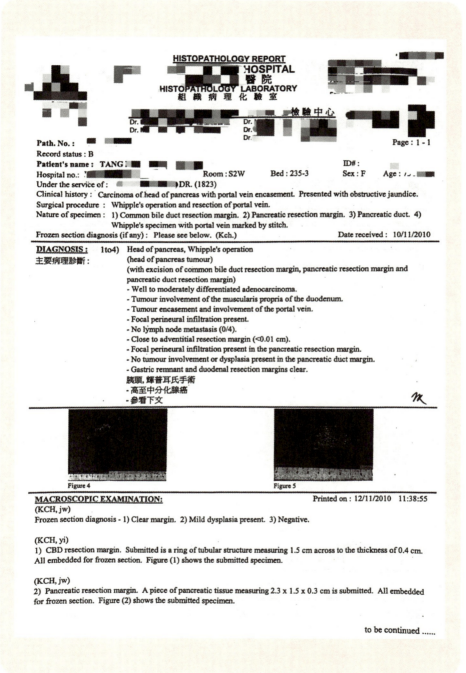

HISTOPATHOLOGY REPORT

HOSPITAL
醫院
HISTOPATHOLOGY LABORATORY
組織病理化驗室

檢驗中心

Dr.   Dr.
Dr.   Dr.
                       Dr.

Page : 1 - 1

Path. No. :
Record status : B
Patient's name : TANG   ID# :
Hospital no.:   Room : S2W   Bed : 235-3   Sex : F   Age :
Under the service of :   DR. (1823)
Clinical history : Carcinoma of head of pancreas with portal vein encasement. Presented with obstructive jaundice.
Surgical procedure : Whipple's operation and resection of portal vein.
Nature of specimen : 1) Common bile duct resection margin. 2) Pancreatic resection margin. 3) Pancreatic duct. 4)
Whipple's specimen with portal vein marked by stitch.
Frozen section diagnosis (if any) : Please see below. (Kch.)   Date received : 10/11/2010

DIAGNOSIS : 1to4) Head of pancreas, Whipple's operation
主要病理診斷 :　　　　(head of pancreas tumour)
(with excision of common bile duct resection margin, pancreatic resection margin and
pancreatic duct resection margin)
- Well to moderately differentiated adenocarcinoma.
- Tumour involvement of the muscularis propria of the duodenum.
- Tumour encasement and involvement of the portal vein.
- Focal perineural infiltration present.
- No lymph node metastasis (0/4).
- Close to adventitial resection margin (<0.01 cm).
- Focal perineural infiltration present in the pancreatic resection margin.
- No tumour involvement or dysplasia present in the pancreatic duct margin.
- Gastric remnant and duodenal resection margins clear.
胰頭. 輝普耳氏手術
- 高至中分化腺癌
- 參看下文

Figure 4   Figure 5

MACROSCOPIC EXAMINATION: Printed on : 12/11/2010   11:38:55
(KCH, jw)
Frozen section diagnosis - 1) Clear margin. 2) Mild dysplasia present. 3) Negative.

(KCH, yi)
1) CBD resection margin. Submitted is a ring of tubular structure measuring 1.5 cm across to the thickness of 0.4 cm.
All embedded for frozen section. Figure (1) shows the submitted specimen.

(KCH, jw)
2) Pancreatic resection margin. A piece of pancreatic tissue measuring 2.3 x 1.5 x 0.3 cm is submitted. All embedded
for frozen section. Figure (2) shows the submitted specimen.

to be continued ......

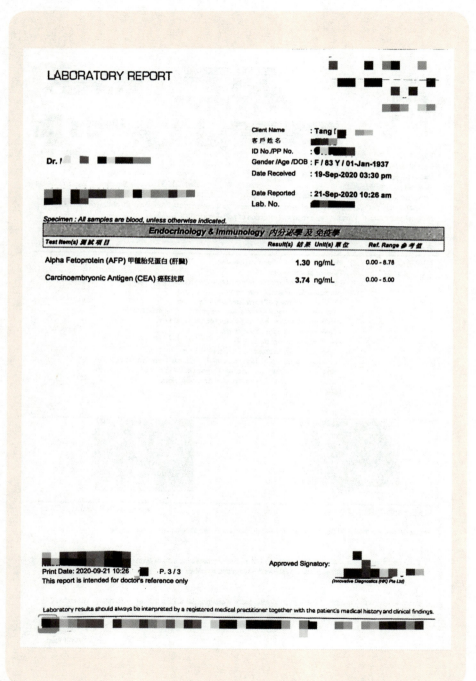

LABORATORY REPORT

Client Name : Tang
客戶姓名
ID No./PP No. : C
Gender /Age /DOB : F / 83 Y / 01-Jan-1937
Date Received : 19-Sep-2020 03:30 pm

Dr.

Date Reported : 21-Sep-2020 10:26 am
Lab. No.

Specimen : All samples are blood, unless otherwise indicated.

Endocrinology & Immunology 內分泌學 及 免疫學

Test Item(s) 測試項目	Result(s) 結果	Unit(s) 單位	Ref. Range 參考值
Alpha Fetoprotein (AFP) 甲種胎兒蛋白 (肝癌)	1.30	ng/mL	0.00 - 8.78
Carcinoembryonic Antigen (CEA) 癌胚抗原	3.74	ng/mL	0.00 - 5.00

Print Date: 2020-09-21 10:26   P. 3 / 3
This report is intended for doctor's reference only

Approved Signatory:

(Innovative Diagnostics (HK) Pte Ltd)

Laboratory results should always be interpreted by a registered medical practitioner together with the patient's medical history and clinical findings.

病案 17

肝癌术后复发康复 18 年

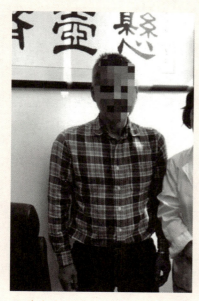

🔊 曾先生 2024 年 1 月前来诊治时
合影留念

曾先生于 2004 年的血液检查中，发现患有乙型肝炎；2005 年又发现肝硬化；2006 年因消瘦、腹胀、腹痛前往医院检查，显示肝癌指数 AFP 明显增高，又进一步做 CT 等检查，证实已患上肝癌。于 2007 年年初做了手术切除肿瘤，之后进行了 1 年的化疗。化疗不良反应严重，令他难以承受，但是他认为既然忍受了这么久，在忍受几次之后就能确保平安，即使再难熬也要忍受下去。没想到化疗结束后，2008 年，他再去医院检查，发现不仅肿瘤已经复发，肝脏也有肿瘤出现，并且得知在这种情况下，肿瘤还会增大，且一般都是多发肿瘤，难以控制。

当时的曾先生每日都感到疲惫不堪、腹部闷胀、食欲消减，经过朋友介绍，他前来接受生命修复的中药治疗，虽然距离他家的路途较远，但他依然风雨无阻的到来。经过 1 年多的治疗后，他的情况良好，连乙型肝炎指标也已恢复正常，没有测出乙肝病毒。如今已经过去18年了，曾先生一直健康快乐地经营着他的生意，开了不止一家餐馆，每日忙忙碌碌，生意火爆。

肝炎与肝癌有密切的联系，乙型肝炎与肝癌的关系则更为密切。据有关报道，两者相关率高达80%，所以重视对乙型肝炎的预防和积极治疗都是非常重要的。对于乙型肝炎的治疗，也是防止肝癌的重要手段。假如乙型肝炎长期不能得到有效治疗，就会演变成肝硬化，之后随着病程进展，也会发生基因突变，HBV增殖复制，部分患者最终引发肝癌。

从确诊患肝癌至今，已经过去了18年，曾先生不仅完全康复，而且经过进一步调理之后，他们喜得贵子，也实现了他们夫妻俩想要孩子的愿望。如今儿子已经12岁，曾先生的人生也早已揭开了新的篇章。

治疗原则

软坚散结，通滞攻毒。

常用中药

1. 龙葵、山慈菇、柴胡、白芍、鳖甲、丹参、石见穿、生大黄、玄明粉、土鳖虫等。
2. 同时服用消瘤丸。

影像学、病理学检查报告及诊疗记录

1. 2007 年 1 月肝癌手术后病理报告，确诊为肝细胞癌。

2. 2009 年 12 月检查报告，肝脏出现新生肿瘤，以往检查中没有，同时有 AFP 升高，肝癌复发。

3. 2014 年 3 月检查报告，肿瘤消失无复发转移。

附：患者检查报告

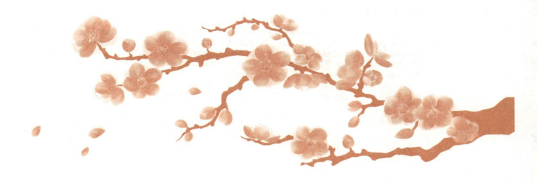

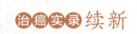
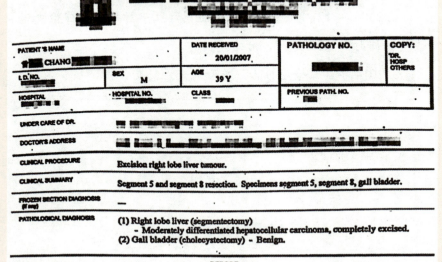

PATIENT'S NAME			DATE RECEIVED 20/01/2007	PATHOLOGY NO.	COPY: DR. HOSP OTHERS
曾▇▇CHANG					
I.D. NO.	SEX M	AGE 39 Y		PREVIOUS PATH. NO.	
HOSPITAL	HOSPITAL NO.	CLASS			
UNDER CARE OF DR.					
DOCTOR'S ADDRESS					
CLINICAL PROCEDURE	Excision right lobe liver tumour.				
CLINICAL SUMMARY	Segment 5 and segment 8 resection. Specimens segment 5, segment 8, gall bladder.				
FROZEN SECTION DIAGNOSIS (if any)	—				
PATHOLOGICAL DIAGNOSIS	(1) Right lobe liver (segmentectomy) - Moderately differentiated hepatocellular carcinoma, completely excised. (2) Gall bladder (cholecystectomy) - Benign.				

REPORT

Macroscopic examination:

(1) "Segment 5 + 8 of liver" - Two pieces of liver tissue altogether 280 grams in weight, 12 x 9 x 5 cm., 7 x 5.5 x 4.7 cm. The larger piece, partly cut-open before receipt, showed a well-defined firm tan-coloured nodular tumour 3 x 1.8 x 1.8 cm. which was 1.1 cm. from the resection margin. The capsular surface of the liver was grossly intact. The smaller piece of liver tissue showed no definite macroscopic lesions on sectioning.

(2) "Gall bladder" - A green-brown smooth-surfaced gall bladder 7.5 cm. long, 3 cm. in diameter. On sectioning the mucosa was green-brown and intact and the wall measured 0.2 to 0.3 cm. thick. No stones were received.

Microscopic examination:

(1) Sections of the tumour show a moderately differentiated hepatocellular carcinoma with trabecular and focal pseudoglandular morphology. The tumour is multinodular, but no definite microsatellite foci are seen in adjacent hepatic parenchyma. Some dilated peritumoural lymphatics show tumour emboli without definite mural invasion. The capsular surface and resection margins are clear. Adjacent liver parenchyma shows an established cirrhosis, with minimal interface hepatitis, and extensive macrovesicular steatosis. The smaller piece of liver tissue shows no evidence of malignancy.

(2) Gall bladder shows no significant pathological abnormalities.

Date Reported: 22/01/2007

Signed: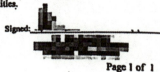

Page 1 of 1

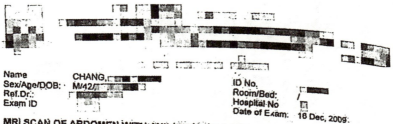

Name   CHANG,   ID No.
Sex/Age/DOB: M/42/   Room/Bed:
Ref.Dr.:   Hospital No
Exam ID   Date of Exam: 16 Dec, 2009.

MRI SCAN OF ABDOMEN WITH AND WITHOUT CONTRAST

Clinical data: Ca liver resected

Technique:
Pre-contrast:
Axial T1, T2, fat-sat T2, fat-sat T1   Post-contrast (Gadolinium):
Coronal T2 weighted   Dynamic Axial fat saturation T1 weighted
Axial long fat-sat T2, in & out-of-phase   Coronal fat saturation T1 weighted

Findings:
Comparison is made with previous MRI dated 26 May 2009.

Evidence of previous right hepatectomy is noted. Left lobe liver remnant is
hypertrophied.

There is a small T1 slightly hyperintense and T2 isointense nodule in anterior aspect
of left lateral segment. It shows signal loss in the opposed-phase image, suggestive
of presence of intralesional fat. After contrast injection, no significant arterial
enhancement is seen. It is hypoenhancing in the portovenous and delayed phase
(series 16 image 40 and series 19 image 17). It is not seen in previous MRI.

No other focal mass lesion in the liver is demonstrated. Portal veins, hepatic veins
and IVC are patent.

Bile ducts are not dilated. Spleen is not enlarged. No focal lesion in spleen is seen.

Both adrenal glands are normal. Left kidney is displaced inferiorly due to
hypertrophied left lobe of liver. Both kidneys are otherwise normal.

No enlarged retroperitoneal lymphadenopathy is seen. No ascites is present.

Impression:
1. Status post right hepatectomy. Hypertrophied left lobe liver remnant.
2. Tiny fat containing nodule without significant arterial enhancement in anterior
aspect of left lateral segment. It is not seen in previous MRI dated 26 May 2009.
DDx include focal fat deposit, regenerative nodule or recurrent hepatocellular
carcinoma. Suggest correlation with AFP and close follow-up MRI for progress.

Department of Diagnostic & Interventional Radiology
MBChB FRCR FHKCR FHKAM (Radiology)

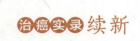

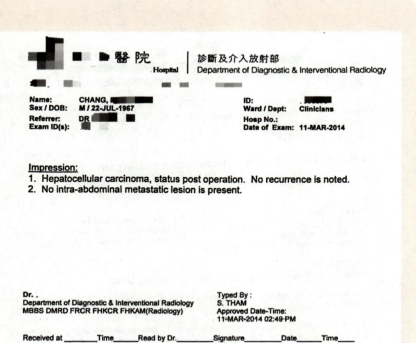

肺癌手术后复发转移者康复 13 年

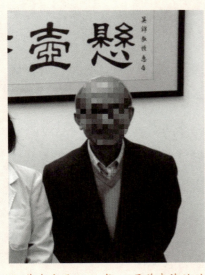

🔊 黄先生于 2022 年 12 月前来诊治时合影留念

黄先生身体一向不错，从来没有得过什么大病，但是在 2011 年，他开始经常咳嗽，甚至有时候会有胸痛及痰中带血的症状。起初他以为只是感冒及喉咙发炎了，没有太在意。但是过了 2 个月，咳嗽并没有好转，甚至越来越频繁，黄先生急忙去医院做检查。经过一系列的检查，确诊他患了肺癌，在右肺下叶有比较大的肿瘤。医院的专家说，现在只有 1 个肿瘤，应在它的体积变得更大之前尽早切除，避免进一步增长、转移和扩散。

在医生的建议和家人的共同商讨之下，黄先生毅然决定尽快动手术切除肿瘤。手术范围比较大，需要切断肋骨，将右肺下半部分全部切除。手术之后，黄先生的身体在逐渐恢复。他非常注重饮食和作息，更勤加锻炼身体。他心想经过这次的教训，一定要好好对待自己，加强锻炼，不要再得病了。就这样大概过了 2 年，2014 年，黄先生又出现了咳嗽、胸痛、气促及多痰的状况。于是他再去医院做检查，这次检查的结果是他万万没想到的，虽然他的右侧肺部连同肿瘤已经切除，但又发生了肿瘤的另一侧肺部转移。左肺经检查后发现了多个肿瘤病灶。在这种情况下，医生建议他尽快再次做手术切除左侧肺部的多个肿瘤，然后做化疗。

黄先生已经没有第1次手术时的决心了，他认为自己的身体在手术之后已经受到了很大的损伤，到现在还没有恢复，如果要再次手术，身体恐怕不能承受。在这种情况下，经过多方打听，他来到了我们的生命修复中心进行治疗。黄先生初来的时候精神很差且非常消瘦，不停地咳嗽，气喘吁吁上不来气，喉中多痰并有血丝状痰咳出，还经常出现胸痛、胸闷的情况。当时经过检查发现，除了有肺癌复发转移的严重情况外，他还有冠心病、冠状动脉狭窄的病症。所以胸闷、胸痛是由两个原因导致，一是肺部的疾病，一侧的肺做了大手术，令肺功能受损，以及多个肿瘤压迫从而令他感到疼痛、胸闷、气短；另一个是冠状动脉狭窄造成的胸闷、气短。

当时的他已经70岁了，仍坚持每天服用中药，非常认真且从不间断。过了数月，他再去医院里做检查，报告显示肿瘤并没有增大，并且有缩小的趋势，医生也不再坚持要求他做手术了。黄先生很高兴亦觉得很受鼓舞，于是他更积极吃中药和治疗。随后，他体内的肿瘤逐渐缩小，病情慢慢稳定下来。到现在过去了13年，他一直很健康，左侧的肺一直也没有再去做手术，这些年来他也从来没有做过化疗、放疗、靶向等治疗。他深切认识到生命修复的中医药疗法最符合大自然的规律，也最适合修复人体的各种疾病。在长期的治疗过程当中，我们发现他有心律不齐等问题，因为他的冠状动脉疾病相当严重，需同时调补心气、心血，所以在治疗中增加了活血通脉的有关方药。现在这么多年过去了，他的心脏功能也很好，能够正常的进行日常生活和工作，他亦没有按照医院的要求去做心脏支架手术，他说之前做过大手术了，现在很怕再动手术。

现在黄先生每隔一段时间就来看一次病，继续做生命修复中药的治疗、继续抗癌和调理心脏。他的病情一直很稳定，每年都去做全身检查，再也没有问题，他也积极地投入自己的工作之中。

治疗原则

祛邪消瘤，活血通脉。

常用中药

1. 瓜蒌、薤白、太子参、黄药子、生地黄、玉竹、石斛、玄参、川贝、浙贝母、生大黄、全蝎等。
2. 同时服用散结丸。

影像学、病理学检查报告及诊疗记录

1. 2011 年右下叶肺癌切除后，于 2015 年 12 月 16 日报告再次活检证实了左下肺叶腺癌。

2. 2018 年 1 月、2019 年 3 月、2019 年 10 月及 2020 年 7 月的检查报告，均显示肺部无新发肿瘤或增大，病情稳定。

附：患者检查报告

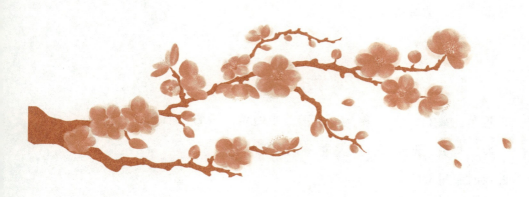

Client's Copy Doctor's Copy

4+25

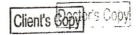

醫院
HOSPITAL
病理報告
PATHOLOGY REPORT

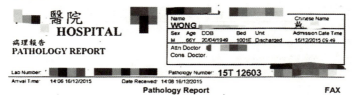

Name WONG				Chinese Name 黃
Sex	Age	DOB	Bed	Unit
M	66Y	20/04/1949	1001E	Discharged
Attn Doctor				Admission Date Time 16/12/2015 09 49
Cons Doctor				

Lab Number: ███████   Pathology Number: **15T 12603**

Arrival Time: 14:06 16/12/2015   Date Received: 14:08 16/12/2015

Pathology Report   FAX

SPECIMEN TYPE
CT guided biopsy apical segment left lower lobe lung lesion.

CLINICAL DETAILS
Adenocarcinoma.
History of Ca lung right lung with previous right lower lobectomy. Now two new ground glass opacities in lingula (next to heart) and in apical segment of left lower lobe.
Previous FNA apical segment LLL lesion shows atypical cells. For CT guided core biopsy of apical segment LLL lesion - to confirm malignancy prior to surgical intervention.

MACROSCOPIC EXAMINATION
Specimen labeled as CT guided biopsy apical segment left lower lobe lung lesion. Received fresh are 3 cores of tan to whitish tissue, measuring 0.1 cm, 0.3 cm and 0.5 cm in length. Specimen is all embedded in 3 frozen blocks.

Frozen section diagnosis: Apical segment left lower lobe lung lesion, CT guided biopsy - Atypical cells seen.

MICROSCOPIC EXAMINATION
The paraffin sections show small area of well differentiated adenocarcinoma composed of irregular malignant glands in a fibrous stroma. The malignant cells have mild nuclear pleomorphism and hyperchromasia, as well as modest amphophilic cytoplasm. There is no lymphovascular permeation. Squamous or spindle cell component is not apparent.

DIAGNOSIS
Apical segment left lower lobe lung lesion, CT guided biopsy - Adenocarcinoma.

Reported by:

Report Time: 08:17 18/12/2015

Dr. ████████
MBBS (HK), FRCPA, FHKCPath,
FHKAM (Path), Grad Dip (Derm) NUS

━━━━━ End of Report ━━━━━

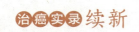

██ Hospital ██ 醫院
MEDICAL IMAGING DEPARTMENT (██ ██ ██

Patient's Name	:	WONG	Unit Record No.	:	██
Sex	:	M	Age	:	68
Examination Date	:	03-JAN-2018	Accession No.	:	
Ward / Class	:		Attending Doctor	:	██ ██

EXAMINATION / PROCEDURE REPORT

Liver has smooth contour and normal size. Portal vein and hepatic veins are patent. Small subcentimeter liver cysts are suggested without significant interval change.

Bilateral adrenals are unremarkable. The spleen is not enlarged. A tiny ~5mm hypoenhancing focus is noted in the spleen which is already seen and being static compared with previous CT in 05/01/2017.

There is no discrete mass along the oesophagus and stomach.

The visualised pancreas appears unremarkable.

No ascites is seen.

Thyroid gland is unremarkable. No enlarged supraclavicular lymph node.

Mild spondylosis along the thoracic spine. There is no destructive bony lesion.

OPINIONS:

1. Status post right lung lower lobectomy and with right side thoracotomy.

2. The previously noted predominantly left lung ground glass opacities are again seen showing no significant interval change. There is evidence of associated volume loss and traction bronchiectasis, they are more suggestive of fibrotic changes than tumour recurrence. Suggest follow up imaging and clinical correlation.

3. Gallstones and gallbladder fundus adenomyomatosis, being static.

4. A subcentimeter splenic hypodense focus, could represent a small splenic cyst, being static.

Thank you for your referral./yc

(Electronically Signed)
Dr. ████████
Specialist in Radiology
MBChB(CUHK), FRCR, FHKCR, FHKAM(Radiology),
MMed(DR)(NUS), MSc(Epidemiology and Biostatistics)(CUHK)

Approved on : 08-JAN-2018 07:14 PM
Page 2 of 2

MR-C101

Hospital 醫院

MEDICAL IMAGING DEPARTMENT

Patient's Name	: WONG	Unit Record No.	:	
Sex	: M	Age	: 69	
Examination Date	: 25-MAR-2019	Accession No.	:	
Ward / Class	:	Attending Doctor	:	

EXAMINATION / PROCEDURE REPORT

bronchi are patent. No other dilated airway or bronchioles suggestive of bronchiectatic changes noted. Heart size is not enlarged.

Gallbladder fundus adenomyomatosis and gallstones are noted. Tiny liver cysts are noted. The scanned part of upper abdomen is otherwise unremarkable. No adrenal mass lesion is seen. No abnormal mass lesion is seen in the scanned part of liver. No other significant bone lesion is noted.

IMPRESSION:

1. Previously noted left lung ground glass opacities remain static.
2. Evidence of right 7th rib lateral aspect defect is seen.
3. Gallbladder fundus adenomyomatosis and gallstones are noted.

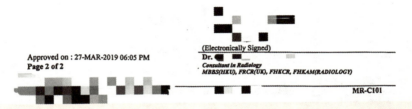

Approved on : 27-MAR-2019 06:05 PM
Page 2 of 2

(Electronically Signed)
Dr.
Consultant in Radiology
MBBS(HKU), FRCR(UK), FHKCR, FHKAM(RADIOLOGY)

MR-C101

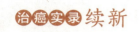

■■■■Hospital ■■醫院
MEDICAL IMAGING DEPARTMENT

Patient's Name	: WONG	Unit Record No.	:
Sex	: M	Age	: 70
Examination Date	: 04-OCT-2019	Accession No.	:
Ward / Class	:	Attending Doctor	:

EXAMINATION / PROCEDURE REPORT

Gallbladder fundus adenomyomatosis and gallstones are noted. Tiny liver cysts are noted.

The scanned part of upper abdomen is otherwise unremarkable. No adrenal mass lesion is

seen. No abnormal mass lesion is seen in the scanned part of liver.

Thoracic spine degeneration is noted.

IMPRESSION:

1. Previously noted left lung ground glass opacities remain static. Suggest interval follow-up CT scan.

2. Evidence of right 7th rib lateral aspect defect is seen.

3. Gallbladder fundus adenomyomatosis and gallstones are noted.

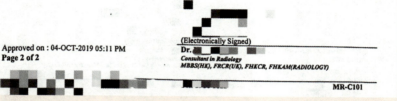

(Electronically Signed)
Dr. ■■■■■
Consultant in Radiology
MBBS(HK), FRCR(UK), FHKCR, FHKAM(RADIOLOGY)

Approved on : 04-OCT-2019 05:11 PM

Page 2 of 2

MR-C101

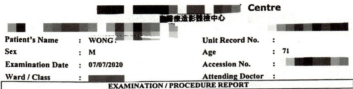

Centre
神醫療造影體檢中心

Patient's Name	: WONG	Unit Record No.	:	
Sex	: M	Age	: 71	
Examination Date	: 07/07/2020	Accession No.	:	
Ward / Class	:	Attending Doctor	:	

EXAMINATION / PROCEDURE REPORT

Right costophrenic angle pleural thickening is noted, likely due to old insult.

There is no other air space consolidation, interstitial thickening or fibrosis seen. No other abnormal lung mass is noted. There is no pleural effusion on both sides.

No enlarged abnormal mediastinal mass or lymphadenopathy identified. Small amount of pericardial recess fluid is seen.

Trachea and bronchi are patent. No other dilated airway or bronchioles suggestive of bronchiectatic changes noted.

Heart size is not enlarged.

Gallbladder fundus adenomyomatosis and gallstones are noted. Tiny liver cysts are noted.

The scanned part of upper abdomen is otherwise unremarkable. No adrenal mass lesion is seen. No abnormal mass lesion is seen in the scanned part of liver. Thoracic spine degeneration is noted.

IMPRESSION:

1. Previously noted left lung ground glass opacities remain static. Suggest interval follow-up CT scan.

2. Evidence of right 7th rib lateral aspect defect is seen.

3. Gallbladder fundus adenomyomatosis and gallstones are noted.

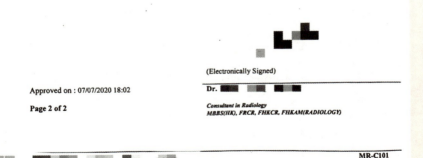

(Electronically Signed)

Approved on : 07/07/2020 18:02

Dr.

Page 2 of 2

Consultant in Radiology
MBBS(HK), FRCR, FHKCR, FHKAM(RADIOLOGY)

129

病案19

鼻咽癌大量颅骨转移康复12年

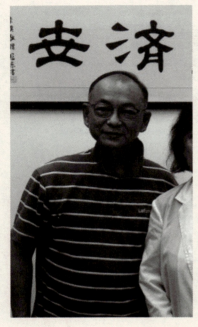

↥ 冯先生于2024年2月前来诊治时合影留念

冯先生49岁时，发现患上鼻咽癌，起初以为是初期肿瘤，只是早期的病变，接受治疗后就会好起来，所以他一直积极进行化疗。经过几个化疗疗程后转为放疗，放疗运用了很大的剂量，而且需要做35次。他认为经过这样大剂量、高强度的现代化治疗，肿瘤肯定没有了，但是放疗后经过检查，发现病情仍然非常严重。他的肿瘤组织已经充斥了鼻腔、上颌窦、蝶窦、颅底、内翼肌、翼腭窝等，头部组织全部充满了肿瘤，锁骨上淋巴及颈部等也有很多的淋巴转移。经过病理学检查，更是确诊了他所得的这种鼻咽癌，是最恶性的未分化癌。

在这种情况下，冯先生来到我们这里，进行中医药和中西医结合的生命修复的治疗。冯先生初来时，非常消瘦，精神萎靡，基本上不能吃饭，只能喝点粥。因为癌组织堵塞了他的鼻孔和周围组织，包括呼吸道，令他呼吸非常困难；没有味觉，鼻涕和痰也有很多，并且有很多的血液在鼻涕和痰中。我们根据他的病情，给他进行了中药排毒、祛浊散结等多方面的治疗。随后他的病情有了好转，经过检查显示，大多数的转移病灶已经消失，可是不幸的是又出现了新的转移灶，这就是鼻咽癌和许多癌症的共同特点。

此后，我们又积极地给他治疗新的转移病灶，直到最后，肿瘤彻底消失，冯先生和家人都很高兴。直到现在，已经过去12年左右，冯先生虽然没有常规的来治疗，但有时候还会来巩固一下治疗效果，再吃一些中药。每次他来的时候总是很高兴，也愿意把他的照片和病例公开，以鼓励更多的患者。鼻咽癌是一种很常见的恶性肿瘤，像他这样所有的鼻窦、鼻腔及周围组织颅底等都有转移，是非常严重的情况。生命修复的中医药治疗，彻底消除了所有的肿块和转移病灶，冯先生现在身体健康，生活及工作也很开心。

治疗原则

解毒化浊，软坚散结。

常用中药

1. 鱼腥草、连翘、金银花、夏枯草、黄药子、半夏、白芥子、乳香、猫爪草等。

2. 同时服用消瘤丸。

影像学、病理学检查报告及诊疗记录

1. 2012 年 4 月 26 日病理报告证实为鼻咽癌，是最恶性的未分化癌。

2. 2012 年 5 月 22 日 PET/CT 检查报告证实鼻咽癌，并有鼻腔、上颌窦、蝶窦、筛窦、颅骨、颅内、淋巴等转移。

3. 2014 年 4 月 3 日 PET/CT 检查报告证实肿瘤无复发，但锁骨上淋巴结有新转移灶。

4. 2019 年 10 月 30 日及 2020 年 10 月 19 日检查结果显示 EBV 病毒检测为阴性。

5. 2021 年 6 月 8 日 CT 检查报告未见肿瘤复发转移。

附：患者检查报告

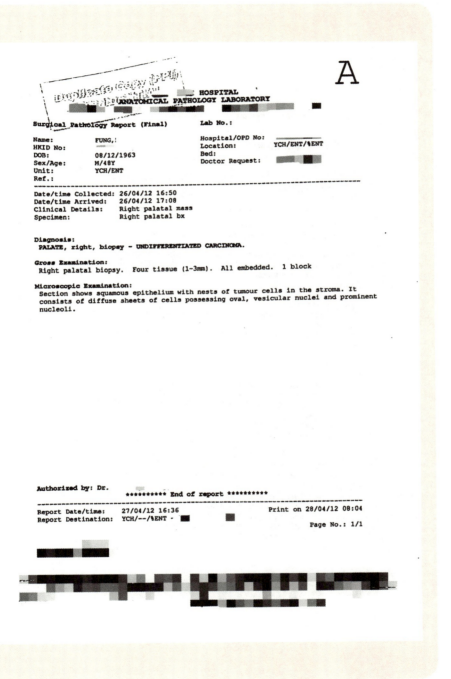

A

HOSPITAL
ANATOMICAL PATHOLOGY LABORATORY

Surgical Pathology Report (Final)   Lab No.:

Name:	FUNG,
HKID No:	
DOB:	08/12/1963
Sex/Age:	M/48Y
Unit:	YCH/ENT
Ref.:	

Hospital/OPD No:
Location: YCH/ENT/%ENT
Bed:
Doctor Request:

Date/time Collected: 26/04/12 16:50
Date/time Arrived: 26/04/12 17:08
Clinical Details: Right palatal mass
Specimen: Right palatal bx

Diagnosis:
 PALATE, right, biopsy - UNDIFFERENTIATED CARCINOMA.

Gross Examination:
 Right palatal biopsy. Four tissue (1-3mm). All embedded. 1 block

Microscopic Examination:
 Section shows squamous epithelium with nests of tumour cells in the stroma. It
 consists of diffuse sheets of cells possessing oval, vesicular nuclei and prominent
 nucleoli.

Authorized by: Dr.
                    ********** End of report **********

Report Date/time: 27/04/12 16:36   Print on 28/04/12 08:04
Report Destination: YCH/--/%ENT -

                                                 Page No.: 1/1

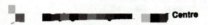

Patient Information

Patient ID: ___
Patient Name: FUNG __
Date of Birth: 8/12/1963
Gender: M

Referring Physician: ___
Examination Date: 22/5/2012
Report Date: 22/5/2012
HKID: ___

These can be identified in images 64 – 116.
On the left neck, the jugulodigastric node measures 1.5 cm in diameter with activity of about 3.2.
These are all consistent with regional metastatic lymphadenopathy.
The thyroid shows no enlargement and no evidence of hypermetabolic lesion.
The left mid and lower neck and supraclavicular region shows no hypermetabolic lesion.

Bony Structures
PET images show no definite hypermetabolic bony lesion to suggest definite bony metastases.
The static images show no destructive bony lesion. There is no definite vertebral collapse.

COMMENT :

1. Large mass centre in the right nasopharynx with invasion of nasal cavity, right maxillary sinus, right sphenoid sinus. The floor of the sphenoid sinus and possibly part of the anterior clivus, the medial pterygoid, pterygo-maxillary fissure have all been eroded by this lesion.
2. There is probably no intracranial invasion.
   This is however best further assess with MRI.
3. Enlarged right retropharyngeal node, enlarged bilateral jugulodigastric node, multiple right posterior jugular lymph nodes enlargement and right supraclavicular metastases. Left jugulodigastric hypermetabolic activity. Appearances are that of significant regional invasion and significant regional metastatic lymphadenopathy.
4. No lung or liver or adrenal metastases. No definite bony metastases.
5. Equivocal increased activity in the right lateral wall of the caecum. The level of activity could still be of physiological nature. However due to rather significant differences compared to the adjacent activity for the rest of the colon, it may be worth considering colonoscopy to exclude a tumour.

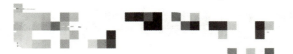

Patient Information

Patient ID:
Patient Name: FUNG
Date of Birth: 8 Dec, 1963
Gender: Male

Referring Physician:
Examination Date: 3 Apr, 2014
Report Date: 3 Apr, 2014
HKID:

COMMENT

1. Status post nasopharyngeal carcinoma post-treatment. Comparison with the PET/CT of 11 December 2013.
2. Residual scarring and effacement of the right fossa of Rosenmuller, due to feature of treatment previous known nasopharyngeal carcinoma. These are not hypermetabolic and findings do not suggest local recurrence.
3. Hypermetabolic mass in the right supraclavicular region is identified. This is a new finding not identified on 11 December 213 and is most likely a new metastatic supraclavicular lymph node.
4. No evidence of lung or liver or adrenal metastasis.

Dr.
MBBS(Syd), FRCR, FRANZCR
FHKCR, FHKAM(Radiology)

Page 3 of 3

135

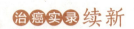

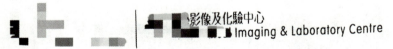
影像及化驗中心
Imaging & Laboratory Centre

Name : FUNG   馮
Sex/Age : M / 56   Collected : 19-Oct-2020 NA
ID No. :   Registered : 19-Oct-2020 19:33
Ref No. :   Reported : 22-Oct-2020 11:59
Lab No. :   Last Print : 22-Oct-2020 11:59

Cumulative Report 累積化驗報告

	Rec. Date:	30/10/2019	19/10/2020				Reference	Unit
	Rec. Time:	18:23	19:33					
化驗項目	Lab. No.:	Y1009757	Z1007079					
EBV 病毒 DNA 數量	EBV DNA, Quantitative	< 20	< 20				See remarks	copies/mL

EBV DNA Quantitative Test Remarks:

1. Negative   : <20 copies/mL

   Low Positive : 20 - 1000 copies/mL

   Positive   : >1000 copies/mL

2. This EBV DNA Quantitative test is a Real-time PCR. The detection limit of the test is 20 copies/mL.

3. This test has a sensitivity of 96% and a specificity of 93% for detecting NPC (Reference: Lo YM, Cancer Res. 1999, Mar 15:59(6):1188-91).

4. EBV DNA Quantitation has been found to be useful for the monitoring of treatment response and prognostication of EBV associated malignancies, such as nasopharyngeal cancer (NPC), infectious mononucleosis (IM), lymphoproliferative disease and lymphoma.

5. Please note that Low Positive results may be expressed in healthy population. Also, Negative result may be encountered in NPC patient due to different disease stage.

6. Cumulative results will be shown when ID number is provided.

THIS REPORT IS INTENDED FOR DOCTOR'S REFERENCE ONLY.
此化驗報告僅供醫生作參考之用

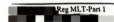

Page: 1 / 1   Reg MLT-Part 1

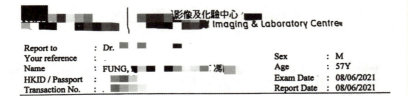

影像及化驗中心
Imaging & Laboratory Centre

Report to	: Dr.		Sex	: M
Your reference	: .		Age	: 57Y
Name	: FUNG, 馮		Exam Date	: 08/06/2021
HKID / Passport	:		Report Date	: 08/06/2021
Transaction No.	: .			

CXR (PA)

FINDINGS:

Lungs are clear with no focal mass lesion or consolidation.

Trachea is central.

Heart size is not enlarged.

No hilar mass lesion and the mediastinum is not widened.

No pleural effusion is seen.

Mild cortical bulging is noted along the right 9th anterolateral rib. ?composite shadow. ?subtle rib fracture. Suggest to correlate clinically for any evidence of previous trauma / tenderness. No destructive bone lesion is noted.

SUMMARY:

1. Lungs are clear. Heart is not enlarged.

2. Mild cortical bulging is noted along the right 9th anterolateral rib. ?composite shadow. ?subtle rib fracture. Suggest to correlate clinically for any evidence of previous trauma / tenderness. No destructive bone lesion is noted.

Thank you for your referral

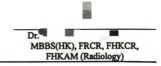

Dr.
MBBS(HK), FRCR, FHKCR,
FHKAM (Radiology)

病案20

成功救治的晚期生殖细胞癌婴儿

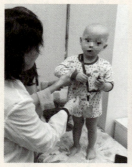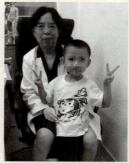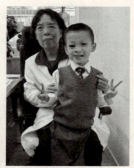

东东在健康成长之中，第三张（最右）拍摄与 2024 年 2 月

　　东东是一位可爱的小男孩，他刚生下来的时候，白白胖胖，家里多了这样一位可爱的小宝贝，大家都感到非常的高兴且满足。但是在他半岁，外婆替他洗澡时，发现他的肚子里面硬硬的，好像是一个肿块。之后孩子逐渐出现了呕吐，不愿意吃奶的情况，外婆和妈妈就急忙抱着他到医院看病。经过检查后发现，他的肚子里有一个非常大的肿瘤，超过 10cm。很难想象一个 6 个月大的小婴儿肚子里面有如此大的肿瘤。

　　肿瘤占据了腹腔的大部分位置，包括肝脏、胰腺、脾脏等都已被压迫。经过更进一步的检查显示，肿瘤是从腹膜后面来的，并且伴有大量的腹水，在腹腔和盆腔里还有几个小一点的肿瘤，但是肿瘤的源头在哪里并不是很清楚。之后经过活组织病理学检查，确诊是生殖细胞恶性肿瘤；骨髓检查显示了有恶性肿瘤侵犯骨髓系统，基因检查显示有染色体异常。于是医院立即开始对东东进行化疗。2018 年 3 月，东东开始做化疗，在完成 6 个化疗疗程后，经过再次检查显示，肿瘤已经缩小，于是 2018 年 11 月进行了肿瘤的切除手术。肿瘤切除之后，又进行了多次的化疗。但在化疗过程中，发生了非常严重的副作用和毒性反应，东东的大便全是血，甚至连肠子都有一尺多脱落了出来，生命垂危。同时，家人多次接到医院的通知，都说这个孩子已经不行了，让他们做好心理准备，但是他们不愿意就此放弃。没过多久，东东再次做检查，在肚子里又发现了新的肿瘤，也就是说手术以后肿瘤又复发了。

他于 2019 年 9 月再次做 CT 检查，显示手术后腹部又长出了 3 个肿瘤，而且又出现大量腹水，孩子的病情日益加重。之后，他的胸部双侧也出现了越来越多的胸腔积液，癌指数亦明显增高。医生连忙找家长商讨病情，表示已用尽方法，这种肿瘤是没有办法再治疗的，也没有治好的可能性。虽然继续做化疗可能会令肿瘤暂时缩小一点，但也只是短期的表现，以后还会再增大。肿瘤没有可能消失，目前也没有办法控制肿瘤的生长情况。东东的妈妈表示，从 6 个月到 1 岁半，孩子在医院治疗的过程中，医院已经 3 次通知说孩子不行了，要他们做好心理准备，东东进入 ICU 进行抢救的情况超过 10 次，医生建议不再做急救处理，因为未必有效。经过多方打听探问及查询，家长抱着奄奄一息的东东来到我们这里，进行一个全新且方式完全不一样的中医药治疗。

当时的东东身体非常虚弱，还不会说话也不会行走，连坐起来的力气也没有。在为他做针灸治疗的时候，因为太虚弱，他连哭都发不出声音，没有任何力气进行反抗和挣扎，只是一动不动地用非常微弱的声音呻吟。经过一段时间的治疗，孩子的精神慢慢好转起来了，面色逐渐红润，也可以吃一些东西了。更可喜的是，他逐渐学会了走路，从开始只能站立几秒钟，然后慢慢增加时间，之后可以迈开小腿，一步步的学走路，很快不但会走，还能慢慢开始跑了。2020 年 3 月东东再次做检查，报告显示他的腹部只剩下一个 1.2cm×1.8cm 的小小肿瘤，其他肿瘤都已经消失了。于是我们继续进行治疗，直到所有肿瘤全部消失。由于东东曾接受长期化疗，造成他的肝脏有些损伤，因此孩子现在仍需要常来进行巩固治疗。

现在的他非常活泼可爱，每次前来在等待治疗的时候，都会发出爽朗的笑声并大声唱歌，每位职员和患者都非常喜欢他。如今东东 6 岁了，他已经康复了。他非常的聪明伶俐，喜欢跑来跑去到处玩耍，与其他同龄孩子没有什么不同。一般人看到他，很难想象他就是那个曾经受过苦难的孩子。待他日后长大了，大概也不会记得这些九死一生的经历，盼望他健康成长，前程无量。

治疗原则

养阴固肾，排毒，散结消瘤。

常用中药

1. 生地黄、玉竹、石斛、玄参、瓜蒌、薤白、太子参、黄药子、浙贝母、桃仁、红花、石见穿、全蝎等。
2. 同时服用散结丸。

影像学、病理学检查报告及诊疗记录

1. 2018 年 3 月 20 日骨髓检查报告显示骨髓癌细胞浸润。

2. 2018 年 3 月 23 日手术后病理报告为生殖细胞癌。

3. 2019 年 9 月 7 日放射检查报告显示手术后肿瘤复发，腹部有 3 个肿瘤，脾脏肿大达 8cm，腹腔、盆腔、胸腔积液，纵隔软组织高密度影等。

4. 2019 年 9 月 17 日医院报告说明：患儿 6 个月时入院，腹部肿瘤最大的为 8.7cm×5.5cm×10.2cm。心包积液、胸腔积液、腹水。2018 年 3 月 29 日开始化疗 6 个疗程。2018 年 9 月 10 日切除肿瘤后又进行化疗。2019 年 9 月 7 日 CT 检查报告显示肿瘤复发，腹部有 3 个肿瘤，脾脏肿大达 8cm，腹水、盆腔积液、双侧胸腔积液，肿瘤细胞骨髓浸润。已跟家长讲明：进一步的化疗有严重不良反应，只能短期缩小肿瘤。尚无资料显示有其他有效的治疗方法。

5. 2020 年 5 月 27 日经生命修复治疗中，CT 检查显示腹部只剩余 1.2cm×1.8cm 肿瘤。

6. 2021 年 3 月 31 日检查报告显示，经生命修复治疗后，肿瘤已全部消失。

附：患者检查报告

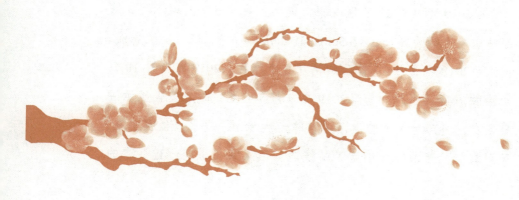

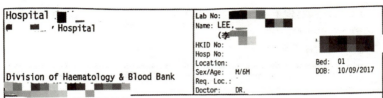

Hospital		Lab No:
' Hospital		Name: LEE,
		(李
		HKID No:
		Hosp No:
Division of Haematology & Blood Bank		Location:
		Sex/Age: M/6M
		Req. Loc.:
		Doctor: DR.

Bed: 01
DOB: 10/09/2017

Date Collected: 19/03/2018 11:24
Date Arrived: 19/03/2018 14:13
Clinical Details: ? neuroblastoma,.suspected lymphoma,abdominal tumour with LN with pericardial and
pleural effusion

BONE MARROW ASPIRATION EXAMINATION

Specimen type: Marrow blood

Report:
Abdominal tumour with lymph nodes, pericardial & pleural effusion.

PBS: Hb 9.9 (anisopoikilocytosis, HcMc, occ targets & fragments, minimal polychromasia)
WBC 13.2 (N65 L28 M6 E1 occ atypical lymphocytes) Plt 533 (occ giant plt)

BM (bilateral): The left marrow aspirate is mildly hypocellular for age. There is a
prominent infiltration by abnormal mononuclear cells, some of which appear to occur in
clusters. These cells are mainly medium-to-large to large in size, with low N/C ratio,
roundish nuclear contour, clumped chromatin, strongly basophilic agranular cytoplasm
with a perinuclear hof. A proportion of these abnormal cells show variable number of
cytoplasmic vacuoles. Erythropoiesis & granulopoiesis are fairly represented.
Maturation is unremarkable. Blasts are not obviously increased. Megakaryopoiesis is
mildly increased. Lymphocytes are prominent but not excessive for age. The right
aspirate is peripheral blood diluted. Stainable iron is demonstrable with paucity of
sideroblasts. Ring sideroblasts are not found.

Conclusion:
Consistent with marrow infiltration by malignant tumour with reactive megakaryocytic
hyperplasia & iron block. To await further investigations for characterization of the
abnormal cells.

Report Date: 20/03/2018   Pathologist: Dr. ▮ ▮ ▮ ▮ ▮ ▮

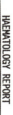

HAEMATOLOGY REPORT

This laboratory is accredited by the College of American Pathologists.
CAP Accreditation Number
*Please retain permanently in patient record to assist in patient care.

Report Date & Time: 20/03/2018 18:36   Generated on: 21/03/2018 07:12
Report Destination: QMH/--/K8 - K8, Paediatrics   Page No.: 1/1

143

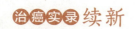

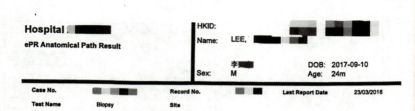

Hospital [REDACTED]

ePR Anatomical Path Result

HKID:	
Name:	LEE, [REDACTED]
	李[REDACTED]
Sex:	M
DOB:	2017-09-10
Age:	24m

Case No.	[REDACTED]	Record No.	[REDACTED]	Last Report Date	23/03/2018
Test Name	Biopsy	Site			

Final Report (20/09/2018)

MICROSCOPIC EXAMINATION:
The tumour cells are weakly positive for PLAP.

DIAGNOSIS:
A-C. PERITONEUM, incisional biopsy - suggestive of GERM CELL TUMOUR

Provisional Report (29/03/2018)

CLINICAL HISTORY:
Abdominal mass with ascites, pleural and pericardial effusion. BM exam showed infiltration by malignant cells.

SPECIMEN(S):
Tissue mass x incisional biopsy

GROSS EXAMINATION:
(Specimen received fresh)
(A) All embedded, 1 piece, 1 x 10 mm. 1 cassette, tan, soft. Frozen for future use.
(B) All embedded, 1 piece, 1 x 2 mm. 1 cassette, tan, soft. Frozen for future use.
(C) All embedded, 1 piece, 1 x 15 mm. 1 cassette, tan, soft.

MICROSCOPIC EXAMINATION:
A-C. The biopsy material of A and C consists of sheets and nests of pleomorphic medium to large polygonal cells that have irregular nuclei, eosinophilic nucleoli and prominent mitotic activity. The cytoplasm is amphophilic with clearing present, and there appears to increased apoptotic body formation noted. In particular there is no evidence of rhabdoid differentiation, blastema appearance, rosette formation or a fibrillary stroma, and no epithelial elements are seen. The tumour cells are negative for desmin, myogenin, MNF116, S100 protein, CD30, CD45, chromogranin, synaptophysin, CD3, CD99, CD20 and ALK, but about 30% of the cells show some cytoplasmic positivity for c-kit.

The appearances are those of a poorly differentiated primitive tumour with a high mitotic activity and no evidence of neural, skeletal muscle, or lymphoid differentiation. The c-kit positivity is suggestive of a seminoma/germ cell tumour, and additional stains will be performed to be incorporated into a final report. No tumour is present in block B.

DIAGNOSIS:
A-C. PERITONEUM, incisional biopsy - suggestive of GERM CELL TUMOUR

醫院

Patient ID:	Case No: .. ...
	Patient Type:
Name: LEE	Referrer: Dr.
	Philip
Sex: M DOB: 10.09.2017	Exam Date: 07.09.2019
Accession No:	

Radiological Examination Report

hepatic veins are normally opacified. Biliary tree not dilated. No calcified gallstone detected in the gallbladder.

Pancreas is unremarkable with no focal mass lesion detected. Pancreatic duct is not dilated. No abnormal pancreatic calcifications seen.

The splenic vein is well opacified. Spleen is prominent in size measuring 8.0cm.

Both adrenals are not enlarged with no focal mass lesion detected.

The coeliac, superior and inferior mesenteric arteries are well opacified.

No hyperdense renal stone detected. No hydronephrosis detected. No focal renal mass lesion detected. Both kidneys showing comparable contrast excretion. No ureteric obstruction detected. Urinary bladder is grossly unremarkable.

Ascites noted in the abdomen and pelvis.

Bilateral pleural effusions noted, more over the left side.

Soft tissue density noted over the anterior mediastinum, may represent rebound thymic hyperplasia in the proper clinical context.

Dr
Consultant Radiologist
MBBS (HK), FRCR, FHKCR, FHKAM (Radiology)

Approved Date: 07.09.2019 13:23

Page 2 of 3

治癌实录续新

Patient ID:

Name: LEE

Sex: M   DOB: 10.09.2017
Accession No:

Case No:
Patient Type:
Referrer: Dr. Philip
Exam Date: 07.09.2019

Radiological Examination Report

IMPRESSION:

1. Germ cell tumour status post-chemotherapy. Three irregular enhancing lesions are noted in the abdomen measuring 1.9x2.5x2.6cm (APxTSxLS) over the left anterior abdomen, measuring 3.3x4.1x3.1cm (APxTSxLS) over the left para-aortic region just anterior to the left kidney and over the right-sided mesentery measuring 1.6x1.9x1.2cm (APxTSxLS). These are suspicious of recurrence.

2. Spleen is prominent in size measuring 8.0cm.

3. Ascites noted in the abdomen and pelvis.

4. Bilateral pleural effusions noted, more over the left side.

5. Soft tissue density noted over the anterior mediastinum, may represent rebound thymic hyperplasia in the proper clinical context.

Dr
Consultant Radiologist
MBBS (HK), FRCR, FHKCR, FHKAM (Radiology)

Approved Date: 07.09.2019 13:23

Hospital

To: Dr

Dear Dr

Re: LEE, ▮ ▮ [▮ **Sex: M Age: 24m**

<u>Reason for referral: relapse metastatic germ cell tumour</u>
<u>Special consideration: Others (upon parents' request)</u>
<u>Reason for priority: Malignancy/ suspected malignancy</u>

I would like to refer this child to you upon parents' request for assessment and opinion on treatment plan.

The child was referred to Queen Mary Hospital at 6 months of age for persistent vomiting. He was found to have abdominal mass with ascites, pleural effusion and pericardial effusion. His first AFP was 20ng/ml and beta-HCG was normal. Subsequently AFP was noted to increased to 57 ng/ml in April 2019.

USS abdomen showed a 8.7 x 5.5. x 10.2 cm lobulated vascular mass over anterior upper abdomen displacing liver, spleen and pancreas. PET-CT scan showed it arising from retroperitoneal , ascites and also a few metabolic nodules near stomach and in pelvis. Primary origin was uncertain. Peritoneal biopsy confirmed germ cell tumour. Bone marrow examination showed infiltration with non-haemic malignancy. Cytogenetics found complex karyotype with multiple trisomies and structural abnormalities.

He was started on HK GCT protocol 94 on 29/3/18 and completed 6 cycles of JEB. BM was cleared. Reassessment CT showed 3 cm residual tumour and OT for tumour excision was done on 10/9/18 and histology confirmed residual tumour. He was given 3 more courses of TIP chemotherapy. Reassessment CT on 27/11/2018 showed significant reduction in tumour size with tiny focus of calcification. There was no other definite abdominal or pelvic metastasis disease.

He underwent auto PBSCT (conditioning with carbopantin and etoposide) in December 2018. He suffered from adenovirus colitis and had severe diarrhea with blood in stool He was treated with cidofovir. His gut conditions gradually improved. He WAs subsequently discharged.

A mass lesion over abdomen was felt last week. He was brought to QMH and was then

請盡早到轉介之診所辦理預約的手續。此轉介信的有效期為發出日起的三個月內。
Please make appointment with the referred clinic as early as possible. This referral letter is valid for 3 months from the date of issue.

Printed on 17/09/2019 09:29   Printed by: ▮

Page 1 of 2

Hospital

transferred to [REDACTED] Hospital for further investigation.

CT scan was done at Gleneagle on 7/9/2019 showing:
1. Germ cell tumour status post-chemotherapy. Three irregular enhancing lesions are noted in the abdomen measuring 1.9x2.5x2.6cm (APxTSxLS) over the left anterior abdomen, measuring 3.3x4.1x3.1cm (APxTSxLS) over the left para-aortic region just anterior to the left kidney and over the right-sided mesenteron measuring 1.6x1.9x1.2cm (Epistaxis). These are suspicious of recurrence.
2. Spleen is prominent in size measuring 8.0cm.
3. Ascites noted in the abdomen and pelvis.
4. Bilateral pleural effusions noted, more over the left side.
5. Soft tissue density noted over the anterior mediastina, may represent rebound thymic hyperplasia in the proper clinical context.

Serum AFP and beta HCG remained normal. Bone marrow showed infiltration by abnormal mononuclear cells, the morphology is similar to those cells at initial presentation.

We have interviewed parents and explained tumor relapse. We have plan to get biopsy of abdominal lesion under anesthesia with imaging guidance on 17 Sept 2019. We explained to parents that the cure rate is low. Further chemotherapy may shrink the tumour for short time but will not be able to clear the tumour. On the other hand, patient may not tolerate chemotherapy well and can develop serious complications.

Palliative approach is probably the more appropriate direction for quality of life. Both parents wish to seek cure and they consider alternative treatment options such as targeted therapy, immunotherapy or Chinese medicine. Targeted therapy (such as use of TKI or PD-1 inhibitor) may be considered if genetic testing on the current tissue biopsy can identify actionable genes. However there are little data in medical literature to show effectiveness. There are also scarce data in using allogeneic transplant or cellular therapy in this type of tumour.

Thank you again for agreeing to accept this patient for review and giving opinions.

Signature:
签名:
Name in Block Letters:
姓名:

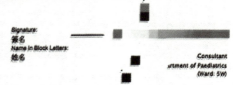

Consultant
...rtment of Paediatrics
(Ward: 5W)

請盡早到轉介之診所辦理預約手續。此轉介信的有效期為簽出日起的三個月內。
Please make appointment with the referred clinic as early as possible. This referral letter is valid for 3 months from the date of issue.

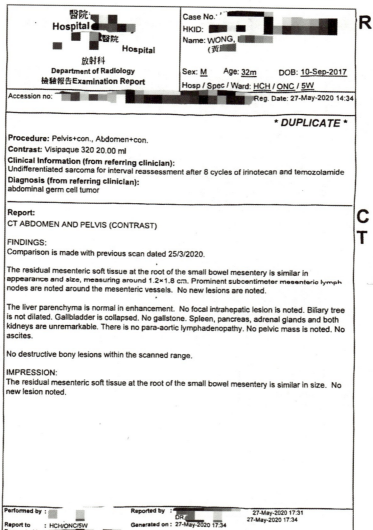

为癌症患者却病延年

COPY

R

醫院 Hospital 醫院 Hospital 放射科 **Department of Radiology** 檢驗報告**Examination Report**	Case No.: HKID: Name: WONG, (黃 Sex: **M** Age: **32m** DOB: **10-Sep-2017** Hosp / Spec / Ward: **HCH** / **ONC** / **5W**

Accession no: Reg. Date: 27-May-2020 14:34

* DUPLICATE *

Procedure: Pelvis+con., Abdomen+con.
Contrast: Visipaque 320 20.00 ml
Clinical Information (from referring clinician):
Undifferentiated sarcoma for interval reassessment after 8 cycles of irinotecan and temozolamide
Diagnosis (from referring clinician):
abdominal germ cell tumor

C

T

Report:
CT ABDOMEN AND PELVIS (CONTRAST)

FINDINGS:
Comparison is made with previous scan dated 25/3/2020.

The residual mesenteric soft tissue at the root of the small bowel mesentery is similar in appearance and size, measuring around 1.2×1.8 cm. Prominent subcentimeter mesenteric lymph nodes are noted around the mesenteric vessels. No new lesions are noted.

The liver parenchyma is normal in enhancement. No focal intrahepatic lesion is noted. Biliary tree is not dilated. Gallbladder is collapsed. No gallstone. Spleen, pancreas, adrenal glands and both kidneys are unremarkable. There is no para-aortic lymphadenopathy. No pelvic mass is noted. No ascites.

No destructive bony lesions within the scanned range.

IMPRESSION:
The residual mesenteric soft tissue at the root of the small bowel mesentery is similar in size. No new lesion noted.

Performed by :   Reported by :   27-May-2020 17:31
                                              DR.   27-May-2020 17:34
Report to   : HCH/ONC/5W   Generated on : 27-May-2020 17:34
Requested by :   Reprinted by   on 15-Jun-2020 15:30

Page 1 of 1

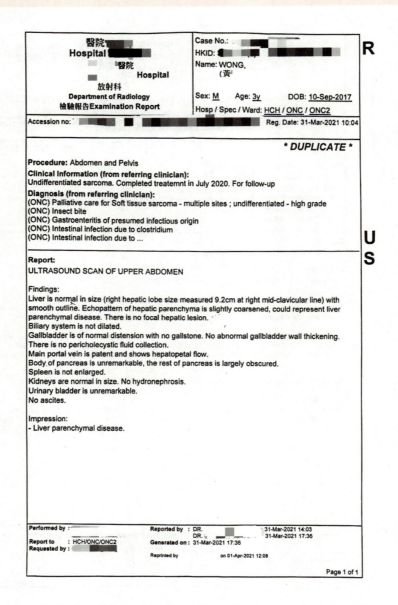

医院
Hospital

医院
Hospital

放射科
Department of Radiology
检验报告**Examination Report**

Case No.:
HKID:
Name: WONG,
(黄

Sex: <u>M</u>   Age: <u>3y</u>   DOB: <u>10-Sep-2017</u>
Hosp / Spec / Ward: <u>HCH</u> / <u>ONC</u> / <u>ONC2</u>

Accession no:

Reg. Date: 31-Mar-2021 10:04

R

U
S

* DUPLICATE *

Procedure: Abdomen and Pelvis
Clinical Information (from referring clinician):
Undifferentiated sarcoma. Completed treatemnt in July 2020. For follow-up
Diagnosis (from referring clinician):
(ONC) Palliative care for Soft tissue sarcoma - multiple sites ; undifferentiated - high grade
(ONC) Insect bite
(ONC) Gastroenteritis of presumed infectious origin
(ONC) Intestinal infection due to clostridium
(ONC) Intestinal infection due to ...

Report:

ULTRASOUND SCAN OF UPPER ABDOMEN

Findings:
Liver is normal in size (right hepatic lobe size measured 9.2cm at right mid-clavicular line) with smooth outline. Echopattern of hepatic parenchyma is slightly coarsened, could represent liver parenchymal disease. There is no focal hepatic lesion.
Biliary system is not dilated.
Gallbladder is of normal distension with no gallstone. No abnormal gallbladder wall thickening. There is no pericholecystic fluid collection.
Main portal vein is patent and shows hepatopetal flow.
Body of pancreas is unremarkable, the rest of pancreas is largely obscured.
Spleen is not enlarged.
Kidneys are normal in size. No hydronephrosis.
Urinary bladder is unremarkable.
No ascites.

Impression:
- Liver parenchymal disease.

Performed by :

Report to   : HCH/ONC/ONC2
Requested by :

Reported by : DR.
DR.
31-Mar-2021 14:03
31-Mar-2021 17:36
Generated on : 31-Mar-2021 17:36

Reprinted by   on 01-Apr-2021 12:08

Page 1 of 1

病案 21

肾脏移植后又患晚期癌症

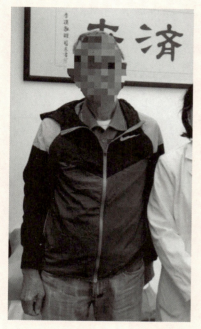

🔊 刘先生于 2022 年 3 月前来诊治时合影留念

刘先生长期患有严重的高血压和糖尿病，并逐渐损害了肾功能，于 2017 年出现严重的肾功能衰竭状况。2018 年 2 月，他做了肾脏移植手术，手术后需长时间服用抗排斥药物。又因同时患有高血压及糖尿病，也需长期服药，所以是一位患有多种严重疾病的患者，每天都需服用多种药物。

更不幸的是，2020 年 1 月，他又发现患上膀胱癌。虽然有积极做化疗，然而又发现在前列腺位置出现多个肿瘤，前列腺癌指数增高，因此他经常感到疲乏，继之出现咯血。于是急忙再次做详细检查，发现膀胱癌的双肺多发转移。因为原有肾脏已被破坏，现在他的肾脏是移植来的，确实承受不了更多化疗带来的副作用。所以他转而求助于我们的生命修复治疗。

刘先生前来时非常虚弱，白细胞、血小板等指数都非常

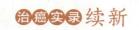

低，全身严重水肿、气喘。由于他的病情非常复杂，一是严重的晚期癌症，需要尽快治疗；二是化疗等造成的严重毒副作用，令他的全身出现严重水肿，同时他体内所移植的肾也难以承受。针对他身体状况的治疗，需要培本固肾与抗癌攻毒双管齐下。

经过数月的治疗，他的严重水肿逐渐减少，直至现在已完全消失；双肺的多发转移瘤亦都逐渐减少，并且大部分已消失。目前刘先生还在治疗之中，大家都很有信心定能使他体内的肿瘤全部消失，恢复健康。

软坚散瘀，通滞攻毒。

常用中药

1. 红参、田七、海马、重楼、土茯苓、薏苡仁、鳖甲、桃仁、淫羊藿、肉苁蓉等。
2. 同时服用化症丸。

影像学、病理学检查报告及诊疗记录

1. 2020 年 3 月检查报告证实曾因肾功能衰竭而进行肾脏移植，膀胱癌治疗后，考虑前列腺癌，肺有结节。

2. 2021 年 7 月检查发现膀胱癌前列腺肿瘤双肺转移。

3. 2021 年 12 月检查报告显示转移病灶已明显好转。

附：患者检查报告

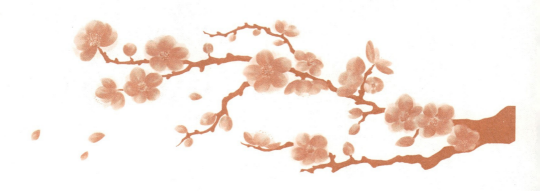

醫院 同位素及正電子掃描部
Department of Nuclear Medicine & Positron Emission Tomography

Tel:
Fax:

Name:	Lau,	劉		Date:	05&09/03/2020
I.D. No.:		Sex:	Male	Ref. Dr.:	
Hosp. No.:	O.P.	Age:	70 Y	Fax:	
Ward/Dept.:		ExamID:		Tel:	

POSITRON EMISSION TOMOGRAPHY
(^{18}F-FDG & ^{18}F-PSMA-1007 ONCOLOGY)

History:

A 70 year-old gentleman had carcinoma of bladder with TURBT done on 22/02/2020. Patient complained of urgency and frequency of urination after operation. Blood test showed elevated PSA (exact level was unknown). PET scan for assessment. Known DM, hypertension and renal failure with renal transplant in 02/2018. No TB or hepatitis. Non-smoker and non-drinker.

Radiopharmaceutical: 8.5 mCi ^{18}F-PSMA-1007 and 11.1 mCi F-18 Fluorodeoxyglucose (^{18}FDG) injected intravenously.

Findings:

On 09/03/2020, limited whole body CT transmission and PET emission imaging began at 83 minutes after radiopharmaceutical administration (blood glucose 5.1 mmol/l), spanning a region from base of skull to upper thigh. 60 mg Spasmonal was given p.o. 15 min before ^{18}FDG administration.

On 05/03/2020, limited whole body CT transmission and PET emission imaging began at 101 minutes after ^{18}F-PSMA-1007 administration spanning a region from base of skull to upper thigh.

^{18}FDG: Liver tissue normal reference uptake has a SUVmax of 2.21
^{18}F-PSMA-1007: Liver tissue normal reference uptake has a SUVmax of 13.15.

The current examination is performed with both ^{18}F-PSMA-1007 and ^{18}FDG PET tracers. The prostate gland is enlarged, ~52 mm LD x 45 mm PD. There are several (at least 3) ^{18}F-PSMA-1007-avid foci in anterior midline base and bilateral posterolateral aspects of prostate at mid level. They are non ^{18}FDG-avid. No hypermetabolic activity in seminal vesicles superiorly, urinary bladder wall anteriorly or rectum posteriorly. No hypermetabolic node in bilateral external iliacs, internal iliacs, around obturator nerve cross level or near pectineal ligaments. The upper retroperitoneum, mesentery and omentum show no suspicious lymphadenopathy. There is normal size and metabolism of the liver, pancreas, spleen, adrenals and kidneys; except small hypometabolic cyst in right kidney. Bowel activities are prominent; can be due to hypertonicity, colitis or related to oral hypoglycemic drugs. No abnormal focal glycolysis can be detected in the bladder on the delayed imaging. No ascites.

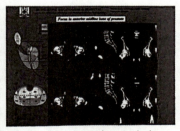

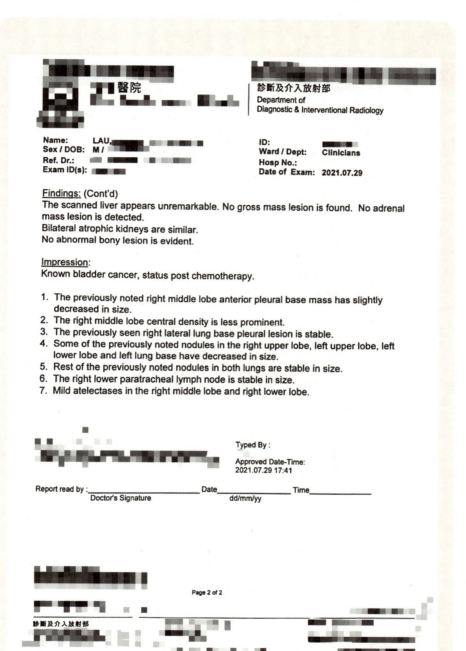

醫院 診斷及介入放射部
Department of
Diagnostic & Interventional Radiology

Name: LAU,
Sex / DOB: M /
Ref. Dr.:
Exam ID(s):

ID:
Ward / Dept: Clinicians
Hosp No.:
Date of Exam: 2021.07.29

Findings: (Cont'd)
The scanned liver appears unremarkable. No gross mass lesion is found. No adrenal mass lesion is detected.
Bilateral atrophic kidneys are similar.
No abnormal bony lesion is evident.

Impression:
Known bladder cancer, status post chemotherapy.

1. The previously noted right middle lobe anterior pleural base mass has slightly decreased in size.
2. The right middle lobe central density is less prominent.
3. The previously seen right lateral lung base pleural lesion is stable.
4. Some of the previously noted nodules in the right upper lobe, left upper lobe, left lower lobe and left lung base have decreased in size.
5. Rest of the previously noted nodules in both lungs are stable in size.
6. The right lower paratracheal lymph node is stable in size.
7. Mild atelectases in the right middle lobe and right lower lobe.

Typed By :

Approved Date-Time:
2021.07.29 17:41

Report read by :_____ Date_____ Time_____
Doctor's Signature   dd/mm/yy

Page 2 of 2

診斷及介入放射部

155

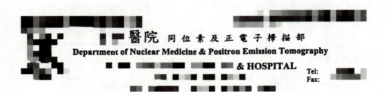

醫院 同位素及正電子掃描部
Department of Nuclear Medicine & Positron Emission Tomography
& HOSPITAL

Tel:
Fax:

In the thorax, several isometabolic lung densities are seen in superolateral RLL, superoposterior RLL and posterolateral RLL. In addition, a small calcified granuloma is identified in anteromedial LUL. No hypermetabolic nodal activity in the mediastinum, both hila, axillae, supraclavicular fossae and jugular lymphatics. No pleural or pericardial effusion. Thyroid gland and nasopharynx are unremarkable. Marrow metabolism in the axial skeleton is within normal limits.

Functional parameters of these lesions are tabulated as below:

LAU,				F-18 PSMA-1007	
		in mm		Standard	Delayed
Site		LD	PD	SUVmax	SUVmax
Focus in anterior midline base of prostate		16.3	11.6	5.2	4.6
Focus in L posterolateral prostate at mid level		16.9	11.9	4.6	6.0
Focus in R posterolateral prostate at mid level		12.7	10.4	4.6	5.4

Note: LD=longest diameter; PD=diameter perpendicular to LD

Impression:

1. Several (at least 3) ^{18}F-PSMA-1007-avid foci in anterior midline base, bilateral posterolateral aspects of prostate at mid level are noted. They are non ^{18}FDG-avid. In view of elevated PSA level, diagnosis of prostatic neoplasm cannot be excluded. Tissue biopsy for correlation may be considered if clinically indicated. No tumor infiltration to seminal vesicles superiorly, urinary bladder wall anteriorly or rectum posteriorly.
2. No abnormal focal glycolysis can be detected in the bladder on the delayed imaging to suggest local recurrence in regard of patient's history of treated carcinoma of bladder.
3. No hypermetabolic node in the abdomen or pelvis.
4. Several isometabolic lung densities in RLL are non-specific and can be due to prior infection. Nonetheless, follow-up study is recommended for serial monitoring if clinically indicated.
5. No abnormal focal metabolism in the remaining body survey.

Thank you very much, , for your referral.

醫院 ___ Hospital

診斷及介入放射部
Department of
Diagnostic & Interventional Radiology

Name: LAU
Sex / DOB: M /
Ref. Dr.:
Exam ID(s):

ID:
Ward / Dept: Clinicians
Hosp No.:
Date of Exam: 2021.12.08

Impression:

1. Previously noted pleural based lesion at anterior aspect of right middle lobe has largely resolved, with residual parenchymal opacity with air bronchograms and traction bronchiectasis; can represent post-treatment changes.
2. Stable subpleural nodules at posterior aspect of right lower lobe, with no hypermetabolic activity on last PET-CT study; can represent residual lesions or post-treatment changes.
3. Newly seen multifocal small ill-defined areas of ground glass density in both lungs, more at right upper lobe; as well as tiny centrilobular nodules at posterior basal segment of right lower lobe; could represent infective or inflammatory changes. Suggest follow up examination, and clinical correlation.
4. New multifocal ill-defined areas of subpleural ground-glass densities and air-spaced densities at posterolateral aspect of left upper and lower lobes, inferior aspect of left lingular segment, and posterior aspect and lung base of right lower lobe; could represent infective or inflammatory changes; however lung metastases cannot be excluded. Suggest follow up examination.
5. Stable left upper lobe calcified granuloma.
6. Stable small thin-walled cystic lesion at anterior segment of right upper lobe, corresponding to the cavitation seen on last PET-CT study.
7. No enlarged mediastinal or hilar lymph node is seen. Stable shotty right paratracheal lymph node.
8. Tiny gallstone.

Typed By :

Approved Date-Time:
2021.12.09 22:08

Report read by : _____ Date_____ Time_____
　　　　　　　　Doctor's Signature　　　　　　　　　　dd/mm/yy

Page 3 of 3

157

病案 22

晚期卵巢癌已渡 25 年

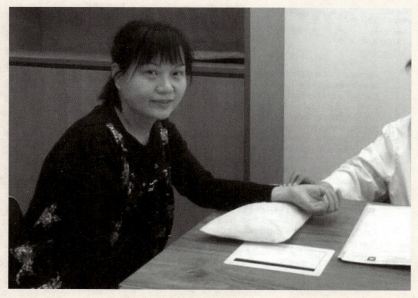

🎧 张女士于 2022 年 10 月前来诊治时合影留念

　　1999 年 3 月，张女士感到腹部疼痛，经过进一步检查，证实患上卵巢癌。于是在 1999 年 5 月做手术切除肿瘤，同时也切除了子宫、卵巢、输卵管、大网膜等，希望彻底切除干净后就不会再复发了。手术后的病理检查报告，亦证实她是患上卵巢癌。

　　无奈的是，2006 年她的卵巢癌再次复发，之后又做了 2 次手术，也进行了多次化疗，但是一直未能控制肿瘤的发展。

2014年，她的腹腔肿瘤转移且生长得很快，已经达到9.6cm，而且每天腹痛严重，令她不能睡觉也不能吃饭。由于肿瘤越来越大，疼痛已经不能够得到控制，所以医院里给她用上吗啡作为治疗药物。当时张女士对此非常疑惑，医院的医生向她解释说，因为她的病是没有办法治疗的，能为她减轻疼痛就已经很好了，至少能够让她过得舒服一点。但是实际上，吗啡上瘾之后剂量越用越大，且有很多副作用，例如恶心、呕吐、大便困难等，且腹痛依然，于是她来到我们的生命修复治疗中心，开始了一种崭新的治疗方法。

经过治疗之后，张女士腹部的肿瘤逐渐得到控制，癌指数明显降低。经过中药的治疗和调理，她逐步减少了吗啡的用量，疼痛也逐渐地减少，到最后不再出现疼痛。2017年1月，她彻底戒除了吗啡和毒瘾。张女士的病情逐渐变得稳定，生活逐渐变得正常。直到现在，已经过去了25年，张女士生活正常且健康快乐。

治疗原则

软坚散瘀，通滞攻毒。

常用中药

1. 龙葵、山慈菇、柴胡、白芍、鳖甲、丹参、石见穿、生大黄、玄明粉、土鳖虫等。
2. 同时服用消瘤丸。

影像学、病理学检查报告及诊疗记录

1. 2014 年 6 月 19 日检查报告显示盆腔肿瘤增大，病情加重，肿瘤有 9.6cm。
2. 2019 年 6 月 10 日检查报告显示小于 1cm 的肿瘤结节。

附：患者检查报告

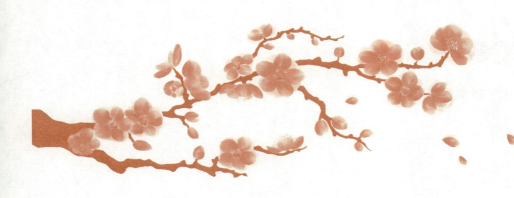

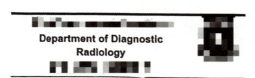

Department of Diagnostic Radiology

There is no pleural nor peri-cardial effusion seen.

Abdomen and pelvis

Multiloculated cystic lesion in the left lower pelvis is noted with mildly increased FDG uptake (SUVmax = 1.5).
It shows interval increase in size (longest dimensions = 9.6cm) and soft tissue component when compared to the previous CT.
Radiologically, features are suggestive of disease progression.

The lesion exerts mass effect onto the urinary bladder anteriorly.

The background FDG uptake of the liver is homogenous without discrete hypermetabolic focus. (SUVmax = 1.9).
Intra-hepatic and common ducts are not dilated.
The gallbladder, pancreas and spleen are unremarkable.
Bilateral kidneys are comparable in contrast excretion. Bilateral renal pelvis are slightly prominent.
Both adrenal glands are normal.
Evaluation of the para-aortic region reveals no hypermetabolic focus.
There is no ascites seen.

Skeletal system

Marrow uptake is unremarkable.
In the corresponding CT images, no osseus lesion is seen.

Opinion :

Multiloculated cystic lesion in the left lower pelvis with interval increase in size and soft tissue component. Radiologically, features are suggestive of disease progression.

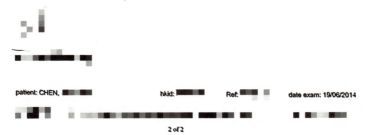

patient: CHEN, ▨▨▨▨▨   hkid: ▨▨▨▨   Ref: ▨▨▨▨   date exam: 19/06/2014

2 of 2

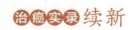

Patient ID:
Name: CHEN
Sex: F   DOB: 04.12.1977
Accession No:

Case No:
Patient Type: OutPatient ()
Referrer:
Exam Date: 10.06.2019

Radiological Examination Report

detected at the expected region in the previous study.

Multiple solid or partially calcific nodes are detected, representative lesions are tabulated:

Site	Size (cm x cm)	SUVmax
Ileocaecal node, solid	0.7 x 0.6	-
Ileocaecal node, calcific	0.8 x 0.6	-
Ileocaecal node, solid	0.6 x 0.3	-
Anterior ileocaecal node, solid	0.5 x 0.5	-
Anterior left external iliac node, partially calcific	1.2 x 1	3.4
Anterior right external iliac node, calcific	0.8 x 0.5	2.2
Aortocaval node	0.6 x 0.4	
Left para-aortic node at left renal lower level, solid	0.6 x 0.4	-
Left paraaortic node at left renal lower level, partially calcific	1.2 x 0.7	2.1
Right caval node	0.9 x 0.4	2.0

Right subphrenic partially calcific nodule abutting segment 7 dome is now 2.5cm x 1.7cm, SUVmax 2.7 (previously 2.5cm x 1.7cm).

Liver shows physiological FDG uptake with no focal area of hypermetabolism. No hyperdense gallstone. Biliary tree is not dilated. No hypermetabolic lesion is seen in pancreas, spleen, adrenals or kidneys. No hydronephrosis.

Bones
A sclerotic focus is detected at the left superior acetabulum, may be non-aggressive bone lesion. No hypermetabolic bone lesion or destruction is detected.

Approved Date: 12.06.2019 20:43

Page 3 of 4

双肺多发癌康复

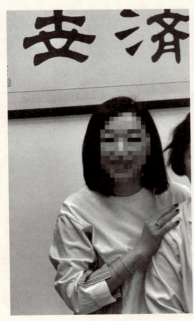

🔊 戴女士于 2024 年 1 月前来诊治时合影留念

2017 年 2 月，戴女士来到我们生命修复治疗中心，那时的她刚做完一侧肺部肿瘤切除手术，但是她的双肺仍残留多数未被切除的肿瘤。于是在 2017 年 1 月 11 日又切除了左肺上叶和左肺下叶的 2 个肿瘤。当时因为肿瘤数量多，无法完全切除，故手术的目的是确诊肿瘤的性质。经过医院的病理学检查后，证实是肺癌。她曾询问负责手术的医生，为什么不把肿瘤全部切除呢？得到的答复是因为切除的面积太大，而且肿瘤分布在 2 个肺上，无法全部切除。因此她非常紧张地来到我们这里。她是想先观察一下，咨询查问能否不必再次动手术治疗。她得悉许多患者都在这里取得良好的治疗效果，才逐渐增加了信心。

在与她谈话和治疗的过程中，我们了解到戴女士的父亲和母亲都有患肺癌的病史，后来，就连她的哥哥也得了肺癌。由于戴女士的肺癌病情非常严峻，我们开始积极地给她做治疗。当时的她常感到胸闷气短、咳嗽有痰、声音低微，动手术以后的身体更是虚弱，伤口仍然感到疼痛。再加上她的精神压力大、睡眠很差、大便干燥、小便不利，针对她的这种情况，我们进行积极的辅助正气和祛除病邪的治疗。

经过数月之后，她再次去做了检查，发现体内肿瘤已经明显缩小，有的甚至已消失。这样的结果令戴女士充满信心，继续认真的治疗。随后又为她增加了一些针灸和疏通经络的治疗，并且按时检查，了解她的病情变化，这样大概又过了2年，她觉得自己身体很好，已没有什么问题，也不觉得有什么不舒服的地方。她更是多次前往大医院做相关先进仪器检查，均显示肿瘤缩小及减少，病情非常稳定，没有任何病变的发展迹象。

自此戴女士生活恢复正常，没有受到疾病的任何影响，直到现在，已经7年多了，她的感觉亦非常良好，认为不需要再吃中药了。加上要顾及孩子学业，全家于半年多前已经远走他乡，过着更加舒适、更加适合的生活。我们仍继续保持联系，不时了解她的现状，目前一切都好，她和丈夫也常陪孩子出门旅游，让孩子扩展视野，增长见识。

治疗原则

扶正祛邪，攻毒抗癌。

常用中药

1. 黄芪、人参、半夏、田七、杏仁、蛤蚧、紫苏子、香附、大黄、芒硝、瓜蒌、沉香、百部等。

2. 同时服用消瘤丸。

影像学、病理学检查报告及诊疗记录

1. 2016 年 12 月 2 日 CT 检查报告显示双肺有多发结节。

2. 2017 年 1 月 12 日手术后病理报告显示左肺下叶：腺癌；肺腺癌。

3. 2019 年 2 月 15 日检查报告显示肺部结节缩小并稳定。

4. 2021 年 3 月 18 日检查报告显示肺部结节缩小稳定无变化。

附：患者检查报告

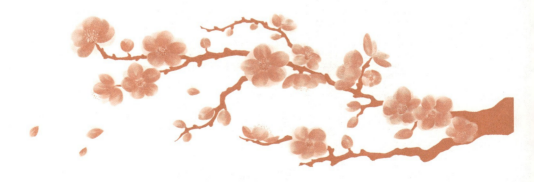

165

中心

MRI Centre

PARTNERSHIP WITH
YOUR HEALTH

COPY

REF./TO : ▮▮▮▮▮ ▮.▮▮

PATIENT NAME : TAI.▮▮ ▮▮

PATIENT ID : ▮▮▮   D.O.B. : 17/12/1963

SEX/AGE : F/52Y   REF. NO. :

EXAM. DATE : 02/12/2016   CASE NO. : ▮ ▮▮ ▮▮

PET/CT REPORT

WHOLE BODY PET-CT SCAN (PLAIN + CONTRAST SCAN)

CLINICAL INFORMATION:
Multiple lung nodules. Increase in size 1.5 year. Dx: ? BAC

IMAGING PROTOCOL:
- 60minutes following 9.4mCi F-18 fluorodeoxyglucose (FDG) injected intravenously.
- Blood glucose level prior to injection was 4.7mmol/l.
- One set of topogram and whole body CT without contrast agent, spanning from skull base level down to upper thigh level.
- One set of whole body PET scanning with emission and transmission (3minutes per bed position) image acquisitions were performed at 7 bed positions to include skull base through upper thigh.
- Another intravenous contrast enhanced CT scanning of the whole body performed.
- Emission and attenuation corrected emission images were reconstructed in trans-axial, coronal and sagittal planes for review.
- Standard uptake values (SUV) were calculated for semiquantitative analysis.

IMAGING FINDINGS:
[HEAD AND NECK]
Included section of brain showed no focal space occupying lesion. No hypermetabolic soft tissue mass is spotted in the nasopharynx. Normal and symmetrical FDG uptakes are seen in both tonsils. No significant enlarged or hypermetabolic nodes are noted in cervical region.

[THORAX]
Multiple hypometabolic ground glass nodules are seen in both lungs. The sizes and locations of the nodules are as below. Possibility of multi-focal bronchoalveolar cell carcinoma or carcinoma in-situ cannot be excluded. Differential diagnosis includes
- Right lung apex, 6.35 x 8.41 x 9.52mm.
- Antero-basal RLL, 6.85 x 7.33 x 4.28mm.
- Lateral-basal LLL, 11.2 x 13.5 x 14.2mm. This is amenable to CT guided FNA or trucut biopsy for definitive cytology/histology diagnosis.
- Antero-basal LLL, 4.5 x 6.56 x 5.64mm.
- Left lung apex, 11.2 x 12.4 x 10.8mm.
- Left upper lobe, 6.2 x 6.28 x 4.53mm.

No hypermetabolic lung mass is detected. No pulmonary collapse or consolidation is discerned. No significant enlarged or hypermetabolic hilar or mediastinal lymph node is observed. Neither pleural or pericardial effusion is present.

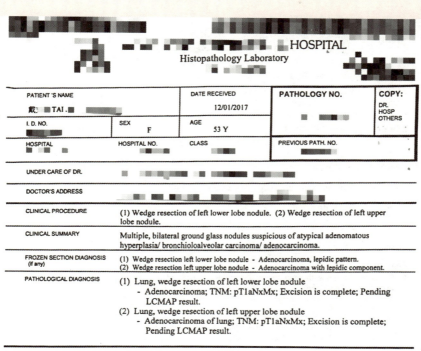

HOSPITAL

Histopathology Laboratory

PATIENT 'S NAME		DATE RECEIVED		PATHOLOGY NO.	COPY:
戴 ■ TAI . ■		12/01/2017			DR. HOSP OTHERS

I. D. NO.	SEX F	AGE 53 Y		
HOSPITAL	HOSPITAL NO.	CLASS	PREVIOUS PATH. NO.	

UNDER CARE OF DR.	
DOCTOR'S ADDRESS	

CLINICAL PROCEDURE	(1) Wedge resection of left lower lobe nodule. (2) Wedge resection of left upper lobe nodule.
CLINICAL SUMMARY	Multiple, bilateral ground glass nodules suspicious of atypical adenomatous hyperplasia/ bronchioloalveolar carcinoma/ adenocarcinoma.
FROZEN SECTION DIAGNOSIS (If any)	(1) Wedge resection left lower lobe nodule - Adenocarcinoma, lepidic pattern. (2) Wedge resection left upper lobe nodule - Adenocarcinoma with lepidic component.

PATHOLOGICAL DIAGNOSIS	(1) Lung, wedge resection of left lower lobe nodule
	  - Adenocarcinoma; TNM: pT1aNxMx; Excision is complete; Pending LCMAP result.
	(2) Lung, wedge resection of left upper lobe nodule
	  - Adenocarcinoma of lung; TNM: pT1aNxMx; Excision is complete; Pending LCMAP result.

REPORT

<u>Macroscopic examination:</u>

(1) Labelled "Wedge resection of left lower lobe nodule" is a reddish smooth wedge of lung weighing 9.0 grams and measuring 5.5 x 2.5 x 2.0 cm. The cut surface shows an ill-defined tan slightly firm lesion causing some retraction of the pleural aspect. The area measures 0.8 x 0.7 x 0.6 cm. and is 1.7 cm. from the stapled resection margin and <0.1 cm. from the overlying pleural surface. The pleural surface is marked with red ink and a stapled margin with blue ink.

Blocks: (1A) Lesion, one piece for frozen section and subsequent paraffin section. (1B) Lesion, one piece. (1C) Two random pieces of lung.

(2) Labelled "Wedge resection of left upper lobe nodule" is a reddish smooth surfaced wedge of lung weighing 11.8 grams and measuring 6.0 x 4.0 x 1.5 cm. The cut surface shows the presence of an ill-defined tan slightly firm lesion 1.0 x 1.0 x 0.6 cm. situated 1.0 cm. away from the stapled resection margin and <0.1 cm. from the overlying puckered pleural surface.

Blocks: (2A) Lesion, one piece for frozen section and subsequent paraffin section. (2B) Lesion, one piece. (2C) Two random pieces of lung tissue.

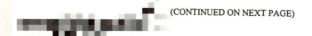

(CONTINUED ON NEXT PAGE)

Page 1 of 2

167

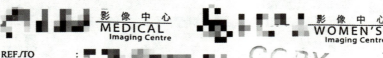

REF./TO   :

PATIENT NAME : TAI,

PATIENT ID :   D.O.B. : 17/12/1963

SEX/AGE   : F/55Y   REF. NO. :

EXAM. DATE : 15/02/2019   CASE NO. :

RADIOLOGY REPORT

There is no pleural effusion.

Heart size is within normal limit. There is no pericardial effusion.

No adrenal mass is detected.

The liver, spleen and pancreas included in this scan are unremarkable.

No destructive bone lesion is found in the skeleton scanned.

COMMENT:
1. Surgical sutures with mild fibrosis in medial aspect of left upper lobe and in lateral aspect of left lower lobe, in keeping with previous wedge resection.
2. Multiple ground glass attenuation nodules in RUL, RLL, LUL and LLL. These are similar to previous scan.
3. A small faint cavitary nodule in RLL. static in size.
4. A small pleural based nodule or granuloma in RLL is unchanged.
5. Follow up scan for monitoring suggested.

Thank you for your kind referral,

2

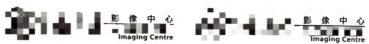

REF./TO :
PATIENT NAME : TAI,
PATIENT ID :   D.O.B. : 17/12/1963
SEX/AGE : F/57Y   REF. NO. :
EXAM. DATE : 18/03/2021   CASE NO. :

RADIOLOGY REPORT

There is no pleural effusion.

Heart size is within normal limit. There is no pericardial effusion.

The liver, adrenal, spleen and pancreas included in this scan are unremarkable.

No destructive bone lesion is found in the skeleton scanned.

COMMENT:
1. Surgical sutures with mild fibrosis in medial aspect of left upper lobe and in lateral aspect of left lower lobe, in keeping with previous wedge resection.

2. Multiple ground glass attenuation nodules in RUL, RLL, LUL and LLL. They show similar in size as compared with previous scan.

3. A small faint cavitary nodule in RLL is static in size.

4. A small pleural based nodule or granuloma in RLL is unchanged.

Thank you for your kind referral !

病案 **24**

晚期皮肤癌已渡 18 年

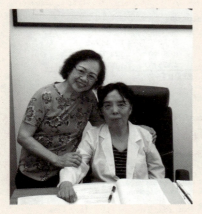

 王太太于 2024 年 1 月前来诊治时合影留念

王太太是位喜爱运动的女士，特别是游泳，这是她多年的爱好。她常去海边游泳，然后躺在沙滩上晒太阳，当热得出汗了，就会再跳进水里多游一会。自退休后，她便经常做这样的运动。

2005 年，王太太经常感到腹痛，而且全身发红，尤其臀部皮肤更严重，但她并没有特别在意。然而，这些不适影响了她的游泳锻炼，因此在这大半年里减少了运动次数。2007 年年初，她的病情加重，臀部皮肤开始发硬并迅速溃烂，王太太才急忙去看医生，非常惊讶地得知自己患上皮肤癌，并且已经有全身多发的淋巴转移，包括腹股沟处、腹腔内肠系膜等，都有多处淋巴转移，医院确诊她是属于皮肤癌 IV 期。医院立即为她安排大面积切除臀部皮肤的手术。

王太太手术后愈合良好，接着又做了化疗。但化疗令她感到疲乏无力，多处可以摸到的淋巴部位仍然肿大质硬，腹痛加重。医生更是告诉她，对于全身大量的淋巴转移，实在没有治愈的办法，癌症还是会复发，并且会在全身多处出现。而她感到腹痛就是因为大量腹腔淋巴转移导致，这种情况下，生命最多只能维持 1 年，医生让她想吃什么就吃什么吧。

王太太不甘心就这样结束一生，于是前来进行生命修复治疗，当时的她骨瘦如柴，精神疲惫不堪，失眠且腹痛严重，因为腹部肿块的压迫，令她的下肢水肿严重。她每周都会前来就诊，按时且认真的接受治疗。随后，她的腹痛逐渐减缓并消失，面色开始转好，肿块消失了，精神也好转了。直至如今，过去了 18 年，她已经 76 岁，但她一点也闲不住，经常参加各种社交活动，例如游泳、唱歌，目前的她已经完全康复了。

皮肤癌在中医学中有着不同的称谓，例如翻花疮、石疔、石疽等。生命修复中医药治疗在皮肤癌当中有一定的优势，我们认为局部性皮肤癌的手术治疗，是不能解决根本性问题的，特别是已经发生在腹股沟处、腹腔内、肠系膜等处的大量淋巴转移。手术只是暂时切除局部已破溃的皮肤，即使做了更深层、更大一些面积的皮肤切除，也不能完全治疗已经全身多处转移的病灶。如果没有进一步的生命修复中医药治疗，王太太的转移病灶会迅速地发展并危及生命。所幸在手术之后，她选择了正确的治疗方法，利用攻毒抗癌，首先控制住了大量腹腔中及肠系膜的肿瘤，使这些转移灶逐渐缩小并消失。

王太太现在大约隔 2 个月就来进行 1 次养生保健，上周她来治疗时，说起生命修复的中医药救了她的命，她永远心存感激，并且说快要去德国旅行了，生活非常开心。

治疗原则

解毒化浊，软坚散结。

常用中药

1. 薏苡仁、土茯苓、败酱草、金银花、猪苓、白芥子、乳香、
   猫爪草、夏枯草等。
2. 同时服用消瘤丸。

影像学、病理学检查报告及诊疗记录

1. 2007 年 4 月 25 日同位素及正电子扫描部报告证实：左腹
股沟区有大量转移性淋巴结肿瘤，下腹部有大量转移性肠系膜
淋巴结肿瘤。

2. 2007 年 8 月 3 日同位素及正电子扫描检查报告显示腹股
沟及肠系膜转移性淋巴结肿瘤消失，连续 2 次 PET 检查未见
异常。

3. 2020 年 1 月检查报告显示肠系膜的复发肿瘤经再次使用
生命修复中医药治疗后得到有效控制，没有局部复发和转移。

附：患者检查报告

醫院 同位素及正電子掃描部

Department of Nuclear Medicine & Positron Emission Tomography

████████████████ HOSPITAL

Name:	Mak.		Date: 25/4/2007
I.D. No.:	AIE	Sex: Female	
Hosp. No.:		Age: 63 Y	Fax:
Ward/Dept.:			Tel:

POSITRON EMISSION TOMOGRAPHY
(¹⁸F-FDG ONCOLOGY)

History:

A 63 year-old lady initially presented with 2 left groin masses. She was diagnosed sebaceous carcinoma of left buttock with excision done on 10/4/2007. One left groin node was excised and confirmed lymph node metastasis. Pre-operative CT scan showed a cluster of enlarged mesenteric lymph nodes up to 2.5 cm in lower abdomen and suspected of metastasis. PET scan for further investigation. DM on oral medication. No history of hepatitis or tuberculosis.

Radiopharmaceutical: 10.8 mCi F-18 Fluorodeoxyglucose (^{18}FDG) injected intravenously.

Findings:

Limited whole body CT transmission and PET emission imaging began at 46 minutes after radiopharmaceutical administration (blood glucose 6.8 mmol/l), spanning a region from vertex to toe. 60 mg Spasmonal was given p.o. 15 min before ^{18}FDG administration.

Liver tissue normal reference uptake has a SUVmax of 3.65 and delayed SUVmax of 2.66.

There are diffuse mild activities in the medial left groin and left buttock regions and likely represent post-operative inflammatory changes. A focally hypermetabolic left groin node is seen more laterally. The right groin appears normal with no abnormal lymphadenopathy. In addition, multiple enlarged hypermetabolic mesenteric nodes are identified in the lower abdomen with the largest one noted at L5 level. These are most consistent with multiple metastatic mesenteric lymphadenopathy. There is no abnormal uptake in the uterine and bilateral adnexal regions. The liver shows uniform uptake without any focal area of hypermetabolism. The adrenal glands and pancreas appear normal. The bowel shows some physiological activity. There is no hypermetabolic intramammary lesion in the breasts. Both lungs reveal no focal abnormal glycolysis. The mediastinum and bilateral hila show normal physiological activities. Bilateral supraclavicular and cervical lymph nodes are unremarkable. There is no abnormal uptake in the nasopharynx. Marrow activities within the axial skeletons are normal. No other suspicious hypermetabolic skin lesion is noted in the remaining regions of the body.

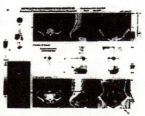

Functional parameters of these lesions are tabulated below:

Mak, Choi Ping Site	in cm			Standard SUVmax	Delayed SUVmax
	X	Y	Z		
Liver (normal)				3.65	2.66
Largest mesenteric node at L5 level	1.9	2.4	2.0	3.81	6.57
Mesenteric node at S1 level	1.3	1.2	1.2	3.20	3.10
Lt groin node	1.0	1.2	1.0	2.52	2.92
Lt buttock activity	2.4	2.8	2.5	1.52	1.95

Impression:

1. Multiple metastatic lymphadenopathy are identified as left groin node and multiple mesenteric nodes in the lower abdomen.
2. Post-operative inflammatory changes in the left buttock and medial left groin regions.
3. No other metabolic evidence of solid organ involvement is noted.

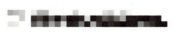

醫院 同位素及正電子掃描部

Department of Nuclear Medicine & Positron Emission Tomography

■■■■■■■■■■■■■■■■■■■■■■■■ HOSPITAL

Name:	Mak, ■■■■■■			Date:	3/8/2007
I.D. No.:	A1■■■■■■	Sex:	Female	Ref. Dr.:	■■■■■■
Hosp. No.:	■■■■■■	Age:	63 Y	Fax:	
Ward/Dept.:	Clinical Oncology			Tel:	

Impression:

1. Resolved mesenteric and left groin nodal metastases. As understood, metabolic quiescence is not equivalent to true tumoricidal effect. At least 2 serial PET studies demonstrating no abnormal metabolism may be considered more confirmative of metabolic remission.

2. Resolved previous post-operative inflammatory changes in the left groin and left buttock activity.

3. No new lesion is seen.

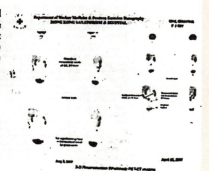

■■■■■■■■■■■■, MBBS(HK), FHKCR, FHKAM (Radiology)
Specialist in Nuclear Medicine, Department of Nuclear Medicine & P.E.T., HKSH

174

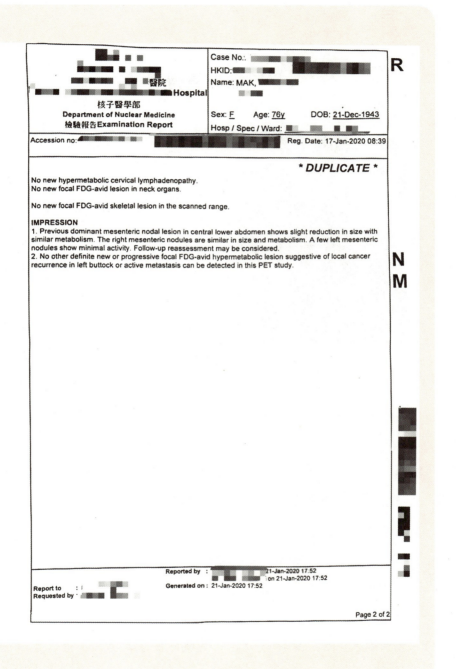

R

Case No.: ▓▓▓▓

HKID: ▓▓▓▓▓▓▓

Name: MAK, ▓▓▓▓

醫院 Hospital

核子醫學部
Department of Nuclear Medicine
檢驗報告 Examination Report

Sex: <u>F</u>   Age: <u>76y</u>   DOB: <u>21-Dec-1943</u>

Hosp / Spec / Ward: ▓▓▓▓

Accession no: ▓▓▓▓▓▓▓   Reg. Date: 17-Jan-2020 08:39

* DUPLICATE *

N

M

No new hypermetabolic cervical lymphadenopathy.
No new focal FDG-avid lesion in neck organs.

No new focal FDG-avid skeletal lesion in the scanned range.

IMPRESSION
1. Previous dominant mesenteric nodal lesion in central lower abdomen shows slight reduction in size with similar metabolism. The right mesenteric nodules are similar in size and metabolism. A few left mesenteric nodules show minimal activity. Follow-up reassessment may be considered.
2. No other definite new or progressive focal FDG-avid hypermetabolic lesion suggestive of local cancer recurrence in left buttock or active metastasis can be detected in this PET study.

Reported by : ▓▓▓ 21-Jan-2020 17:52
             on 21-Jan-2020 17:52

Report to   : ▓▓▓
Requested by : ▓▓▓

Generated on : 21-Jan-2020 17:52

Page 2 of 2

鼻咽癌康复得贵子

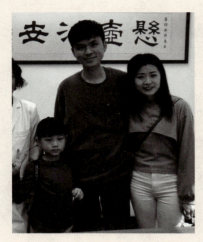

↑ 马先生于2024年2月前来诊治时全家合影留念

2014年，马先生只有32岁，当时的他工作非常忙碌，精神非常紧张、压力很大。忙碌的工作也导致他常感到浑身无力、失眠及焦虑。于是他前往医院看病，医生给他处方抗焦虑药和精神科药以治疗。这样的情况持续了1年多，随后他经常感到口干舌燥、咳嗽痰多、鼻塞流涕。起初以为是服食精神科药物所造成的，所以没有理会。但是，他的症状逐渐加重，口水渐多且带有血丝，鼻涕增多和痰中带血。马先生仍然工作忙碌，每天都有很多应酬，既抽烟又喝酒，所以他认为只是上火（即热气）所致而已。由于情况一直没有改善，持续了2个多月，他才决定去医院就诊。

经过医院的检查，确定他是患了鼻咽癌，并且已经有淋巴、颅内等转移。在鼻咽部的活组织病理检查亦显示，他患的是未分化癌，这种肿瘤是没有分化的，恶性程度亦属于最高的。马先生非常紧张，要求用最快、最强的治疗方法，于是医院给他安排了放疗。在放疗的过程中，他感到非常痛苦，口干舌燥的他不能饮水，更无法进食，而且出现严重呕吐、胃肠胀满、口腔溃烂及失眠消瘦的状况。随着放疗的次数增多，他每天都会呕吐不已，导致口腔糜烂出血，胃痛不能进食，连喝水都难以下咽。

马先生非常尽力，终于坚持到放疗全部完成，经过一段时间的恢复和休息，医院要求他再做检查，看看治疗后的情况。经过多次检查显示，他的鼻咽部肿瘤有部分缩小，但还是有不少残留的肿瘤，在他双侧的筛窦、上额窦、双侧鼻咽部淋巴结、双侧颈部等都有淋巴转移。马先生知道这种癌症的复发率相当高，并且经过治疗后，仍有多个部位的癌组织残留，实在担心不已。

经过朋友的介绍，他来到我们这里进行生命修复的治疗。当时马先生非常消瘦，咽喉部、双侧颈部都可以见到肿大的淋巴结，持续有咳嗽痰多、鼻子堵塞，鼻腔及口水中常有血丝及血块。根据他的病情，我们给他定下了治疗方案，他也很快地在抗癌过程中恢复过来。经过 2 个月的治疗，他的病情明显减轻，面部逐渐红润，身体一天天地好起来了。

马先生从患癌至今，已经有 10 年的时间，现在已经恢复健康了。他觉得已没有问题，就不再坚持认真地服用中药。但每隔一段时间，也会前来进行一些巩固性治疗。现在的马先生家庭幸福美满，前些日子更是带着太太和儿子来到我们的研究中心，和大家一起拍照留念，并希望把他的全家福照片分享给大家看，借以鼓励其他患者。

治疗原则

驱毒化瘀，散结消瘤。

常用中药

1. 柴胡、黄芩、僵蚕、海浮石、八月炸、浙贝母、鱼脑石、半夏、鱼腥草、山慈菇等。
2. 同时服用消瘤丸。

影像学、病理学检查报告及诊疗记录

1. 2014 年 9 月 5 日鼻咽部活组织病理组织学检查证实为未分化癌。

2. 2014 年 9 月 5 日 CT 检查证实为鼻咽癌，并有颅内骨转移灶、淋巴转移。

3. 2015 年 4 月放射治疗之后，CT 检查鼻咽部颅骨内、双侧筛窦、上颌窦、乳突部仍有多处残留病灶，双侧鼻咽后及双侧颈部淋巴结转移。

附：患者检查报告

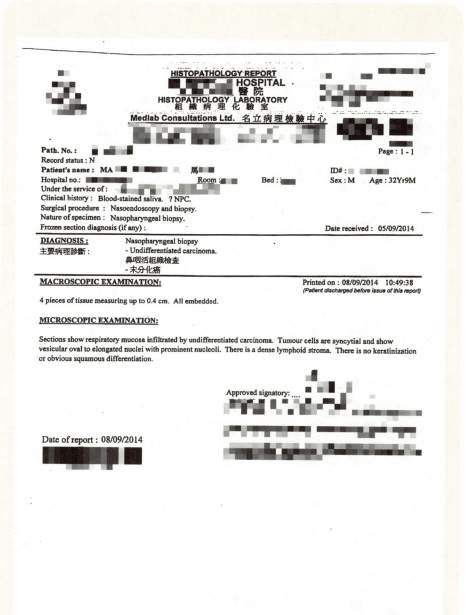

HISTOPATHOLOGY REPORT
HOSPITAL
醫院
HISTOPATHOLOGY LABORATORY
組織病理化驗室
Medlab Consultations Ltd. 名立病理檢驗中心

Path. No. :
Page : 1 - 1

Record status : N

Patient's name : MA ████ 馬█   ID# :

Hospital no. :   Room :   Bed :   Sex : M   Age : 32Yr9M

Under the service of :

Clinical history : Blood-stained saliva. ? NPC.

Surgical procedure : Nasoendoscopy and biopsy.

Nature of specimen : Nasopharyngeal biopsy.

Frozen section diagnosis (if any) :   Date received : 05/09/2014

DIAGNOSIS :   Nasopharyngeal biopsy
主要病理診斷 :   - Undifferentiated carcinoma.
                          鼻咽活組織檢查
                          - 未分化癌

MACROSCOPIC EXAMINATION: Printed on : 08/09/2014 10:49:38
                                        (Patient discharged before issue of this report)

4 pieces of tissue measuring up to 0.4 cm. All embedded.

MICROSCOPIC EXAMINATION:

Sections show respiratory mucosa infiltrated by undifferentiated carcinoma. Tumour cells are syncytial and show vesicular oval to elongated nuclei with prominent nucleoli. There is a dense lymphoid stroma. There is no keratinization or obvious squamous differentiation.

Approved signatory: ....

Date of report : 08/09/2014

179

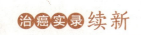

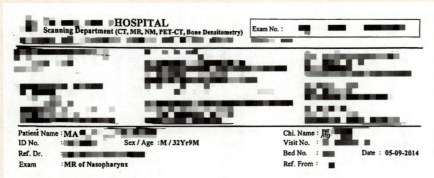

HOSPITAL
Scanning Department (CT, MR, NM, PET-CT, Bone Densitometry)

Exam No. :

Patient Name : MA	Chi. Name : 馬
ID No. :	Visit No. :
Sex / Age : M / 32Yr9M	
Ref. Dr. :	Bed No. : Date : 05-09-2014
Exam : MR of Nasopharynx	Ref. From :

Clinical Information / History:

Blood stained post-nasal drip for two months. Left tinnitus. P/E showed ? NP swelling. ? NPC.

Radiological Report:

Imaging Technique:

Sagittal scans : SE T1 weighted 4 mm.
Axial scans : TSE T1 weighted 4 mm, TSE T2 weighted with fat saturation 4 mm,
         TSE T1 weighted post-contrast with fat saturation 4 mm.
Coronal scans : STIR 4 mm, TSE T1 weighted 2 mm,
         GRE T1 weighted post-contrast with fat saturation 2 mm.

Imaging Findings:

Enhancing soft tissue mass is noted occupying the roof and posterior wall of right nasopharynx, obliterating the right fossa of Rosenmuller. Mild extension across midline to the left side is seen. Nasopharyngeal carcinoma has to be considered. Please correlate with endoscopy and biopsy to confirm its nature. There is no extension of lesion to the right parapharyngeal space. Anteriorly, the lesion reaches the posterior border of the nasal septum. No definite invasion of the posterior nasal space is noted. No invasion of the pterygo-palatine fossae and pterygo-maxillary fissures. No inferior extension to oropharynx. Posteriorly, the longus capitus muscle appears intact. Bilateral carotid spaces posterolaterally are not involved.

Superiorly, the floor of the sphenoid appears intact with no definite marrow signal change or erosion. Small area of T2 hyperintense signal with corresponding contrast enhancement is seen at central clivus, suggestive of invasion (IM 20 SE 23 film 18). Signal intensity of the petrous bone is normal. Meckel's cave is clear. No perineural spread along the foramen ovale and foramen rotundum. No enhancing nodule within both parotids.

			(DD/MM) (HH/MM)		
NO. OF FILMS 19 14" x 17"				REPORT & FILMS SENT OUT :	
NO. OF COLOR PRINTS	NO. OF CDR 1	'WET FILMS: SENT		06-09-2014	PM OK
Remark :		RETURNED			

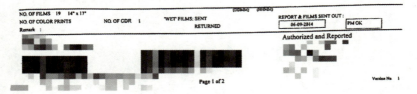

Authorized and Reported

医院 Hospital

放射科
Department of Radiology
检验报告 **Examination Report**

Case No.:	
HKID:	
Name: MA,	
(马	
Sex: **M** Age **33y** DOB: **17-Nov-1981**	
Hosp / Spec / Ward:	

R

M R I

Accession no.: ▨   Reg. Date: 01-Apr-2015 14:00

Procedure: NP (w/ neck)+con., NP plain, DWI (extra-cranial), Brain+con.
Contrast: Dotarem 20ml/bot 10.00 ml
Clinical Information (from referring clinician):
NPC with T1N1 with RT completed, would like a MRI
Diagnosis (from referring clinician):
(RTU) Cancer of nasopharynx , stage I (c T 1 N 0 M 0) ; histology: undifferentiated carcinoma (
Baseline EBV DNA - 12) (147.9)Baseline EBV DNA - 12

Report:
MRI NASOPHARYNX & NECK (CONTRAST):

PROTOCOL:
Pre-Gd: T1_SE_SAG, T1_SE_TRA, T2_TSE_TRA_FS
Post-Gd: DWI ADC, T1_TSE_COR_FS+C, T1_SE_TRA_FS+C, T1_SE_TRA_FS+C (NECK),
T1_MPR_COR_ISO_WE+C

FINDINGS:
Correlation is made with prior private MRI dated 8.9.2014.

Previously noted nasopharyngeal tumour has largely resolved. Mild T2 hyperintensities are seen in
the nasopharynx, may represent post-treatment changes and mucosal thickenings.

Equivocal T2 hyperintense changes with mild enhancement are seen at the prevertebral muscles
and anterior aspect of the clivus, may be due to post-treatment changes +/- residual disease.

The pterygopalatine fossa, pterygo-maxillary fissures, pterygoid muscles, pterygoid processes,
parapharyngeal spaces, nasal cavities and orbits are unremarkable. No intracranial tumour
involvement is seen.

T2 hyperintensities are noted in bilateral ethmoid, maxillary sinuses and mastoids, may represent
retention / inflammatory changes.

Small bilateral retropharyngeal lymph nodes measuring up to 3x7mm are noted. Small non-
enlarged bilateral cervical lymph nodes up to 5mm are seen.

IMPRESSION:
Correlation is made with prior private MRI dated 8.9.2014.
Known NPC with RT given.
1. Previously noted nasopharyngeal tumour has largely resolved. Mild T2 hyperintensities seen in

Reported by : ▨ ▨ on 02-Apr-2015 13:19

Report to :
Requested by : ▨   Generated on : 02-Apr-2015 13:19

Page 1 of 2

181

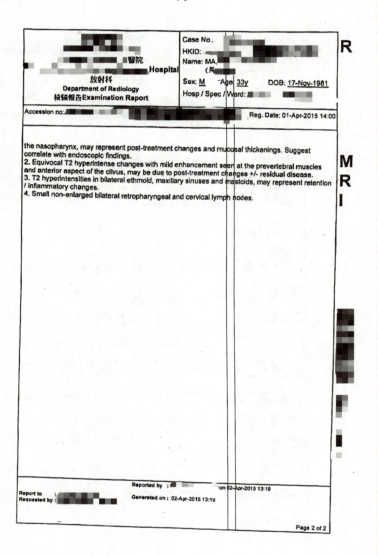

Case No.:
HKID:
Name: MA,
（馬
Sex: M   Age 33y   DOB: 17-Nov-1981
Hosp / Spec / Ward:

R

医院 Hospital
放射科
Department of Radiology
检验报告 Examination Report

Accession no.:   Reg. Date: 01-Apr-2015 14:00

MRI

the nasopharynx, may represent post-treatment changes and mucosal thickenings. Suggest correlate with endoscopic findings.
2. Equivocal T2 hyperintense changes with mild enhancement seen at the prevertebral muscles and anterior aspect of the clivus, may be due to post-treatment changes +/- residual disease.
3. T2 hyperintensities in bilateral ethmoid, maxillary sinuses and mastoids, may represent retention / inflammatory changes.
4. Small non-enlarged bilateral retropharyngeal and cervical lymph nodes.

Reported by :   on 02-Apr-2015 13:19

Report to   :
Requested by :   Generated on : 02-Apr-2015 13:19

Page 2 of 2

甲状腺癌双肺转移骨转移康复 15 年

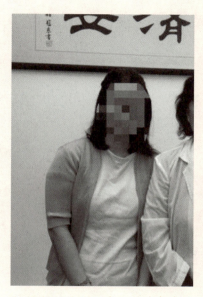

🔈 孙女士于 2022 年 6 月前来诊治时合影留念

2009 年，孙女士只有 33 岁，当时的她却发现患上了甲状腺癌，并且有双肺多发转移和全身多发性骨转移。于是她在 2010 年动手术切除全部甲状腺及肿瘤周围组织，手术后的病理检查亦证实是乳头状甲状腺癌。在甲状腺周围组织切除了的 17 个淋巴结中，有 14 个已发生转移；左肺组织切除的 13 个淋巴结中，有 8 个发生转移，右肺组织切除的 25 个淋巴结中，有 20 个已发生转移。手术后，她的癌症发展仍非常迅速，在 2010 年 4 月的 CT 透视检查中，发现右颈部和左锁骨都有多发的肿瘤，并有双肺转移、髂骨转移等多发转移灶，于是再做放疗。

从发现晚期癌症后，孙女士在 2 年的时间内，完成了医院要求做的所有治疗，例如手术、放疗等，但她的癌指数仍不断升高，转移灶增多、增大。无奈之下，只能前来求助于我们的生命修复中医药治疗。自从用生命修复治疗后不久，她的癌指数

逐渐下降，已转为正常状态。

更可喜的是，15年过去了，她并没有再去做有放射性损伤的检查，因为她觉得身体已恢复正常，每天都忙于照料丈夫、女儿，为女儿做功课辅导，一家人常一起去旅游，生活非常幸福美满。

化瘀通滞，散结攻癌。

常用中药

1. 三棱、莪术、海带、昆布、半夏、牡蛎、桃仁、红花、瓦楞子、青皮、陈皮等。
2. 同时服用消瘤丸。

影像学、病理学检查报告及诊疗记录

2011年12月16日检查报告证实，曾于2010年2月做甲状腺癌切除手术，并有大量颈部淋巴结，双肺转移和骨转移，本次检查无肿瘤复发和转移。

附：患者检查报告

184

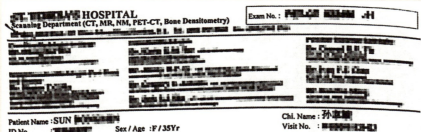

Patient Name : SUN █████████
ID No. : ███████   Sex / Age : F / 35Yr
Ref. Dr. : ██████████████
Exam : PET-CT of Whole Body Trunk PET-CT

Chi. Name : 孙████
Visit No. : ████████ ███████
Bed No. :
Ref. From : CLINIC   Date : 16-12-2011

Clinical Information / History:

Ca thyroid with totally thyroidectomy done in February 2010. Multiple left neck lymph node metastases and bilateral lung and bone metastases at right ilium. 2 times radioactive iodine treatment. External RT to pelvis and thyroid bed given. Good general condition. Initially palpable left supraclavicular fossa lymph node was no long palpable. Chest X-ray clear. Serum thyroglobulin slowly rising.

Blood glucose level is 5.1 mmol/l.

Radiological Report:

RADIOPHARMACEUTICAL:

10.5 mCi F-18 deoxyglucose.

FINDINGS:

Whole body trunk PET-CT scan was performed from the base of skull to the upper thighs. Serial tomographic images of the whole body trunk were presented in transaxial, coronal and sagittal projections.

Evidence of total thyroidectomy is noted. No evidence of residual active tumour is noted in the thyroid bed. A prominent inactive lymph node is present at the left upper neck, measuring 7.5 x 7.5 x 12.1 cm. SUV max = 1.0, most likely reactive in nature. There is no hypermetabolic lymph node in bilateral neck and supraclavicular fossae. Focal uptake is noted at the left laryngeal area, near the posterior aspect of the left vestibular fold. SUV max = 4.6. This is a non-specific finding and may represent focal inflammatory, physiological uptake or less likely recurrent tumour. Endoscopic correlation is recommended.

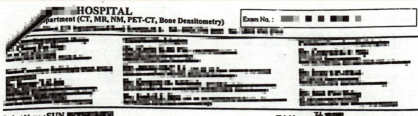

HOSPITAL
Department (CT, MR, NM, PET-CT, Bone Densitometry)

Exam No. :

Patient Name : SUN		Chi. Name : 孙
ID No. :	Sex / Age : F / 35Yr	Visit No. :
Ref. Dr. :		Bed No. : Date : 16-12-2011
Exam : PET-CT of Whole Body Trunk PET-CT		Ref. From : CLINIC

No active lesion is present in the mediastinum and hila. A 7.9 x 6.4 x 9.3 mm nodule is present in the left lung lower lobe apical segment. SUV max = 0.6, worrisome for early pulmonary metastasis. A tiny nodule is also present in the right lung lower lobe, that is too small for accurate characterization. This may represent a granuloma or early metastasis. There is no disease activity in bilateral breasts and axillae.

The liver shows uniform physiological activity. The spleen, adrenals, pancreas, GI tract and other abdominal and pelvic visceral organs are normal.

No active lesion is present in the axial skeleton. In particularly, no abnormal uptake is noted in the right iliac bone.

(SUV = Standardized Glucose Uptake Value.)

IMPRESSION :

No recurrent tumour is identified in the thyroid bed. No hypermetabolic lymph node is present in bilateral neck and supraclavicular fossae. Focal activity at the left laryngeal area may represent focal inflammation, physiological uptake or less likely recurrent disease. Endoscopic correlation is recommended.

Small nodule in the left lung lower lobe is worrisome for early pulmonary metastasis. The tiny nodule in the right lung lower lobe is too small for accurate characterization.

No disease activity is present in the abdomen and pelvis.

No active lesion is present in the axial skeleton.

Thank you for your referral.

(This examination does not include the brain.)

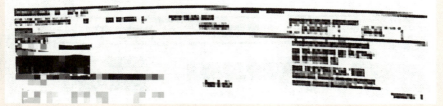

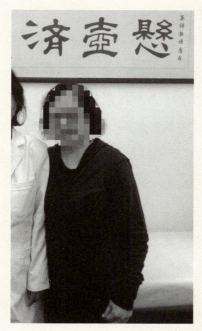

病案27

肠癌肝转移康复 13 年

2011 年，李太太 58 岁，因大便习惯改变，多日不能排便，于是去医院做检查，发现患上了结肠癌。于 2011 年 4 月 14 日做了结肠癌手术。手术后的病理检查报告证实，属于中分化结肠腺癌 Ⅲ 期。手术后经过休息和恢复，李太太以为没事了，但总是觉得疲累，腹部亦有胀气不适，进食少、胁下隐痛。于是她在 2012 年 4 月，也就是手术后刚满 1 年，再次做检查，发现了肝脏的转移肿瘤。全家对这样

○李太太于 2022 年 3 月前来诊治时合影留念

的结果都很紧张，决定于 2012 年 5 月再次做手术，切除右肝叶 4.5cm×5cm 肿瘤。

当时她的肝脏转移癌肿瘤靠近门静脉，有门静脉淋巴及周围淋巴等转移。手术后，她在恢复期间，CEA 癌指数升高，在化疗过程中仍然增高，同时化疗的副作用令她的白细胞、红细胞指数降低，于是急忙前来寻求生命修复的中医药治疗。当时

李太太有腹痛、恶心、呕吐的症状，而化疗药物导致过敏，更是令她有全身出皮疹、手足麻痹、不能进食及失眠等情况，整个身体状态很差。经过生命修复的细心调理，她恢复得很快。

2013 年 5 月，她与家人去日本旅游，回来后还兴高采烈地说，她尝试爬上了两千多米高度的雪山。然后她继续认真调理 3 个月，身体恢复得很好。她又去爬了泰山，还说了她坐缆车到山的一半时下来，然后自己爬到了泰山山顶的经历。随后，她再治疗一段时间便放松下来，没有再认真服药，导致血液检查 CEA 等癌指数升高和反复，她吸取了教训之后，不敢再停药，继续坚持认真治疗，终于恢复了健康。

从患上癌症至今，已经 13 年过去了，在这段时间，她每年都有做身体检查，一直良好，没有再发生复发或转移，当感到身体不适时就会前来诊治调整。目前已有 4～5 年的时间没有每日吃药了，李太太每日开心快乐，健康地生活着。

治疗原则

解毒化湿，散结消瘤。

常用中药

1. 夏枯草、山慈菇、土茯苓、生大黄、薏苡仁、桃仁、败酱草、槐角等。
2. 同时服用散结丸。

影像学、病理学检查报告及诊疗记录

1. 2012 年 4 月 19 日 PET/CT 报告证实，2011 年曾做结肠癌手术，发现肝转移肿瘤。

2. 2012 年 5 月 10 日手术后病理报告证实为结肠癌肝转移，转移性腺癌，并有肝门淋巴结转移，为转移性中分化腺癌。

3. 2014 年 5 月 5 日 PET/CT 检查报告证实无肿瘤复发转移。

4. 2015 年、2016 年及 2017 年检查报告均证实无肿瘤复发转移。

附：患者检查报告

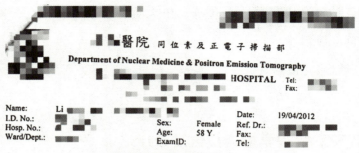

醫院 同位素及正電子掃描部

Department of Nuclear Medicine & Positron Emission Tomography

HOSPITAL   Tel:
Fax:

Name:	Li		Date:	19/04/2012
I.D. No.:			Ref. Dr.:	
Hosp. No.:		Sex: Female	Fax:	
Ward/Dept.:		Age: 58 Y	Tel:	
		ExamID:		

POSITRON EMISSION TOMOGRAPHY
(¹⁸F-FDG ONCOLOGY)

<u>History</u>:

A 58 year-old lady, carcinoma of transverse colon with right hemicolectomy in 04/2011. Pathology showed moderately differentiated mucinous adenocarcinoma with no lymph node metastases. Colonoscopy performed today's morning showed mild proctitis. PET-CT for evaluation. Non-diabetic. No TB. No hepatitis.

<u>Radiopharmaceutical</u>: 10.2 mCi F-18 Fluorodeoxyglucose (¹⁸FDG) injected intravenously.

<u>Findings</u>:

Limited whole body CT transmission and PET emission imaging began at 72 minutes after radiopharmaceutical administration (blood glucose 4.6 mmol/l), spanning a region from base of skull to upper thigh. 60 mg Spasmonal was given p.o. 15 min before ¹⁸FDG administration.

Liver tissue normal reference uptake has a SUVmax of 1.35.

Patient is status post right hemicolectomy for primary colonic malignancy. Survey of the remaining colon demonstrates no suspicious focal hypermetabolic lesion to suggest local colonic recurrence. There is no hypermetabolic focal lesion at the anastomotic site as marked by the surgical hyperdensities. There is, however, a hypermetabolic segment VI liver lesion. It carriers a functional size of 52.4 mm LD x 41.1 mm PD and SUVmax 6.6. It has hypometabolic centre suggestive of central necrosis and internal calcific densities. There is a 9.4 mm segment II liver cyst with no abnormal metabolism. No other hypermetabolic focal pathology in the remaining liver parenchyma. There is normal size and metabolism in the adrenal glands, pancreas and spleen. A 2.5 cm left renal cyst is seen in upper pole of left kidney and rest of the kidney configuration is unremarkable. No hypermetabolic focal pathology in presacral peritoneum or bilateral ischiorectal fossae. There is no isolated hypermetabolic lymph node in bilateral groins, along the iliac lymphatics or retroperitoneum. The root of mesentery and omentum, portal, celiac and superior mesenteric stations are unremarkable. No hypermetabolic focal pathology in the uterus or bilateral adnexal regions. There is no ascites.

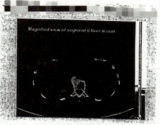

Magnified view of segment 6 liver lesion

In the thorax, there is a subcentimeter RML subpleural nodule with no abnormal metabolism. Normal parenchymal and pleural activity is seen in the rest of bilateral lung segments. No lymphadenopathy is identified in bilateral hila, mediastinum, supraclavicular fossae or jugular lymphatics. Thyroid gland and nasopharynx are unremarkable. Skeletal survey shows spondylolytic spine with osteophytic growth in

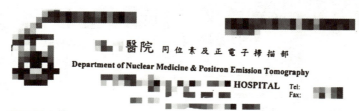

Department of Nuclear Medicine & Positron Emission Tomography

HOSPITAL Tel:
Fax:

T10 to L2 vertebrae, suggestive of degenerative change. Marrow metabolism in the axial skeleton is within normal limits.

Functional parameters of these lesions are tabulated as below:

Li, Site	in mm		Standard
	LD	PD	SUVmax
Segment 6 liver lesion	52.4	41.1	6.6

Note: LD=longest diameter; PD=diameter perpendicular to LD

Impression:

1. A 52.4 mm LD x 41.1 mm PD hypermetabolic segment VI liver lesion with hypometabolic centre and internal calcifications is suggestive of aggressive liver neoplasm with central necrosis. In the present clinical context, it is most consistent with liver metastasis from colonic malignancy.
2. No ^{18}FDG PET-CT evidence of local recurrence or regional metastatic lymphadenopathy in regard to patient's history of treated primary colonic malignancy.
3. Segment II liver cyst and left upper pole renal cyst.
4. No other focal hypermetabolic pathology in the rest of body survey to suggest other ^{18}FDG-avid primary malignancy that responsible for the metabolically active liver tumor.

Thank you very much, ▮▮▮ ▮▮▮ for your referral.

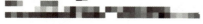

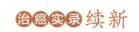

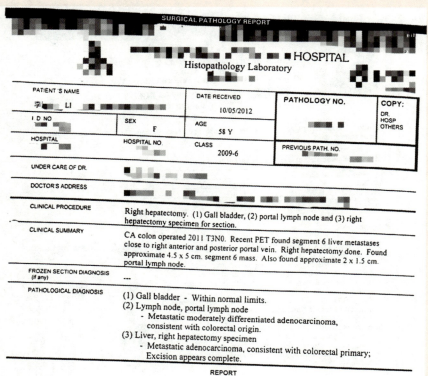

SURGICAL PATHOLOGY REPORT

.... HOSPITAL

Histopathology Laboratory

PATIENT'S NAME		DATE RECEIVED		PATHOLOGY NO.		COPY:
李... LI ...		10/05/2012		...		DR. HOSP OTHERS
I D NO	SEX F	AGE 58 Y				
HOSPITAL	HOSPITAL NO.	CLASS 2009-6		PREVIOUS PATH. NO.		

UNDER CARE OF DR.	
DOCTOR'S ADDRESS	
CLINICAL PROCEDURE	Right hepatectomy. (1) Gall bladder, (2) portal lymph node and (3) right hepatectomy specimen for section.
CLINICAL SUMMARY	CA colon operated 2011 T3N0. Recent PET found segment 6 liver metastases close to right anterior and posterior portal vein. Right hepatectomy done. Found approximate 4.5 x 5 cm. segment 6 mass. Also found approximate 2 x 1.5 cm. portal lymph node.
FROZEN SECTION DIAGNOSIS (if any)	...
PATHOLOGICAL DIAGNOSIS	(1) Gall bladder - Within normal limits. (2) Lymph node, portal lymph node 　　- Metastatic moderately differentiated adenocarcinoma, 　　　consistent with colorectal origin. (3) Liver, right hepatectomy specimen 　　- Metastatic adenocarcinoma, consistent with colorectal primary; 　　　Excision appears complete.

REPORT

<u>Macroscopic examination:</u>

(1) Specimen labelled as "Gall bladder". Present is a smooth-surfaced gall bladder measuring 7.5 cm. in length and 3 cm. in greatest external diameter. The gall bladder is filled with green bile and the mucosa appears unremarkable. The wall varies from 0.25 to 0.5 cm. in thickness. No stones are present. A lymph node 0.8 x 0.4 x 0.3 cm. is present at the cystic duct. Blocks: (1) Six pieces in one block.

(2) Specimen labelled as "Portal lymph node". Present is a tan-coloured firm mass 2.5 x 1.5 x 1.2 cm. which contains two lymph nodes one measuring 1.5 x 1.5 x 1 cm. and the other measuring 0.7 x 0.4 x 0.4 cm. Blocks: (2A) The larger lymph node, trisected and all embedded. (2B) The smaller lymph node, bisected and all embedded.

(3) Specimen labelled as "Right hepatectomy specimen". Present is a mass of liver, which is brownish and wedge-shaped measuring 15.2 x 11.5 x 6 cm. and weighing 534 grams. The liver has been partly incised before receipt. The capsular surface is smooth with a raw area measuring 14 x 6.4 cm. A whitish depressed area 2 x 1.3 cm. in area and 0.4 cm. below the adjacent surface is situated 2.8 cm. from the surgical resection margin. On sectioning, an underlying tumour nodule 4.2 x 3.3 x 3 cm. is present. This is

(CONTINUED ON NEXT PAGE)

Page 1 of 2

192

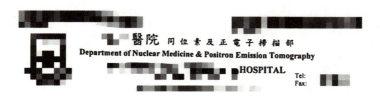

In the thorax, there is a stable subcentimeter RML subpleural nodule with no interval increase in metabolism. There is normal parenchymal and pleural activity in the rest of bilateral lung segments. No pleural or pericardial effusion noted. No hypermetabolic lymphadenopathy in bilateral hila, mediastinum, supraclavicular fossae or jugular lymphatics. Thyroid gland and nasopharynx are unremarkable. There is no hypermetabolic focal intramammary lesion in both breasts and no hypermetabolic lymphadenopathy in bilateral axillae.

Spondylitic spine with no hypermetabolic focal marrow lesion in axial and proximal appendicular skeleton in skeletal survey. An interval diffuse hypermetabolic activity at L3/4 interspinous process is suggestive of degenerative change.

Impression:

1. No ^{18}FDG PET/CT evidence of local recurrence or regional metastatic lymphadenopathy in regard to patient's history of treated primary colonic malignancy.
2. No hypermetabolic focal lesion in the liver remnant to suggest liver metastasis.
3. No other suspicious activity in the remaining body survey to suggest distant metastasis.
4. In summary: metabolic remission.

Thank you very much, ▆▆ for your referral.

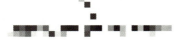

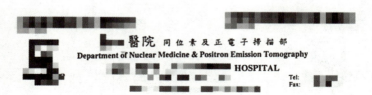

醫院 同位素及正電子掃描部
Department of Nuclear Medicine & Positron Emission Tomography
HOSPITAL

Tel:
Fax:

In the thorax, there is a stable subcentimeter RML subpleural nodule with no interval increase in metabolism. There is normal parenchymal and pleural activity in the rest of bilateral lung segments. No pleural or pericardial effusion noted. No hypermetabolic lymphadenopathy in bilateral hila, mediastinum, supraclavicular fossae or jugular lymphatics. Thyroid gland and nasopharynx are unremarkable. There is no hypermetabolic focal intramammary lesion in both breasts and no hypermetabolic lymphadenopathy in bilateral axillae.

Spondylitic spine with no hypermetabolic focal marrow lesion in axial and proximal appendicular skeleton in skeletal survey.

Impression:

1. No ^{18}FDG PET/CT evidence of local recurrence or regional metastatic lymphadenopathy in regard to patient's history of treated primary colonic malignancy.
2. No hypermetabolic focal lesion in the liver remnant to suggest recurrent liver metastasis.
3. No other suspicious activity in the remaining body survey to suggest distant metastasis.
4. In summary: metabolic remission.

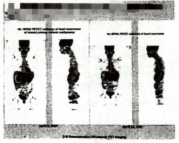

Thank you very much, ▮ ▮ for your referral.

病案28

肝癌肝硬化康复 16 年

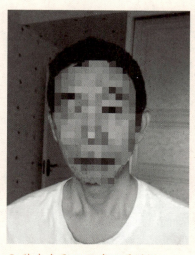

🔊 陈先生于 2022 年 3 月近照

2004 年，陈先生经血液检查发现患上乙型肝炎，他在医院就诊时表示并不知道什么时候得的这病，但因他知道患乙肝的人比较多，自己身体并没有什么太大不适，也就没有当回事。2006 年，他开始经常腹胀、胃口差，并逐渐发生明显消瘦等症状，急忙前去医院做详细检查，结果发现患有肝癌和肝硬化。按照医院的安排，他于 2007 年做了右侧肝叶的切除手术，手术后报告证实为中分化肝细胞癌。完成切除手术后紧接着连续做化疗，整个疗程长达 1 年时间。他认为经过手术及化疗后，身体应该恢复健康了。

但没想到在 2009 年复查时，发现他的左侧肝叶又出现了新的肿瘤，是以前检查中所没有的，证实肝癌已经复发，同时肝癌指数 AFP 也明显增高。尽管他已经做了手术切除，化疗也结束了，肝癌却还是复发。在这种非常困难的情况下，经朋友介绍，他前来求助于生命修复的治疗。

当时的陈先生经常觉得疲劳无力、面色暗黑、双下肢水肿、腹部膨胀，完全没有食欲。经过1年多的治疗后，现在的他已完全恢复健康，不仅肝脏的肿瘤完全消失，而且有关乙型肝炎的指数也都全部恢复正常。

生命修复的中医药在预防和治疗乙型肝炎，以及在治疗各阶段肝病、肝癌中的疗效备受肯定，对于控制癌组织生长、发展，以及对晚期患者、失去西医治疗时机的患者，仍然可提供很多机会和方法，为他们进行抗癌治疗。

治疗原则

攻毒祛瘀，行气通滞化瘤。

常用中药

1. 石见穿、生大黄、重楼、土鳖虫、三棱、莪术、当归、桃仁、红花、九香虫等。
2. 同时服用消瘤丸。

影像学、病理学检查报告及诊疗记录

1. 2014 年 1 月 7 日肝脏手术后病理报告证实为肝细胞癌，癌旁肝组织为结节性肝硬化。

2. 2019 年 9 月 6 日检查报告证实慢性肝病，无肝癌复发。

附：患者检查报告

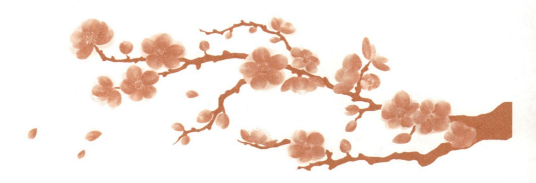

197

病理诊断报告单

送检医院：本院

病理号：

基本信息

姓名：陈██	性别：男	年龄：64岁	住院号：██
科室：肝移植9楼病区	床号：9		门诊号：
收到日期：2014-01-07	送检医师：██		ID 号：██

标本信息

肉眼所见：1. 不整形组织，4.2*4*2.5cm，切面见一灰白色结节，大小0.8*0.7*0.5cm，紧邻肝脏切缘。
2. 不整形肝组织，2.5*1.5*1.2cm，切面见淡黄色结节，直径1cm，质中，距切缘0.5cm。

镜下所见：

病理诊断： "肝脏左内叶"肿瘤0.8*0.7*0.5cm一个，生长方式：小癌型；病理分型：肝细胞癌，脉管癌栓（-）；组织类型：实体型；中分化，包膜侵犯（-），卫星灶（-），手术切缘（肿瘤紧挨切缘）；癌旁肝组织：结节性肝硬化；
"肝尾状叶"结节性肝硬化；
免疫组化结果：Ki67（约30%阳性），CEA（-），AFP（+），Hep-1（+），CK18（+），CK19（-），CK7（-），CA19-9（-），TS（个别细胞阳性），HBs（-），HBc（-），HCV（-），CK8（+），CD34（血管阳性）。

诊断医师：██████   报告日期：2014-01-10

姓　名：陈▒▒　　　性　别：男　　　出生日期：1953-03-12　超声号：J▒▒▒▒
科　别：门诊内科　　住院号：　　　　床　号：
检查部位：肝|胆|胰|脾|双肾　　　　　　　　　　　仪器名称：Sequoia-512

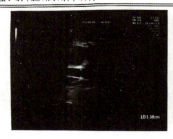 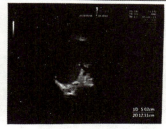

超声描述：【肝脏】肝脏表面欠光整，右肝最大斜径100mm，肋下刚及，肝内血管网欠清，肝
　　　　　光点增粗分布不均匀，在肝内散见多枚高回声结节，其中右肝近膈顶一枚大小约
　　　　　24*20mm稍高回声区，境界欠清，在肝内可见几枚强光斑，其中一枚大小约5*
　　　　　4mm。在肝内可见多枚囊性团块，其中一枚大小约13*12mm，边界清，有包膜，团
　　　　　块后方伴增强效应。门静脉宽约14mm。
　　　　　【胆囊】胆囊大小正常，胆囊壁毛糙、增厚，囊内透声性好，囊内可见一枚强
　　　　　回声，大小约4*5mm，其后伴声影，变动体位未见移动。胆总管宽6mm，显示部分
　　　　　管内未见占位性病变。
　　　　　【胰腺】胰腺部分因气体影响显示不清，所见部分大小、形态正常，胰内未见明
　　　　　确占位性病变。胰管未见扩张。
　　　　　【脾脏】脾肿大，脾厚约50mm，脾长约121mm，回声欠均，脾静脉增宽，胰腺后
　　　　　方脾静脉宽约8.9mm。
　　　　　【肾脏】双肾大小、形态未见异常，肾盂未见积水，二肾内散见少许点状强回
　　　　　声。

超声诊断：慢性肝病伴结节
　　　　　肝内钙化斑、肝多发囊肿
　　　　　胆囊壁毛糙、增厚，胆囊结石
　　　　　脾肿大、回声欠均
　　　　　二肾小结晶

检查结束：2019-9-6 8:37:20　　　检查医师：▒▒▒▒　　　审核医师：▒▒▒
▒▒▒▒▒　　　▒▒　　　　　　　　　　　　　　　　　　书写员：▒▒

199

病案 29

肺癌加中风、脑肿瘤康复

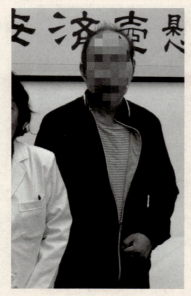

❶ 黄先生于 2023 年 12 月前来诊治时合影留念

2017 年，黄先生 61 岁，是一家企业的老板，日理万机，即使是星期日也在工作。8 月的一天清晨，他突然感到起床困难，身体不能活动，家人看到他面部口唇歪斜、说话不清，于是急忙叫救护车送往医院就诊。经过检查后，证实他患了急性脑梗死，紧急住院治疗。

接下来的几个月时间，他都有咳嗽、气短、胸闷、多痰的症状，在家人的催促下再去医院做更进一步的身体检查，祸不单行的是，他被确诊为非小细胞性肺癌，并有纵隔与肺门淋巴转移。于是黄先生在 2017 年 11 月开始做放疗。但在治疗过程中，他于 2017 年 11 月，再次中风，左侧上下肢完全瘫痪，同时发现了脑垂体肿瘤。三种重病突然集于一身，且黄先生在短时间内还有 2 次中风脑梗死，令他深受打击。

经过 5 次化疗后，他在家人的陪同下前来接受生命修复治疗。目前的他，肺癌、脑肿瘤及脑梗死三种重病均全部康复了。

治疗原则

化瘀通脉，祛邪消瘤。

常用中药

1. 黄芪、红花、桃仁、地龙、姜黄、威灵仙、蜈蚣，土鳖虫等。
2. 同时服用散结丸。

影像学、病理学检查报告及诊疗记录

1. 2017年10月25日病理学检查报告证实为非小细胞型肺癌。

2. 2018年10月8日MRI脑、颈部扫描报告证实肺癌、脑梗死复发伴左侧偏瘫，脑垂体瘤。

3. 2020年9月23日PET/CT报告证实左肺癌并纵隔，肺门淋巴转移，经生命修复治疗后肿瘤消失，转移病灶消失。

4. 2021年9月29日PET/CT报告证实病情稳定，无肿瘤复发转移。

附：患者检查报告

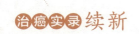

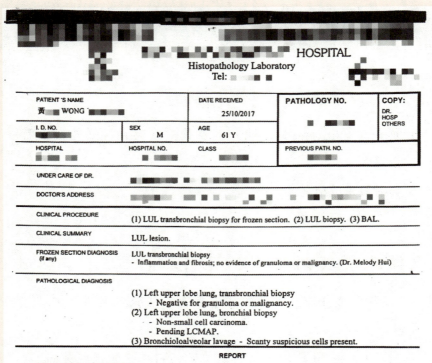

HOSPITAL

Histopathology Laboratory
Tel: ▮ ▮ ▮

PATIENT 'S NAME		DATE RECEIVED		PATHOLOGY NO.		COPY:
黄 ▮ WONG ▮		25/10/2017		▮ ▮		DR. HOSP OTHERS
I. D. NO.	SEX M	AGE 61 Y				
HOSPITAL	HOSPITAL NO.	CLASS		PREVIOUS PATH. NO.		

UNDER CARE OF DR.	▮ ▮
DOCTOR'S ADDRESS	▮ ▮ ▮
CLINICAL PROCEDURE	(1) LUL transbronchial biopsy for frozen section. (2) LUL biopsy. (3) BAL.
CLINICAL SUMMARY	LUL lesion.
FROZEN SECTION DIAGNOSIS (if any)	LUL transbronchial biopsy - Inflammation and fibrosis; no evidence of granuloma or malignancy. (Dr. Melody Hui)
PATHOLOGICAL DIAGNOSIS	(1) Left upper lobe lung, transbronchial biopsy 　- Negative for granuloma or malignancy. (2) Left upper lobe lung, bronchial biopsy 　- Non-small cell carcinoma. 　- Pending LCMAP. (3) Bronchioloalveolar lavage - Scanty suspicious cells present.

REPORT

Macroscopic examination:

(1) Specimen labelled "Left upper lobe transbronchial biopsy" consists of seven pieces of firm tan tissue, the largest piece measuring 2 x 1 x 1 mm. and the smallest 1 mm. in diameter. All embedded in one block for frozen section.

(2) Specimen labelled "Left upper lobe biopsy x 11" consists of eleven pieces of firm tan tissue, the largest piece measuring 2 x 1 x 1 mm. and the smallest 1 mm. in diameter. All embedded in one block.

(3) Specimen labelled "BAL x 1" consists of approximately 4 ml. of reddish and slightly turbid fluid. One cell block and one CytoRich are prepared.

Microscopic examination:

(1) Sections show multiple pieces of bronchial mucosa with biopsy artefact. Mild chronic inflammation with some pigmented macrophages are found in the lamina propria. Scanty lung parenchymal tissue is also included. There is no granuloma or malignancy.

(CONTINUED ON NEXT PAGE)

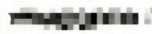

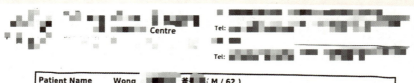

Patient Name	Wong 黄 (M / 62)		
Referring Doctor			
Our Patient Code		Date of Exam	2018-10-08
Exam ID		Date of Report	2018-10-08 Pg 1of3

Your Patient Code

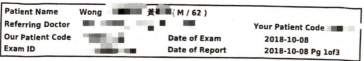

MRI BRAIN AND MRA NECK WITH CONTRAST

CLINICAL HISTORY:
CA lung NSCLC. Recurrent cerebral infarction with left hemiplegia. For reassessment.

IMAGING PROTOCOL:
Axial   T2W TSE, T1W SE, T2W FFE, DWI SENSE,T1W SE+C
Sagittal   T1W SE, T1W SE+C
Coronal   T2W FLAIR, T1W SE + C
Contrast enhanced MRA and TOF Circle of Willis

FINDINGS:
Cerebral atrophy is noted with prominent cerebral sulci associated. T2W and FLAIR hyperintense foci are seen in subcortical white matter, compatible with small vessels ischemia. These show no significant interval change from previous MRI dated 29/09/2017 apart from the right frontal periventricular one now appearing larger and cystic suggesting previous infarction between the two studies. In addition, a large area of cystic encephalomacia is now seen in the right frontal and parietal lobes lateral to the right lateral ventricle, with some internal septations associated. No enhancement or restricted diffusion is seen. This is compatible with a large old infarct. There is perilesional T2 hyperintense signal associated, suggestive of adjacent white matter ischemia. Volume loss is associated with dilatation of the underlying right lateral ventricle. The old infarct in the right temporal lobe with adjacent white matter ischemia shows no significant interval change from previous MRI. The previously seen right occipital lobe lesion is smaller than previous scan and now appears more T2 hyperintense with no enhancement. This may represent post-treatment change or another old infarct. Volume loss associated with dilatation of the occipital horn of the right lateral ventricle.

Abnormal curvilinear T2/ FLAIR hyperintensity is seen extending from the right frontal-parietal infarct down along the posterior limb of the right internal capsule to the right cerebral peduncle and pons. Mild atrophy of right side of midbrain and pons associated. No enhancement, restricted diffusion or mass effect is seen. It is suggestive of Wallerian degeneration secondary to the cerebral infarct.

A hypoenhancing lesion is noted in the pituitary gland, measuring 0.3 x 0.2cm in size. No pituitary gland enlargement is associated. This pre-existed on previous MRI and shows no interval change. It may represent a pituitary microadenoma.

Otherwise, no other focal lesion or abnormal signal intensity is seen in the rest of the brain. Cerebellum appears unremarkable. No abnormal GRE signal is seen to suggest chronic haemorrhagic products. No abnormal contrast enhancement noted in the brain or meninges.

No extra-axial lesion or collection noted.

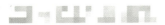

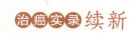

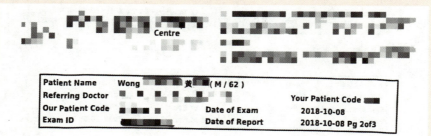

Patient Name	Wong ███ 黃██ (M / 62)		
Referring Doctor	██ ██ ██ ██ ██		Your Patient Code ███
Our Patient Code	██████	Date of Exam	2018-10-08
Exam ID	███████	Date of Report	2018-10-08 Pg 2of3

About 3mm shift of the midline to the right is detected, new to previous study, likely due to right cerebral hemispheric volume loss from the infarct.

No intraventricular lesion detected.

The cavernous and dural venous sinuses are patent.

Both orbits is unremarkable.

Previously seen left maxillary mucus retension cyst has decreased in size, measuring 1.6 x 1.2 x 1.1cm. Rest of the paranasal sinuses is clear.

MRA NECK
On the MR angiogram of the neck, no significant stenosis is seen in the brachiocephalic trunk, bilateral subclavian, bilateral extracranial carotid and vertebral arteries of the neck.

A 9mm segment of moderately severe stenosis (~60%) is noted in M1 segment of right middle cerebral artery (MCA) with distal obliteration. Paucity and markedly attenuated MCA branches are seen distal to this. This likely resulted in the right cerebral hemispheric infarcts seen. Left M1 segment is narrowed (about 60-70%; 6.4mm in length) but left M2 to M4 branches are patent and unremarkable. Rest of the cerebral arteries included appears unremarkable with no significant stenosis.

The intracranial ICAs, vertebral and basilar arteries and their major cerebral and cerebellar branches are patent with no significant stenosis seen.
No intracranial AVM or aneurysm seen.

IMPRESSION:
1. Old infarcts in right temporal lobe with no interval change.
2. Old infarct in the right frontal parietal lobe has increased in size from previous MRI with brain volume loss, dilatation of underlying right lateral ventricle and 3mm ipsilateral midline shift. Curvilinear non-enhancing T2 hyperintense signals extending from this infarct to the pons, suggestive of Wallerian degeneration.
3. Previously seen rim-enhancing right occipital lesion has decreased in size with no more enhancement. Volume loss is associated with dilatation of occipital horn of right lateral ventricle. This could represent an old infarct as well.
4. Periventricular and subcortical white matter small vessels ischemia show no significant change from previous MRI apart from evolution of right frontal periventricular one into infarction. No acute infarction seen.
5. Hypoenhancing lesion in pituitary gland with no interval change, may represent

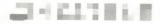

Centre

Patient Name	Wong 黄 (M / 62)		
Referring Doctor			Your Patient Code
Our Patient Code		Date of Exam	2018-10-08
Exam ID		Date of Report	2018-10-08 Pg 3of3

a pituitary microadenoma.

6. Right MCA attenuation and occlusion at its M1 segment with paucity and markedly attenuated distal branches.

7. Moderately severe narrowing of left M1 segment.

8. Decreased size of left maxillary mucus retention cyst.

Thank you for your referral.

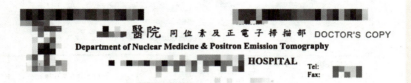

醫院 同位素及正電子掃描部 DOCTOR'S COPY
Department of Nuclear Medicine & Positron Emission Tomography

HOSPITAL

Tel:
Fax:

Name:	Wong, ★			Date:	23/09/2020
I.D. No.:		Sex:	Male	Ref. Dr.:	
Hosp. No.:		Age:	64 Y	Fax:	
Ward/Dept.:	Comprehensive Oncology Centre	ExamID:		Tel:	

POSITRON EMISSION TOMOGRAPHY
(¹⁸F-FDG ONCOLOGY)

<u>History</u>:

A 64 year-old gentleman who was admitted for CVA with left hemiparesis in 08/2017. PET/CT scan on 17/08/2017 found a 3.6 cm hypermetabolic left apical lung mass suggestive of malignancy and slightly prominent mediastinal and left hilar lymph nodes. CT-guided biopsy showed no evidence of malignancy. LUL bronchial biopsy in 10/2017 showed non-small cell carcinoma suggestive of squamous cell differentiation. Status post Cyberknife therapy in 11/2017. PET in 01/2019 showed resolved lesion. No history of DM, hepatitis or TB. Smoker. PET scan for surveillance.

<u>Radiopharmaceutical</u>: 10.2 mCi ¹⁸F-FDG injected intravenously.

<u>Findings</u>:

Limited whole body CT transmission and PET emission imaging began at 60 minutes after radiopharmaceutical administration (blood glucose 6.5 mmol/l), spanning a region from base of skull to upper thigh. 60 mg Spasmonal was given p.o. 15 min before ¹⁸F-FDG administration.

Liver tissue normal reference uptake has a SUVmax of 2.8.

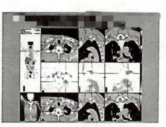

Comparison is made with the previous PET scan performed here on 16/01/2019. The left apical lung tumor is persistently resolved with non-specific activity in the residual scarring. Stable tiny lingular and RML lateral segment subpleural nodules are seen without significant uptake. Stable bilateral bullae are noted. No suspicious new lung nodule is seen bilaterally. Persistent minimal right pleural effusion is noted. There is no evidence of left pleural effusion or pericardial effusion. The mediastinum, bilateral hila and bilateral supraclavicular fossae show normal metabolism. Mildly hypermetabolic left axillary node, right submandibular node and right jugulodigastric node are seen. Focal activity is seen around the right lower molar tooth. Stable small left maxillary sinus retention cyst is seen. The nasopharynx appears unremarkable. Right thyroid shows calcification and no abnormal metabolism.

The liver shows normal metabolism with decrease in size in the large liver cyst. The spleen, pancreas, both adrenals and both kidneys appear unremarkable with stable small right renal cyst noted. There is no abnormal metabolism in the lymphatic of the abdominal and pelvic cavities. The stomach and bowel showed physiological activity. The prostate shows no ¹⁸FDG-avid lesion. Skeletal survey shows no hypermetabolic bone lesion. There is persistent hypodense area in right brain on limited view of brain and in keeping with the patient's known CVA.

醫院 同位素及正電子掃描部
Department of Nuclear Medicine & Positron Emission Tomography

HOSPITAL

Tel:
Fax:

Functional parameters of these lesions are tabulated as below:

WONG,			F-18 FDG
	in mm		Standard
Site	LD	PD	SUVmax
L axillary node	10.3	6.8	2.3
R jugulodigastric node	7.2	5.6	3.7
R submandibular node	10.9	6.8	3.6

Note: LD=longest diameter; PD=diameter perpendicular to LD

Impression:

1. Persistently resolved primary left apical lung tumor with non-specific activity in the residual scarring. No suspicious focal lesion is seen to suggest recurrent tumor.
2. No metabolic evidence of metastatic lymphadenopathy or solid organ distant metastasis.
3. Focal activity around the right lower molar tooth may represent dental disease.
4. Mild activities are seen in left axillary node, right submandibular node and right jugulodigastric node and appear inflammatory in origin.
5. Large liver cyst and small right renal cyst.

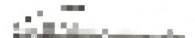

Thank you very much, ■ ■ for your referral.

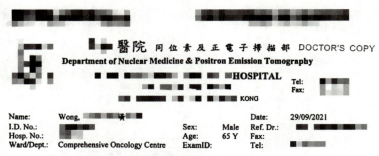

醫院 同位素及正電子掃描部 DOCTOR'S COPY

Department of Nuclear Medicine & Positron Emission Tomography

HOSPITAL
Tel:
Fax:
KONG

Name:	Wong, ██████			Date:	29/09/2021
I.D. No.:		Sex:	Male	Ref. Dr.:	██████
Hosp. No.:		Age:	65 Y	Fax:	
Ward/Dept.:	Comprehensive Oncology Centre	ExamID:		Tel:	██████

POSITRON EMISSION TOMOGRAPHY
(¹⁸F-FDG ONCOLOGY)

<u>History</u>:

A 65 year-old gentleman, known carcinoma of lung (LUL). PET/CT scan in 08/2017 found a 3.6 cm hypermetabolic left apical lung mass suggestive of malignancy and slightly prominent mediastinal and left hilar lymph nodes. LUL bronchial biopsy showed non-small cell carcinoma suggestive of squamous cell differentiation. Status post Cyberknife therapy in 11/2017. PET in 01/2019 showed resolved lesion and no recurrence in 09/2020. Clinically well. Past history of CVA with left hemiparesis in 08/2017. No DM, hepatitis or TB. Smoker. PET scan for surveillance.

<u>Radiopharmaceutical</u>: 10.0 mCi ¹⁸F-FDG injected intravenously.

<u>Findings</u>:

Limited whole body CT transmission and PET emission imaging began at 63 minutes after radiopharmaceutical administration (blood glucose 6.2 mmol/l), spanning a region from base of skull to upper thigh. 60 mg Spasmonal was given p.o. before ¹⁸F-FDG administration.

Liver tissue normal reference uptake has a SUVmax of 2.79.

Comparison is made with the previous PET scan performed here on 23/09/2020. The left apical lung tumor is persistently resolved with non-specific activity in the residual scarring. Stable tiny lingular and RML lateral segment subpleural nodules and RLL posterior tiny nodules with tree-in-bud pattern are seen without significant uptake. Stable bilateral bullae are noted. No suspicious new lung nodule is seen bilaterally. Persistent minimal right pleural effusion is noted. There is no evidence of left pleural effusion or pericardial effusion. The mediastinum, bilateral hila and bilateral supraclavicular fossae show normal metabolism.

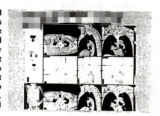

Mildly hypermetabolic left axillary node, bilateral submandibular nodes and right jugulodigastric node are seen with interval increase uptake in the left axillary node. Focal activity is seen around the right denture. Stable small left maxillary sinus retention cyst is seen. The nasopharynx appears unremarkable. Right thyroid shows calcification and no abnormal metabolism.

The liver shows normal metabolism with persistent liver cyst. The spleen, pancreas, both adrenals and both kidneys appear unremarkable with stable small right renal cyst noted. There is no abnormal metabolism in the lymphatic of the abdominal and pelvic cavities. The stomach and bowel showed physiological activity. The prostate shows no ¹⁸FDG-avid lesion. Skeletal survey shows decreased marrow activity in cervicothoracic spine and may be related to the previous radiation therapy. No

醫院 同位素及正電子掃描部
Department of Nuclear Medicine & Positron Emission Tomography

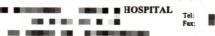 **HOSPITAL**

Tel:
Fax:

hypermetabolic bone lesion is seen. There is persistent hypodense area in right brain on limited view of brain and in keeping with the patient's known CVA.

Functional parameters to compare these 2 studies are tabulated below:

WONG,			29-Sep-2021			23-Sep-2020			
	in mm		F-18 FDG		in mm		F-18 FDG		
Site	LD	PD	SUVmax	TLG	LD	PD	SUVmax	TLG	TLG %change
L axillary node	10.5	8.2	4.3	0.9	10.3	6.8	2.3	0.5	80.0%

Note: LD=longest diameter; PD=diameter perpendicular to LD; TLG=total lesion glycolysis (vol x SUVmean)

Impression:

1. Persistently resolved primary left apical lung tumor with non-specific activity in the residual scarring. No suspicious focal lesion is seen to suggest recurrent tumor.
2. No metabolic evidence of metastatic lymphadenopathy or solid organ distant metastasis.
3. Interval increased uptake in left axillary node and persistent uptake in bilateral submandibular nodes and right jugulodigastric node and appear inflammatory in origin in view of only mild progression in 1-year interval.
4. Focal activity around the right denture and may represent dental disease.
5. Liver cyst and small right renal cyst.

Thank you very much, ■ ■■■ for your referral.

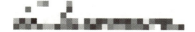

甲状腺癌软骨和肺转移康复 10 年

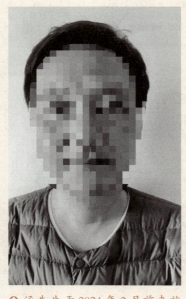

👆 汤先生于 2024 年 2 月前来就诊时照片

42 岁的汤先生是一位工程师，在 2014 年不幸患上了甲状腺癌。他于 2014 年 1 月做了双侧甲状腺全切除手术，以为从此没事了，但在同年的 12 月，就发现有颈部软骨转移，以及肺部淋巴等转移，随后又发现了胸腺瘤，需要再次动手术。反复的发生肺炎，令汤先生有大量咯痰、咯血等严重症状，于是他在 2015 年刚过了新年后就前来就诊。

当时他的肺部本身已患有慢性疾病，如慢性支气管炎、支气管扩张等，再加上甲状腺癌的淋巴转移，以及甲状腺癌手术之后的肺部淋巴、颈部等转移病灶，更是雪上加霜。他要求采用全新的生命修复治疗，希望能够绝处逢生。汤先生风雨无阻的坚持治疗，使得他的病情逐渐得到控制，严重咳嗽及大量咯痰、咯血的情况逐渐减少，精神状态明显好转，并恢复了工作。正当大家都松了一口气之时，万万想不到的事情又发生在他身上，他的身体出现了大面积密集的红疹和水疱，不仅痒还非常痛，病情严重，他急忙去离家近处的急诊住院治疗。经医院使用大量激素治疗，皮肤问题才有所缓解，但是停用激素后，他又开始反复发作，大量水疱除了令他感到痛痒，还很容易破裂，医院认为反复发作的原因是免疫功能受损导致。

经过认真观察及分析，我们认为皮肤问题是由于药物过敏引起的。原来他因癌症将甲状腺全部切除以后，医院里按照常规给予补充甲状腺激素的药物，并且每日均需服用。如不给予补充此类药物（从一般情况来说是不可能的）人体没有甲状腺激素，会影响许多至关重要的身体功能，例如心率、身体热能、消化吸收、水液代谢、血液循环等，均可导致严重后果。

经过我们的仔细辨证分析，为他制订了培补脾肾，养护后天弥补先天的治疗原则，并进行促进机体内分泌代谢，气血通畅、功能健全的治疗，他也在逐渐恢复正常。从患癌到现在已经有 10 年时间了，汤先生没有再做手术，他战胜了癌症。而且也有 6 年多没有服用补充剂了，现在的他生活和工作都很好，身体亦健康正常。

软坚散瘀，化毒消瘤。

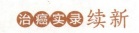

常用中药

1. 柴胡、黄芩、丹参、虎杖、猕猴梨根、牡丹皮、鱼腥草、半夏、山慈菇等。
2. 同时服用消瘤丸。

影像学、病理学检查报告及诊疗记录

1. 2013 年 12 月 27 日甲状腺病理检查报告确诊为甲状腺乳头状癌。

2. 2014 年 12 月 11 日扫描检查报告证实有颈部肺部癌组织残存和转移。

3. 2016 年 5 月 31 日病理检查报告证实全身皮肤疱疹为表皮下大疱。

附：患者检查报告

病 理 图 文 报 告

病人ID: ■■■■ 病理号: ■■■■

姓名: 汤■■■	性别: 男	年龄: 40 岁	床号:		住院号:
送检单位: 本院		送检科室: 内分泌外科门诊		门诊号: ■ ■ ■■	
送检医师: ■■■		接收日期: 2013-12-26		取材日期: 2013-12-27	

临床诊断: 甲状腺左叶肿物,甲状腺癌?
送检组织: 甲状腺左叶FNA

肉眼所见:

　　细胞包埋蜡块切片及离心涂片各一张:镜下见较多乳头状腺体排列,部分滤泡上皮细胞异型,细胞核大小不等、拥挤及深染;可见核内包涵体及核沟,核仁明显。形态符合甲状腺乳头状癌。

附图:

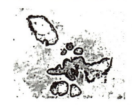 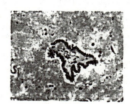

诊断意见:

　　"甲状腺左叶FNA"
　　　——　甲状腺乳头状癌。

Left lobe of THYROID, Fine needle aspiration:
- THYROID PAPILLARY CARCINOMA

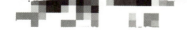

报告医师: ■■■　　审核医师 ■■■
报告日期: 2013-12-30

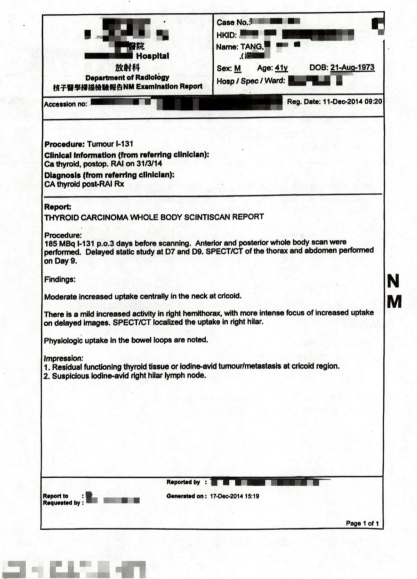

Case No.: ▓▓▓▓

HKID: ▓▓▓▓

Name: TANG, ▓(▓)

Sex: M   **Age:** 41y   **DOB:** 21-Aug-1973

醫院
Hospital

放射科
Department of Radiology
核子醫學掃描檢驗報告NM Examination Report

Hosp / Spec / Ward: ▓▓▓

Accession no: ▓▓▓▓   **Reg. Date:** 11-Dec-2014 09:20

Procedure: Tumour I-131
Clinical Information (from referring clinician):
Ca thyroid, postop. RAI on 31/3/14
Diagnosis (from referring clinician):
CA thyroid post-RAI Rx

Report:
THYROID CARCINOMA WHOLE BODY SCINTISCAN REPORT

Procedure:
185 MBq I-131 p.o.3 days before scanning. Anterior and posterior whole body scan were
performed. Delayed static study at D7 and D9. SPECT/CT of the thorax and abdomen performed
on Day 9.

Findings:

Moderate increased uptake centrally in the neck at cricoid.

There is a mild increased activity in right hemithorax, with more intense focus of increased uptake
on delayed images. SPECT/CT localized the uptake in right hilar.

Physiologic uptake in the bowel loops are noted.

Impression:
1. Residual functioning thyroid tissue or iodine-avid tumour/metastasis at cricoid region.
2. Suspicious iodine-avid right hilar lymph node.

N
M

Reported by : ▓▓▓▓

Report to : ▓▓▓
Requested by : ▓▓

Generated on : 17-Dec-2014 15:19

Page 1 of 1

病 理 图 文 报 告

病人号：██████   病理号：

姓名：汤██	性别：男	年龄：42 岁		床号：25
送检单位：住院	病区：██		送检科室：皮肤科	
送检医师：█████	接收日期：2016-05-31	取材日期：2016-05-31	

临床诊断：皮肤水疱查因：大疱性类天疱疮？多形红斑？其他
送检组织：躯干水疱

肉眼所见：

带皮组织1块，大小0.6 cm×0.5 cm×0.6 cm，切开，全取1盒。

光镜所见：

切片显示部分表皮坏死及表皮下大疱形成，坏死组织见中性粒细胞及蓝染细菌样物，大疱内见红染分泌物及中性粒细胞；真皮浅层小血管周围见中性粒细胞及少许嗜酸性粒细胞浸润；表皮未见明显棘层松解及大疱形成。免疫荧光结果示：IgA(基底膜线性+)，IgG(−)，IgM(−)，C3 (−)，C1q(−)。形态符合表皮下大疱，结合免疫荧光特征提示线状IgA大疱性皮病。

附图：

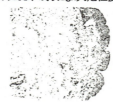 

诊断意见：

"躯干水疱"
—— 表皮下大疱。（详见描述）

SKIN, trunk, biopsy :
- SUBEPIDERMAL BULLE (please see description)

本报告仅供临床参考，如有
不符请及时联系病理科。   报告医师：████   审核医师：

██████   1/1   报告日期：2016-06-03

患有三种肿瘤的康复患者

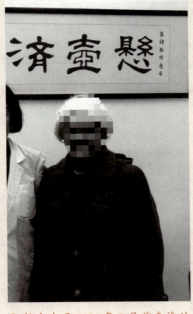

❶ 杨太太于 2024 年 2 月前来诊治时合影留念

杨太太早年曾做过甲状腺癌的手术切除。2016 年杨太太 83 岁，时常感到腹部不适，因此进食减少，人亦变得消瘦，起初她认为只是年龄大了、人老了，当然跟年轻时不一样，所以即使感到很疲累、腹胀及大便困难，也没有去看医生。这样过了数月后，她的大便里有时会见到血，大便的颜色也越来越黑，就好像柏油马路般黑的颜色。她不得已只好把这个情况告诉儿子，儿子立即陪同她到医院看病并做了肠镜检查。几天后检查报告出来，证实她患了直肠、结肠癌，医院便为她安排手术。2016 年 11 月，杨太太做了手术切除肿瘤及部分肠组织。手术后的病理报告诊断为中分化腺癌，并有血管壁的侵犯。

杨太太在手术后，身体仍然非常虚弱，呼吸困难、心悸气喘、水肿、全身无力，经医院再次检查，发现她有胸腔积液、心包积液，更严重的是在她的胰腺体部位又发现了胰腺内分泌肿瘤。因为胰腺肿瘤发展很快，需要尽快动手术切除，否则预后很差，但是她的身体已非常虚弱了，根本不可能再次承受手术。医生告知没有什么好办法了，她的儿子很孝顺，希望能延长母亲的生命，于是在 2017 年 1 月，在其母亲手术后 1 个多月，就带她前来就诊，寻找生命修复中医药的治疗希望。

当时杨太太的病情已经非常严重，两种癌症都做过手术，当前甲状腺部位又出现肿瘤，并有肠癌术后血管壁侵犯、胰腺肿瘤、心包积液、胸腔积液等。加上杨太太已是 83 岁高龄老人，行动困难且呼吸急促，我们便对她进行了全面的以扶正祛邪、阴阳双补为原则的治疗，她的身体也一天天好起来，精神状态逐渐改善，一步步渡过了生命的难关。

如今 8 年过去了，杨太太已经 91 岁了，现在她的精神很好，心情亦很愉快。2017 年 CT 检查报告显示胰腺的肿瘤没有增大，处于稳定状态；2019 年 CT 检查发现已没有胰腺肿瘤，且肠道肿瘤没有复发；2020 年 10 月检查显示甲状腺肿瘤也已消失。杨太太与全家人都感到非常高兴，目前的她正享受愉快、安乐的晚年生活。

 治疗原则

双补阴阳，扶正祛邪。

常用中药

1. 红参、鹿茸、山药、茯苓、鳖甲、夏枯草、牡蛎、龟板、山慈菇等。
2. 同时服用消瘤丸。

影像学、病理学检查报告及诊疗记录

1. 2016 年 11 月 26 日病理学检查报告证实为直肠乙状结肠肿瘤、腺癌。

2. 2017 年 11 月 11 日复查无肿瘤复发，胰腺神经内分泌瘤稳定。

3. 2019 年 4 月 9 日检查报告显示无肿瘤复发，无肺转移及其他转移，未见到胰腺神经内分泌瘤。

附：患者检查报告

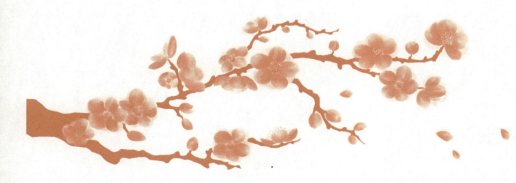

Diagnostic Centre

Testing Laboratory :

Pathologist-in-Charge :

PATIENT NAME YUEN		DATE RECEIVED 26/11/2016	PATHOLOGY NO.
I.D. NO.	SEX F	AGE 83 Y	
HOSPITAL	HOSPITAL / CLINIC NO.	WARD / CLASS	PREVIOUS PATH. NO.

UNDER CARE OF	
DOCTOR'S ADDRESS	
CLINICAL SUMMARY & PROCEDURE	Colonoscopy done. (1) Hepatic flexure polyp and (2) rectosigmoid tumour biopsy for histology.
FROZEN SECTION DIAGNOSIS	---
PATHOLOGICAL DIAGNOSIS	(1) Colonic polyp at hepatic flexure 結腸右曲息肉 (polypectomy 息肉切除術) - Hyperplastic polyp 增生性息肉 - No evidence of malignancy 無發現惡性病變 (2) Rectosigmoid tumour 直腸乙狀結腸腫瘤 (biopsy 活組織檢查) - Adenocarcinoma 腺癌 (please see description)

Macroscopic Examination:

(1) Specimen labelled as "hepatic flexure polyp". Received in formalin are 2 pieces of pale tan-coloured to brownish polypoid mucosal tissue ranging from 0.2 cm to 0.55 cm in greatest dimension (Figure 1). All embedded.

(2) Specimen labelled as "rectosigmoid tumour biopsy". Received in formalin are 3 pieces of irregular pale tan-coloured mucosal tissue ranging from 0.3 cm to 0.45 cm in greatest dimension (Figure 2). All embedded.

Microscopic Examination:

(1) Sections show polypoid pieces of minimally inflamed colonic mucosa with mild goblet cell hyperplasia (Figure 3). There is no evidence of significant dysplasia or malignancy. The overall features are consistent with hyperplastic polyp.

(2) Sections show pieces of inflamed and focally eroded colorectal mucosa infiltrated by moderately differentiated adenocarcinoma cells (Figure 4). The tumour cells show moderate degree of nuclear pleomorphism and are arranged in irregular glandular structures or cribriform pattern. The surrounding stroma shows desmoplastic reaction.

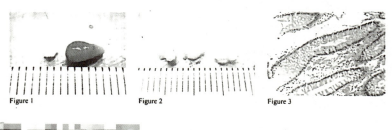

Figure 1   Figure 2   Figure 3

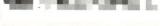

219

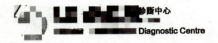

Diagnostic Centre

REF./TO	: ▓▓ ▓ ▓▓▓ ▓▓▓ ▓▓▓			
PATIENT NAME	: YUEN, ▓			
PATIENT HKID	: ▓▓▓▓	D.O.B.	: 01/01/1933	
SEX/AGE	: F/84Y	REF. NO.	:	
EXAM. DATE	: 11/11/2017	CASE NO.	: ▓▓ ▓▓▓	

RADIOLOGY REPORT

Adrenals, Spleen & Pancreas:
Both adrenal glands are of normal sizes and have no focal masses.
No splenomegaly or splenic infiltration found.
Known early arterial enhancing nodule at proximal pancreatic body measuring 9 mm is static.
Normal rest of the pancreas. Pancreatic duct is not dilated.

Kidneys, Ureters & Urinary bladder:
Both kidneys have normal sizes, contour and have comparable enhancement.
No calcified renal stones or renal masses is detected. No hydronephrosis.
No abnormal perinephric fat stranding found.
Simple small bilateral renal cysts are present.
Both ureters are not dilated and contain no calcified stone.

Bone
No aggressive osseous lesions within the scanned range.

IMPRESSION:
1. Post anterior resection. No local recurrence at the colorectal anastomosis. No metachronous colonic tumour is present.
2. There is no sizable abdominal, retroperitoneal or pelvic lymphadenopathy.
3. No distant metastasis in the scanned range.
4. Others:
   - Gallstones are known.
   - Pancreatic proximal body small early arterial enhancing nodule is static, likely indolent neuroendocrine tumour.

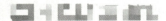

RADIOLOGY REPORT

Ref. / To	:	████████████████			
Patient	:	YUEN, ██ ██			
Attending Dr.	:	Referring Doctor	ID	:	████
Sex / Age	:	Female / 86Y 3M	PRN	:	████
Exam. Date	:	09-Apr-2019 10:40	DOB	:	01-Jan-1933

COMMENT:

- No interval change with CT on 11.11.2017.
- No CT evidence of lung metastasis.
- Static benign bilateral chronic lung changes.
- Cardiomegaly with thin pericardial effusion are unchanged.
- No nodal or distant metastasis in the scanned range.

病案 **32**

晚期恶性脂肪肉瘤康复

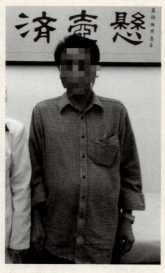

● 宋先生 2022 年 4 月前来诊治时合影留念

宋先生患有多种慢性疾病，冠心病病史 20 多年，走路稍快一点就会心慌气短，另外还患有糖尿病 10 多年。他每天都要服用多种药物来治疗。2014 年，他经常感到腹部疼痛，起初没太注意。但此后疼痛加重，发作频繁。经过医院检查后，得知腹部长了恶性肿瘤。于是在 2016 年做了腹部肿瘤的切除手术，经检查确诊为恶性程度很高的脂肪肉瘤。手术后，他心想肿瘤已被切除，可以放心了。但是仅过了半年，就出现腹腔内多发的肿瘤复发和转移。肿瘤生长迅速，2021 年 7 月复查时，腹腔中已有很多肿瘤，大的约 9cm，并且紧贴肾脏。医院要求他尽快再次手术，并评估了心脏功能，考虑做介入治疗。宋先生认为他的身体状况实在不能再做手术了，于是前来寻求生命修复的中医药治疗。他很认真的服药，并坚持做治疗，肿瘤很快被控制并逐渐消失了。

脂肪肉瘤是一种恶性程度很高的软组织肿瘤，生长快速，复发率高，即使再次手术，也仍有很大风险，更加上腹腔已有大量转移，是非常危险的。宋先生用生命修复治疗取得了很好的治疗效果。

治疗原则

解毒化浊，软坚散结。

常用中药

1. 薏苡仁、土茯苓、牡蛎、鳖甲、重楼、没药、蜈蚣、猫爪草、夏枯草等。
2. 同时服用消瘤丸。

影像学、病理学检查报告及诊疗记录

1. 2021 年 7 月 21 日检查报告显示腹腔肿瘤大量转移，并达 9cm 之大。

2. 2021 年 8 月 11 日报告证实，宋先生长期吸烟，患有糖尿病、冠心病。2016 年恶性肿瘤切除后复发。再次手术前评估并发症后心脏状态，考虑做心脏介入治疗。

附：患者检查报告

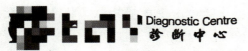 **Diagnostic Centre** 诊断中心

COPY

Report to	: Dr. ■■ ■■		
Name	: SUNG, ■ 宋■		
HKID/Passport	: ■ ■	Age/Sex	: 59Y/M
Date	: 21/07/2021	Other Ref.	:
Our Ref.	: ■■■	Ref.	:

CLINICAL INFORMATION: Suspected recurrent abdominal sarcoma.

EQUIPMENT: GE Discovery IQ Gen2 Clarity Edition PETCT System with 16-slice CT.

TECHNIQUE: Attenuation corrected coronal, axial and sagittal PET scans and CT scan were obtained from base of skull to the upper thigh 1 hour after 9.5 mCi of F18-FDG was injected via the right hand. Blood glucose level prior to injection was 8.1mmol/l.

REPORT:

<u>**Whole Body PET-CT Scan:**</u>
No previous imaging is available for comparison.

<u>**Abdomen & Pelvis:**</u>
Background liver uptake = SUVmean 2.2
At the left side of the peritoneum (including the perirenal space) there are multiple soft tissue masses measuring upto 9cm with SUVmax upto 2.7. There is some associated peritoneal stranding with coarse calcifications. Features are suggestive of peritoneal metastases. The largest nodule is in direct contact with the posterior surface of the left kidney and renal origin could also be considered.

The right kidney is of normal shape. No hydronephrosis or hydroureter is found.

There is no hypermetabolic node found at the pelvis or abdomen.
No ascites or peritoneal deposit is found.

The liver is not enlarged. No focal hypermetabolic hepatic lesion is present. The biliary tract is not dilated. The gallbladder is unremarkable.

Dr. ■■■
Specialist in Radiology
MBChB (Birm), BMedSc (Hons), FRCR,
FHKCR, FHKAM (Radiology)

Page 1 of 3

Medical and Endoscopy Centre
■ ■醫療及內視鏡中心

MBChB, MD, FRCSEd, FCSHK, FHKAM(Surgery)

To :
From :
11th August, 2021

Dear ■■■

Re : **SUNG** ■ ■■■ ■ ■■■ ■ ■

Please kindly assess Mr Sung for fitness for major surgery +/- pre-op intervention for optimization.

Mr Sung is a chronic smoker, also known to have DM and IHD. He was diagnosed to have retro-peritoneal sarcoma with resection in 2016. The disease was known to have recurred and grew slowly.

After recent assessment, the patient and family are considering debulking surgery for the tumour. Please assess if pre-op cardiac intervention is indicated.

Thank you.

Remarks:

Regards,

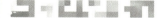

病案 **33**

颅脑肿瘤康复 19 年

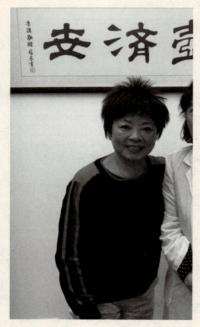
🔊 许女士 2024 年 1 月前来诊治时合影留念

2005 年，许女士 52 岁，当时的她长期头痛、眼痛，并且越来越重，以后又出现经常恶心、视力减退、走路常失去平衡并且摔倒。经在医院做病理学检查，发现是脑肿瘤，为脑膜瘤和硬脑膜肿瘤，许女士得知需要做脑部手术以切除肿瘤，但这种肿瘤非常容易复发，她非常恐惧，急忙前来治疗。

当时她的精神状态很差，记忆力下降很快，还伴有严重失眠。来诊后，她坚持服药，经过 2 年治疗后，她的情况良好。脑膜瘤是一种很容易复发的颅脑肿瘤，经过生命修复的治疗后，19 年了，许女士的脑肿瘤都没有复发。如今她每天都神采奕奕，还在她的花园中种了许多植物，如蔬菜和花草等，并经常送给亲朋好友。

治疗原则

扶阳补肾，软坚消瘤。

常用中药

1. 制附片、蜥蜴、肉桂、牡蛎、杜仲、续断、海藻、夏枯草等。
2. 同时服用消瘤丸。

影像学、病理学检查报告及诊疗记录

1. 2006 年 11 月 22 日病理检查报告证实为脑膜瘤。
2. 2022 年 12 月 23 日 MRI 检查报告证实无肿瘤复发。

附：患者检查报告

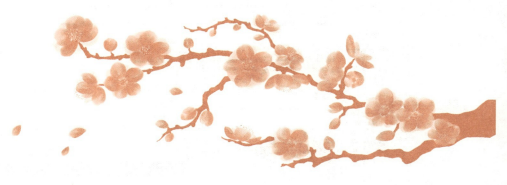

治癌实录续新

Department of Pathology and Clinical Biochemistry
Hospital, Hong Kong

Histopathology

Lab No:

HKID No:	
Name:	HUI,
Hosp No:	
DOB:	22/01/1953
Sex/Age:	F/53Y
Ref:	

Hospital:	Hospital
Unit/Ward/Bed:	QMH/NEU/A7 / 04
Request Loc:	QMH/NEU/A7
Requesting Dr:	

Date Requested: 22/11/06
Date Arrived: 22/11/06

Final Report

COPY

CLINICAL HISTORY:
Right clinoidal meningioma. Presented with headaches. MRI shows a 2 cm in diameter tumour.

PRE-OPERATIVE DIAGNOSIS/OPERATION:
Meningioma.

SPECIMEN(S):
(A) Brain tumour; (B) Dura.

GROSS EXAMINATION:
(A) Received is a lobulated tan-coloured tumour which measures 1.5 x 1.5 x 1 cm. Focally it appears to be covered by dura. Bisected and all embedded. 2 blocks.

(B) Received is a piece of tan-coloured firm tissue which measures 1.5 x 0.7 cm in area and 0.7 cm in thickness. All embedded. 1 block.

MICROSCOPIC EXAMINATION:
(A) Sections show a meningioma of which the tumour cells are arranged in lobules or whorls. The tumour cells show mildly pleomorphic, round or oval nuclei containing fine chromatin pattern, inconspicuous or small nucleoli. Mitotic figures are infrequent. Frequently identified within the tumour lobules are bright eosinophilic globules of pseudopsammoma bodies present in intracellular lumina. Adjacent brain tissue is seen focally but tumour invasion is not seen. The pseudopsammoma bodies are strongly periodic acid-Schiff (PAS) positive and diastase resistant.

Immunohistochemical stains show the tumour cells are positive for epithelial membrane antigen and the tumour cells surrounding the pseudopsammoma bodies are positive for cytokeratin CamS.2 and polyclonal carcinoembryonic antigen (CEA).

The overall features are consistent with secretory meningioma (WHO grade I).

(B) Sections show a piece of dura mater with tiny foci of detached meningothelial cells.

DIAGNOSIS:
(A) BRAIN, tumour; biopsy - Secretory MENINGIOMA (WHO grade I).
(B) DURA, biopsy - MORPHOLOGICAL DESCRIPTION ONLY.

Reported by:
Authorized by:

Report Destination: QMH/--/A7 - A7, Surgery, QMH
Reported on: 28/11/06 16:03
Printed on: 29/11/06 10:12

2 9 NOV 2006

Page No: 1/1

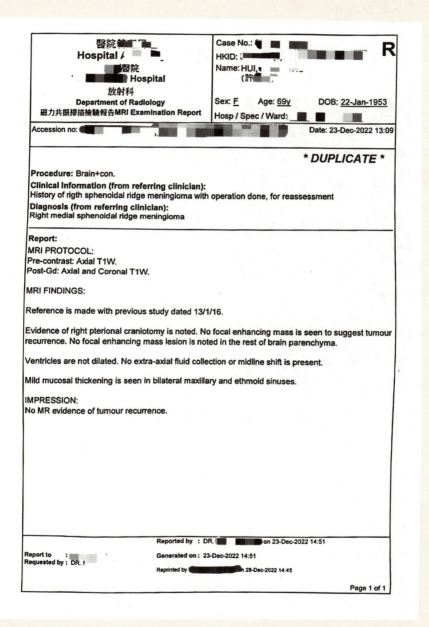

醫院 ███ ███
Hospital ███ ██
██ ██院
██████ **Hospital**
放射科
Department of Radiology
磁力共振掃描檢驗報告MRI Examination Report

Case No.: ███ ███
HKID: ███ ██████
Name: HUI, ██ ████
(許 ██)

Sex: **F**   Age: **69y**   DOB: **22-Jan-1953**

Hosp / Spec / Ward: ██ ██

R

Accession no: ████████████

Date: 23-Dec-2022 13:09

* DUPLICATE *

Procedure: Brain+con.

Clinical Information (from referring clinician):
History of rigth sphenoidal ridge meningioma with operation done, for reassessment

Diagnosis (from referring clinician):
Right medial sphenoidal ridge meningioma

Report:
MRI PROTOCOL:
Pre-contrast: Axial T1W.
Post-Gd: Axial and Coronal T1W.

MRI FINDINGS:

Reference is made with previous study dated 13/1/16.

Evidence of right pterional craniotomy is noted. No focal enhancing mass is seen to suggest tumour recurrence. No focal enhancing mass lesion is noted in the rest of brain parenchyma.

Ventricles are not dilated. No extra-axial fluid collection or midline shift is present.

Mild mucosal thickening is seen in bilateral maxillary and ethmoid sinuses.

IMPRESSION:
No MR evidence of tumour recurrence.

Report to   : ███
Requested by : DR. ██

Reported by : DR. ███ ████ on 23-Dec-2022 14:51

Generated on : 23-Dec-2022 14:51

Reprinted by ████████ n 28-Dec-2022 14:45

Page 1 of 1

229

病案 34

晚期胆管癌肝转移康复 17 年

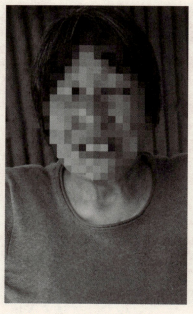

🔊 赵太太 2022 年 4 月拍照留念

赵太太今年 81 岁了，在家照看孙儿，忙里忙外，任谁也看不出她曾是晚期癌症患者，更想不到她的癌症是非常险恶的，是俗称"癌王"的胆管癌。

17 年前，也就是从 2006 年年初开始，赵太太常感右侧肋部、腹部疼痛，去医院检查后，医生告知她有胆管炎，需要消炎治疗，但治疗后疼痛还是越来越严重。2006 年 5 月，她去医院做了胆囊切除手术，心想手术后应该很快就能痊愈，但事与愿违。她右侧腹部与肋部的疼痛没有因做了手术而缓解，反而逐渐加重，常常痛得不能睡觉，也不能吃饭。

无奈之下，2006 年 9 月儿子再次带她去医院做详细检查，其中 CT 检查，诊断为胆管癌，并因拖延了时间，已经发生了肝脏的转移。医院说因她年岁已高，又已发生肝转移，故目前没有什么良好的治疗方法。赵太太疼痛越来越重，伴随而来的是频繁发热，逐渐出现黄疸症状，并很快加重。医生建议先做个支架暂时缓解一下，并解释说，这样可使胆汁流出更畅顺一点，暂时缓解黄疸。除此之外，已无法可医。于是在 2006 年 12 月 30 日行胆道支架手术。

术后赵太太的症状未见明显好转，万般无奈之下，只能求助于生命修复治疗。2007 年 1 月 9 日，赵太太的儿子带她前来就诊。当时她有全身严重黄疸、腹痛严重、不停呻吟、气短不续和下肢水肿的症状。治疗 1 年后再次做 CT 等检查，显示肝内转移灶已全部消失。如今过去了 17 年，赵太太虽然已 81 岁高龄，但身体状况良好，不仅包揽着全部家务还照料着孙儿。

胆管癌素有"癌中之王"的称呼，赵太太发病急，疼痛严重，黄疸持续加重，并反复感染发热，再加上已发生肝转移，十分危险。生命修复的中医药治疗，取得了非常理想的治疗效果。

解毒化湿，祛邪消瘤。

常用中药

1. 党参、丹参、田基黄、猪苓、虎杖、全蝎、蜈蚣、鳖甲、延胡索、田七、茵陈等。
2. 同时服用消瘤丸。

影像学、病理学检查报告及诊疗记录

1. 2006 年 12 月 21 日检查报告显示胆管癌胆管堵塞并发肝脏转移。

2. 2007 年 12 月 13 日检查报告显示肝脏转移病灶等完全消失。

附：患者检查报告

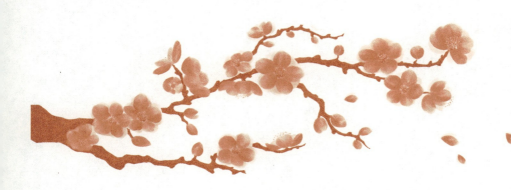

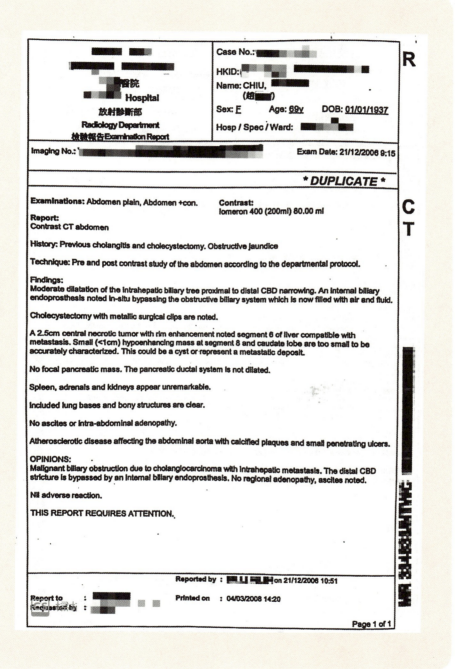

	Case No.: ▓▓▓▓
	HKID: ▓▓▓▓
医院 Hospital	Name: CHIU, ▓▓ (赵▓▓)
放射診斷部 Radiology Department 檢驗報告 Examination Report	Sex: _F_ Age: _69y_ DOB: _01/01/1937_ Hosp / Spec / Ward: ▓▓▓

Imaging No.: ▓▓▓▓▓▓▓   Exam Date: 21/12/2006 9:15

* DUPLICATE *

C
T

Examinations: Abdomen plain, Abdomen +con.   **Contrast:** Iomeron 400 (200ml) 80.00 ml

Report:
Contrast CT abdomen

History: Previous cholangitis and cholecystectomy. Obstructive jaundice

Technique: Pre and post contrast study of the abdomen according to the departmental protocol.

Findings:
Moderate dilatation of the intrahepatic biliary tree proximal to distal CBD narrowing. An internal biliary endoprosthesis noted in-situ bypassing the obstructive biliary system which is now filled with air and fluid.

Cholecystectomy with metallic surgical clips are noted.

A 2.5cm central necrotic tumor with rim enhancement noted segment 6 of liver compatible with metastasis. Small (<1cm) hypoenhancing mass at segment 8 and caudate lobe are too small to be accurately characterized. This could be a cyst or represent a metastatic deposit.

No focal pancreatic mass. The pancreatic ductal system is not dilated.

Spleen, adrenals and kidneys appear unremarkable.

Included lung bases and bony structures are clear.

No ascites or intra-abdominal adenopathy.

Atherosclerotic disease affecting the abdominal aorta with calcified plaques and small penetrating ulcers.

OPINIONS:
Malignant biliary obstruction due to cholangiocarcinoma with intrahepatic metastasis. The distal CBD stricture is bypassed by an internal biliary endoprosthesis. No regional adenopathy, ascites noted.

Nil adverse reaction.

THIS REPORT REQUIRES ATTENTION.

Reported by : ▓▓ U ▓▓ on 21/12/2006 10:51

Report to : ▓▓▓ ▓ ▓   Printed on   : 04/03/2008 14:20
Requested by :

Page 1 of 1

医院
Hospital
放射診斷部
Radiology Department
檢驗報告 **Examination Report**

Case No.:
HKID:
Name: CHIU,
(趙　　)
Sex: F　　Age: **70y**　　DOB: **01/01/1937**
Hosp / Spec / Ward:

R

Imaging No.:　　　　　　　　　　　　　　　Exam Date: 13/12/2007 9:45

* DUPLICATE *

**C
T**

Examinations: Abdomen plain, Abdomen +con.　　**Contrast:**
Iomeron 400 (200ml) 80.00 ml

Report:
CT SCAN ABDOMEN

CLINICAL HISTORY :
Previous cholangitis and cholecystectomy.
Radiological diagnosis of cholangiocarcinoma with liver metastasis treated with chemotherapy.

TECHNIQUES :
Noncontrast and triple phase postcontrast study

FINDINGS :
A metallic biliary stent is in-situ astride distal common duct and second part of duodenum. The biliary tract
is partially decompressed and the common duct measures 17mm in maximal width. Pneumobilia is still
present, mostly in the left lobe of liver.
The previously noted nodule in segment VI of liver cannot be discerned in current study, suggestive of
regression.
The small cysts in segments IV and VIII show no interval change in appearance. There is no newly arised
hepatic mass.
The portal veins are patent.
Pancreas, spleen and adrenal glands are normal.
The left renal artery is occluded with thrombi and the left kidney is small with absence of normal
perfusion. This is a recent development since last CT scan. The right kidney is normal.
No ascites or intra-abdominal adenopathy is discerned.

OPINIONS:
The previously noted intrahepatic metastasis has regressed completely on imaging.
Thrombi in left renal artery causing chronic infarction and atrophy of left kidney.

ADVERSE REACTION:
Nil reported.

Reported by :　　　　　　　　on 13/12/2007 11:41

Report to　　:
Requested by　　　　Printed on　: 26/02/2008 10:08

Page 1 of 1

病案 35、36

夫妻抗癌康复 18 年

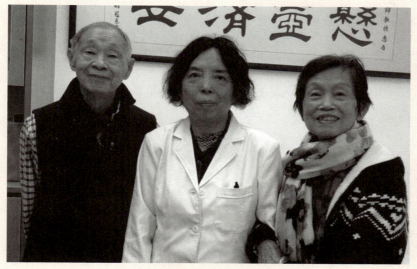

❶ 赵先生与太太于 2022 年 12 月前来诊治时合影留念

从 2007 年开始，赵先生就一直陪着太太看病。当时赵太太得了胃癌，经过手术切除了一半多有癌变的胃，后来又做了化疗和放疗。之后他们夫妻和儿女都以为没有事了。但是过了 3 年，赵太太又诊断出了肠道癌。当时医生说，在这种情况下，她的生命大概也就只能维持半年到 1 年的时间，并会很快发生肝转移。当时赵太太身体非常虚弱，不停地呕吐，只要一进食就会呕吐出来。随后又经常不停地咳嗽、胸痛，发现有肺部的转移。医院里都认为已经走到了最后的关头，但是赵太太没有放弃，她坚持每周都来我们这里做治疗，赵先生每次也都陪着她前来。

经过了数月的治疗之后，她逐渐好转了。当时医院已经下了病危通知，但是经过我们的治疗之后，赵太太每天都在好转。慢慢地，她的精神越来越好了，进食也越来越正常，不再出现呕吐，并且严重的腹痛也越来越少，直至最后完全没有腹痛症状了。直到现在，她已经康复了18年，生活得非常快乐和健康。18年来她到医院只是做常规的检查，了解身体状况，但从来没有吃过其他药物。现在她还能每天早上去游泳，锻炼身体。这对于一位86岁的老人来说，真的是很不容易的。

当时还没有发现疾病的赵先生，一直陪着他太太看病，按理说，应该对中医药、对我们的治疗有相当的了解和认识。很不幸地，他在2018年也得了病。他的身体出现了大大小小的肿瘤，多次检查后，都无法确定肿瘤的来源，随后经过病理学和组织学检查，确诊为恶性淋巴瘤。赵先生对于中医药治疗有很好的认识，他本应该及早地选择前来治疗，但是他在自己生病以后却没有这么想，他认为太太的病是在无法可医，走投无路的情况下才来治疗的。而他自己的病暂时没有到走投无路的程度，并认为现代医学是最先进的，应该用现代化的方法治好自己。于是他积极的到医院里去进行最好、最新的化疗、靶向和免疫治疗，坚信这样就能够消除全身的肿瘤。但经过1年左右的治疗，病情加重，事与愿违。

他先是做化疗，及后又做靶向治疗，经过 1 年左右的治疗，再次做检查时发现有个别地方的肿瘤缩小了，但是在头部和颈部又出现了很多新的肿瘤，特别是在颈部和锁骨上，就连腹股沟的区域也出现了很多肿瘤，腰椎也有肿瘤细胞的扩展和浸润，这使他每日都非常痛苦。在这种情况下，赵先生又转到私人医院继续治疗，并按照医生的建议，选择了当今抗癌更先进和更高级的免疫治疗。但是肿瘤仍然没有得到控制，癌指数上升的更快，他的身体越加虚弱。同时还出现发热、腹痛、腹胀、全血细胞降低、血小板降低等毒副作用。经过多次的靶向和免疫治疗之后，赵先生感觉到身体太虚弱了，确实无法再坚持下去了。他对每次陪伴他去医院的女儿说，他不想再做化疗、靶向和免疫治疗了，他想来我们这里。

自此以后，赵先生就到我们的诊所来治疗，吃中药、做针灸，随后他的身体逐渐恢复。他刚来的时候，即便穿着高领衣服，两侧颈部苹果大小的肿瘤，大家也都看得非常清楚。随后肿瘤逐渐地缩小直至消失。他的癌指数一直很高，大多在 400 多居高不下，即使在接受免疫治疗、靶向治疗的时候，也一直降不下来。经过生命修复的治疗，他的癌指数明显降低并逐渐正常。对此并不信服的医生也不得不承认事实，连说非常神奇。

现在，赵先生已经恢复了正常的生活，并在继续巩固效果的治疗中。他太太常陪他一起来，每次都很高兴，心情舒畅，并反复感叹造福大众的传统中医药学的伟大与神奇。

赵太太治疗原则

解毒化浊，祛邪治癌。

常用中药

1. 白头翁、蜂房、浙贝母、半枝莲、土茯苓、败酱草、夏枯草、蒲公英等。
2. 同时服用散结丸。

赵先生治疗原则

扶阳驱毒，散结消瘤。

常用中药

1. 制附子、吴茱萸、补骨脂、鹿茸、猫爪草、山慈菇、桃仁、红花、大黄等。
2. 同时服用消瘤丸。

影像学、病理学检查报告及诊疗记录

赵太太

1. 2006 年 10 月 31 日胃癌切除手术的病理报告，证实为胃低分化腺癌。

2. 2009 年 7 月第二种癌症，做肠癌手术后病理报告，为肠中分化腺癌，分期为 PT_3N_1 第Ⅲ期有淋巴转移。

赵先生

1. 2018 年 7 月 11 日病理检查报告证实为 B 细胞恶性淋巴瘤。

2. 2018 年 11 月 8 日检查报告证实，虽然经过化疗、靶向、免疫等治疗，但是恶性淋巴瘤增多、增大，全身出现大量新的肿瘤。

3. 2020 年 7 月 28 日检查报告显示经生命修复治疗后全身大量恶性淋巴瘤消失，治疗效果很好。

附：患者检查报告

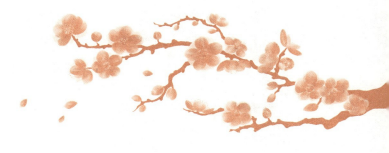

239

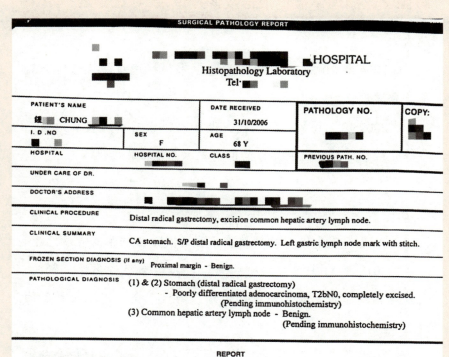

SURGICAL PATHOLOGY REPORT

HOSPITAL

Histopathology Laboratory
Tel·

PATIENT'S NAME	DATE RECEIVED	PATHOLOGY NO.	COPY:
鍾 CHUNG	31/10/2006		

I. D .NO	SEX F	AGE 68 Y	

HOSPITAL	HOSPITAL NO.	CLASS	PREVIOUS PATH. NO.

UNDER CARE OF DR.

DOCTOR'S ADDRESS

CLINICAL PROCEDURE

Distal radical gastrectomy, excision common hepatic artery lymph node.

CLINICAL SUMMARY

CA stomach. S/P distal radical gastrectomy. Left gastric lymph node mark with stitch.

FROZEN SECTION DIAGNOSIS (if any)   Proximal margin - Benign.

PATHOLOGICAL DIAGNOSIS

(1) & (2) Stomach (distal radical gastrectomy)
- Poorly differentiated adenocarcinoma, T2bN0, completely excised.
(Pending immunohistochemistry)
(3) Common hepatic artery lymph node - Benign.
(Pending immunohistochemistry)

REPORT

Macroscopic examination:

(1) "Proximal margin" - A light-brown piece of tissue 3.2 x 1.4 x 0.7 cm.

(2) "Distal stomach" - Specimen consisted of distal stomach, lesser curve 11 cm. long, greater curve 14.2 cm. long, proximal margin 5 cm. in diameter, distal margin 1.5 cm. in diameter, cut-open before receipt. The serosal surfaces were indurated at the greater curve. 5.2 cm. from the distal margin was an ulcerated light-brown firm tumour 2.2 x 1.6 cm. in area, 0.2 cm. deep with necrotic base. Cut surfaces showed infiltration into thickened muscular wall (1.2 cm. thick), adjacent to the greater curve posteriorly. Greater omental fat measured 21 x 19.5 x 1.5 cm., lesser curve fat 9.3 x 3.7 x 1.4 cm. There were eight proximal lesser curve lymph nodes adjacent to the stitch on the lesser curve, largest 0.7 x 0.3 x 0.2 cm., smallest 0.2 cm. in diameter, and twelve distal greater curve lymph nodes, largest 1.2 x 0.8 x 0.4 cm. and smallest 0.2 cm. in diameter.

(3) "Common hepatic artery lymph node" - A brownish-yellow piece of tissue 2.1 x 1.3 x 0.4 cm. with four lymph nodes, largest 1.3 x 0.6 x 0.5 cm. and smallest 0.3 x 0.2 x 0.1 cm.

Microscopic examination:

(1) Paraffin section confirms the frozen section diagnosis and shows gastric mucosa without dysplasia or malignancy.

(PLEASE TURN OVERLEAF)

■HOSPITAL

ANATOMICAL CELLULAR PATHOLOGY

S

CHUNG.   Ward PWH/SUR/11EF - DISCHARGED   F/71Y

Date Collected: 30/07/09 11:00   By:
Date Arrived: 30/07/09 12:42

the muscularis propria. Serosa is not involved. Resection margins, including the apical mesenteric, circumferential, proximal and distal margins are clear. Two out of 14 paracolic lymph nodes show metastasis. The 10 apical and 9 ileal lymph nodes are negative for malignancy.
The perforation site at the base of appendix is noted and accompany with abscess formation and inflamed fibrosing granulation tissue. No malignant gland is seen at the perforation site. A sessile serrated adenoma is noted at the tip of appendix.

DIAGNOSIS
Right hemicolectomy:
-Moderately-differentiated Adenocarcinoma of cecum.
-Invades through muscularis propria.
-Serosa is not involved.
-Two out of 33 lymph nodes show metastasis.
-Resection margins are clear.
-pT3N1.
-Perforation at base of appendix with abscess and granulation tissue formation.
-Sessile serrated adenoma of appendix noted.

Pathology Report   Authorized By: ■ ■■■■■   06/08/09 10:29
                       *** This Laboratory is NATA & RCPA accredited ***

                       ********** End of report **********

Report Destination: ■ ■■ ■■■

13/07/18 ·08:08PM ▩ 頁面 2

7/13/2018 17:08:14 PAGE 2/002 Fax Server

醫 院
HOSPITAL

Histopathology

Name : 趙██CHIU ██	Ward/Bed :
Sex/Age : M/81 Y	Doctor:
Patient No :	Specimen Received: 11/07/2018
Episode No. :	Lab Episode No.

HISTOPATHOLOGY REPORT

Accession No.

Specimen
Right retrocrural lymph node biopsy

Clinical Summary
? Lymphoma

Gross Description
Four cores, 7 mm, 11 mm, 11 mm and 12 mm in length, each 0.5 mm in width, all embedded in block (A). (NMH)

Microscopic Description
Section shows cores of lymph node tissue and extranodal soft tissue involved by sheets and focal nodules comprising small lymphoid cells. Extension to extranodal soft tissue is seen. Immunohistochemically, the abnormal lymphoid cells are positive for CD20 and negative for CD5, CD23 and cyclin D1. In-situ hybridization shows kappa light chain restriction.

Diagnosis
Right retrocrural lymph node biopsy
- Malignant lymphoma, consistent with B cell lymphoma.
- Further immunostains (some are performed in other laboratory) are in progress and a supplementary comment will follow.

Copy to ██ ██ ██

H I S T O P A T H O L O G Y

Print Date : 13/07/2018 15:56
Page 1 of 1

Histopathology

DISCHARGED PATIENT

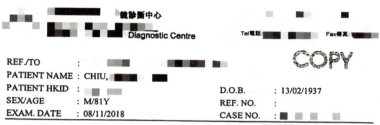

REF./TO : ▮▮▮ ▮▮▮ ▮

COPY

PATIENT NAME : CHIU, ▮▮▮ ▮▮

PATIENT HKID : ▮▮ ▮▮▮▮   D.O.B. : 13/02/1937

SEX/AGE : M/81Y   REF. NO. :

EXAM. DATE : 08/11/2018   CASE NO. : ▮ ▮ ▮ ▮

RADIOLOGY REPORT

18F-FDG PET-CT WHOLE BODY (PLAIN)

CLINICAL HISTORY: Follicular lymphoma. On rituximab done. ? Response.

IMAGING FACTORS:

PET Radiopharmaceutical	8.0 mCi of 18F-FDG IVI
Fasting Blood Glucose Level	5.3 mmol/L
Uptake Time	60 minutes
Body Region Cover (CT)	Dedicated PET-CT diagnostic images from the skull base to the groin
Post-processing	PET, CT & Fusion images reconstructed in axial, coronal and sagittal
SUVmax References	Normal liver: 2.59 ; Mediastinal blood-pool: 1.46

COMPARATIVE STUDY: Whole Body PET-CT on 10.07.2018 (▮ ▮▮ Hospital)

REPORT:

Nodes

Known lymphoma has progressive metabolic disease with increased sizes, number and FDG-avidity of the nodes. There are multiple new FDG-avid nodes at both sides of the diaphragm. Previous infra diaphragmatic nodal disease have increased sizes and metabolism. Their SUVmax were lastly up to 16.5 and now up to 22.03.

- For head and neck regions, multiple new FDG-avid bilateral cervical and bilateral (L>R) supraclavicular nodes with SUVmax up to 11.84 are present. Waldeyer's ring, both parotid, pre-auricular and occipital nodal stations are spared.
- For thoracic region, new hypermetabolic bilateral level I axillary (L>R), left sided mediastinal, bilateral interlobar and right lower posterior sub visceral pleural nodes have SUVmax up to 13.95. Bilateral internal mammary nodes are spared.
- For abdominal to groin regions, known extensive upper to lower retroperitoneal nodes are metabolically worsened. Their SUVmax are increased from 16.5 to 22.03. They are also larger with new extension into right L2/3 foramen with near spinal canal invasion. Extranodal penetration into L2 vertebral body causes new mild fracture collapse. New FDG-avid mesenteric, porta hepatis, portocaval, gastrohepatic, right common iliac, and bilateral external iliac nodes are found. Both groins and femoral nodes are spared.

Extranodal

FDG-avidity at proximal ascending colon is worsened with SUVmax increased from 4.9 to 12.62, considered as extranodal disease.

Spleen measures 109 mm in longest dimension. Liver measures 167 mm in vertical span at right mid-clavicular line. Liver and spleen show diffuse physiological activity with no focal FDG-avid lesion.

Rest of the bone marrows in imaged skeleton then show physiological FDG distribution.

243

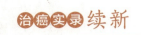

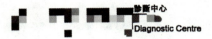 診斷中心
Diagnostic Centre

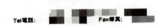 Tel電話: Fax傳真:

REF./TO :

PATIENT NAME : CHIU,

PATIENT HKID :   D.O.B. : 13/02/1937

SEX/AGE : M/81Y   REF. NO. :

EXAM. DATE : 08/11/2018   CASE NO. :

RADIOLOGY REPORT

It is overall progressive metabolic disease (Deauville score 5) and Ann Arbor stage IV (colon and L2 marrow).

Others
Skull Base and Neck
Physiological uptakes over scanned part of the brain and skull base.
No abnormal soft tissue uptake in nasopharynx, tonsil, hypopharynx or larynx.
Fossae of RosenMuller are symmetrical. Paranasal sinuses are clear.
Pharyngeal lymphoid FDG activity are within physiological limits. No focal FDG-avid thyroid lesion.

Thorax
No metabolic or CT evidence of pulmonary involvement. No pleural effusion seen.
Bilateral post infective changes with scars, atelectasis and calcified granulomata are non FDG-avid.
No FDG-avid lesion at oesophagus. Mild cardiomegaly. No pericardial effusion.

Abdomen and Pelvis
No calcified gallstone. Intrahepatic ducts and common duct are not dilated.
No FDG-avid mass can be seen at the ampulla, adrenals, pancreas and spleen.
Rest of gastrointestinal FDG activity within physiological limits. No intestinal dilatation on CT.
Excretory FDG activity in urinary system within physiological limits. No obstructive uropathy or renal stone seen.
No focal FDG-avid lesion in the prostate and seminal vesicles. Prostatic enlargement noted.
No sizable FDG-avid peritoneal, omental or mesenteric deposit. No ascites. No abdominal aortic aneurysm.

The parameters of the mentioned lesions are summarized as below:

Site	LD x PD (mm)	SUVmax
R level II cervical LN	15.0 x 8.5	9.76
L supraclavicular LN	19.1 x 15.7	11.84
L level I axillary LN	12.3 x 8.6	4.32
L mid-para oesophageal LN	8.3 x 6.5	6.67
RLZ pleura	19.9 x 14.6	13.95
R retrocrural LN	74.1 x 35.3	22.03
L para-aortic LN	69.8 x 45.1	16.65
Aortocaval LN	79.0 x 47.1	19.79
R common iliac LN	28.7 x 20.6	19.96
Ascending colon	-	12.62
L2 body and right L2/3 foramen	-	-
Liver background	167.2	2.59
Spleen background	109.0	2.00

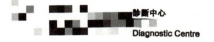 诊断中心
Diagnostic Centre

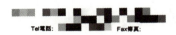

Tel電話: Fax傳真:

REF./TO   :

PATIENT NAME : CHIU,

PATIENT HKID :   D.O.B.   : 13/02/1937

SEX/AGE   : M/81Y   REF. NO.   :

EXAM. DATE   : 08/11/2018   CASE NO.   :

RADIOLOGY REPORT

(SUV = Standardized Uptake Value; LD = largest diameter; PD = perpendicular diameter)

IMPRESSION:

- Known lymphoma has progressive metabolic disease with increased sizes, number and FDG-avidity of the nodes. There are multiple new FDG-avid nodes at both sides of the diaphragm. Previous infra diaphragmatic nodal disease have increased sizes and metabolism. Known extensive upper to lower retroperitoneal nodes are metabolically worsened. They are also larger with new extension into right L2/3 foramen with near spinal canal invasion. Extranodal penetration into L2 vertebral body causes new mild fracture collapse.
- FDG-avidity at proximal ascending colon is worsened, considered as extranodal disease.
- New mild hepatomegaly is present. Normal splenic sizes. Liver, spleen and rest of the marrow (except L2) have no focal FDG-avid lesion.
- It is overall progressive metabolic disease (Deauville score 5).
- Ann Arbor stage IV (colon and L2 marrow).

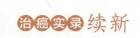

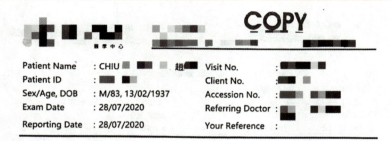

Patient Name	: CHIU 　　　趙	Visit No.	:
Patient ID	:	Client No.	:
Sex/Age, DOB	: M/83, 13/02/1937	Accession No.	:
Exam Date	: 28/07/2020	Referring Doctor	:
Reporting Date	: 28/07/2020	Your Reference	:

PET-CT WHOLE BODY (PLAIN AND CONTRAST)

Musculoskeletal

Diffuse prominent uptake is seen throughout the skeleton, could be due to marrow hyperplasia and recent intake of colony-stimulating factors.

Decrease in FDG uptake is seen in the lower thoracic and lumbar spine, could be due to previous irradiation. Collapse of L2, L3 and L4 vertebral bodies is seen. This appears more marked as compared with previous scan.

No other focal hypermetabolic bony lesion is otherwise seen. No lytic or sclerotic density is seen in the scanned skeleton.

IMPRESSION

- As compared with previous PET-CT scan on 08.02.2020, the hypermetabolic lymphadenopathies in the neck have metabolically resolved.
- Minimally active lymph nodes are again seen in the left interlobar region and the right hilar region, similar to previous scan. These are non-specific.
- The hypermetabolic mesenteric lymphadenopathies noted previously show reduction in size and metabolic activity.
- Mildly prominent uptakes are seen in bilateral adrenal glands, appears less masses as compared with previous scan.
- Diffuse prominent uptake is seen throughout the skeleton, probably due to marrow hyperplasia and recent intake of colony-stimulating factors.
- Collapsed L2, L3 and L4 vertebral bodies are seen.
- Overall features indicate good response to treatment.

(Electronic signature)

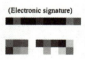

Authorized and Reported: 28/07/2020 01:16:42 PM
Printed: 29/07/2020 10:10:57 AM
Daisy Ng

子宫内膜癌双侧卵巢盆腔等转移康复

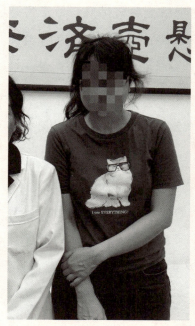

🎧 刘女士 2023 年 12 月前来诊治时合影留念

　　刘女士身体一直很健康，不仅经常晨练，有时还会带女儿去爬山或者全家三口在假期时去旅行，一家人其乐融融。但在 2016 年年初，刘女士 37 岁时，常感腹部不适并可触摸到肿块，丈夫陪她去医院检查，发现了左侧卵巢癌，并于 2016 年 5 月行左侧卵巢癌切除手术，医生说为了切的彻底一些，需要将左侧输卵管附件一并切除，以防复发。手术后她身体在逐渐恢复中，认为肿瘤已全部切除了，从此平安无事，可以好好安心过日子了。但天有不测风云，2019 年年初，手术后刚 3 年，她又时常感到腹部不适，月经失调，急去医院检查，发现了右侧卵巢癌，于 2019 年 6 月开始做放疗，希望可以控制病情，但是治疗无效，肿瘤生长迅速。2020 年 7 月检查时发现腹部隆起肿瘤已达 11cm，2020 年 8 月再次进行手术，将盆腔所有附件子宫全部切除。经过 2 次大手术后，尽管刘女士身体虚弱了很多，但在手术后的恢复期中，医生就要求尽快做化疗。刘女士问可否晚些再做，因为体力很差担心不能承受，遭到医生严词拒绝，还告诉她这种情况非常危险，很快就会出现全身大量转移，危及生命。医院和医生明确讲明：她患的是子宫内膜癌，并且：1.已侵犯到大部分的子宫基层以及子宫浆膜层；2.有大量严重的淋巴血管浸润，盆腔淋巴转移，并已有严重的双侧卵巢转移，虽双侧卵巢已手术切除，但原发病灶在子宫（因开始并未发现子宫的问题，在第2次手术分别切除双侧卵巢及子宫后，才发现子宫是原发的罪魁祸首），全部盆腔淋巴血管都有大量转移，如果不做化疗，后果是不可想象的。

因刘女士十分惧怕化疗所带来的各种可怕的副作用，故转向我们的生命修复中医药治疗寻求帮助。刘女士刚来的时候身体非常虚弱，腹部手术虽然瘢痕累累，但仍可摸到多个色块，并且伴有严重疼痛，不思饮食，经常恶心，经分析后给予扶正祛邪，软坚驱毒的治疗方法，逐渐好转，面色红润，进食逐渐恢复正常，腹部色块彻底消失，腹痛减轻至消失，精神面貌焕然一新。她自2020年10月来诊，在大约1年的时间中认真服药治疗，以后自以为无事，因疫情故半年没有来看诊。后又继续前来看诊，继续服药，目前她的身体状况良好，经复查至今没有复发。

治疗原则

扶正祛邪，软坚散结，化瘀去毒。

常用中药

1. 黄芪、续断、当归、土鳖虫、枳实、白芍、桂枝、全蝎、白花蛇等。
2. 同时服用消瘤丸、攻毒散。

影像学、病理学检查报告及诊疗记录

2020 年 8 月 21 日第 2 次手术病理检查报告证实为子宫内膜癌，并有淋巴血管侵入。

附：患者检查报告

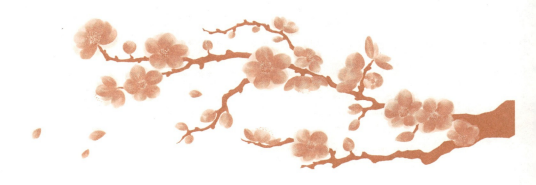

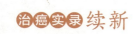

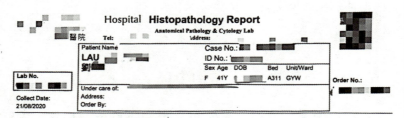

Hospital **Histopathology Report**

Anatomical Pathology & Cytology Lab

Address:

Patient Name	Case No.:
LAU	ID No.:
劉	Sex Age DOB Bed Unit/Ward
	F 41Y A311 GYW

Lab No.

Under care of:

Address:

Collect Date:
21/08/2020

Order By:

Order No.:

CLINICAL SUMMARY & PROCEDURE
Recurrent CA ovary
Conservative LSO and staging 2016 received
Gold grain implant 2019 Rt ovarian tumour
Clinical diagnosis: Recurrent Ca ovary

PATHOLOGY DIAGNOSIS
A. Right ovary, right tube and uterus, total hysterectomy and right salpingo-oophorectomy:
- Right OVARY: ENDOMETRIOID ADENOCARCINOMA 子宮內膜樣腺癌, Grade 2; capsule opened, but
no tumour seen on capsular surface; lymphovascular invasion not identified; right fallopian tube uninvolved.
- UTERUS: Two separate ENDOMETRIOID ADENOCARCINOMAS 子宮內膜樣腺癌；
  Left parametrium involved by tumour; cervix uninvolved
- Tumour 1 (endometrial cavity): Endometrioid adenocarcinoma, Grade 3 with less than 50% myometrial
  invasion.
- Tumour 2 (posterior wall): Endometrioid adenocarcinoma, Grade 2 with peritumoural lymphovascular
  invasion and serosa involvement.
- Other pathological finding: Endometriosis near uterine serosa; low-grade squamous intraepithelial lesion
  of the cervix

B. Tumour in PELVIS:
- ENDOMETRIOID ADENOCARCINOMA 子宮內膜樣腺癌

C. Adhesion on posterior pelvic peritoneum:
- Fibrosis; No malignancy

COMMENT
Right ovarian tumour, pelvic tumour and uterine tumour 1 and tumour 2 represent probably synchronous
endometrioid adenocarcinoma due to field effect.

MACROSCOPIC EXAMINATION
A. Specimen designated uterus and right tube and right ovarian tumour. The capsule of the right ovarian
tumour is cut opened before submission. The ovarian tumour measures 150 x 55 x 50 mm. The tumour
capsule appears smooth with no exophytic papillary tumour on capsular surface. The tumour is cystic solid
with multiple variably sized solid mural nodules covered by necrotic exudates. The largest mural nodule
measures 50 mm in diameter. Elsewhere, the cyst wall is uneven in thickness with papillary plaques and
nodular projections. The fallopian tube is identified on ovarian capsule; it measures 40 mm in length, 8 mm
in external diameter. The uterus is cut opened from its anterior wall. It measures 70 mm from fundus to
external os, 25 mm across cornu and 25 mm from anterior to posterior. The endometrium appears thickened
at fundus. The thickened area measures 18 mm longitudinally, 15 mm across. The endometrium in the lower
segment is smooth and thin. Mucus retention is noted in the endocervical canal. The cervix measures 25
mm in diameter, 25 mm in length. Further sectioning shows a fleshy nodular lesion measuring 18 mm in
greatest dimension, located in posterior myometrium extending to serosa. It is not connected with the
endometrial tumour.

Cassette Summary: A01-06: Right ovarian tumour; A07: Ovarian tumour and fallopian tube; A08: Tubal
fimbria; A09-13: Thickened endometrium, all submitted (posterior wall fleshy nodular lesion included);
A14,15: Anterior and posterior lip of cervix; A16,17: Left and right parametrium.

B. Specimen designated tumour in pelvis. Recieved in formalin is a piece of tan yellowish nodular tissue
measuring 29 x 14 x 5 mm. Cut surface shows a tan coloured lesion 11 x 6 mm across. A cystic cavity 2 mm
in diameter is also noted. Bisected and embedded in 1 cassette B01.

Page 1 of 3

If there is any inconsistency or ambiguity between the English version and the Chinese version, the English version shall prevail.

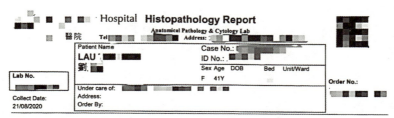

Histopathology Report

Anatomical Pathology & Cytology Lab

医院   Tel: Address:

Patient Name	Case No.:
LAU	ID No.:
劉	Sex Age DOB Bed Unit/Ward
	F 41Y

Lab No.

Collect Date:
21/08/2020

Under care of:
Address:
Order By:

Order No.:

C. Specimen designated adhesion on posterior pelvic peritoneum. Received in formalin are 3 pieces of tan reddish tissue, measuring 4, 6 and 9 mm in greatest dimension. All submitted in 1 cassette C01.

MICROSCOPIC EXAMINATION

A. Right salpingo-oophorectomy and total hysterectomy

Ovarian tumour

Tumour site:	Right ovary
Tumour size:	150 mm in maximum dimension
Histologic tumour type:	Endometrioid adenocarcinoma
Tumour grade:	Grade 2
Borderline tumour:	Not apparent
Histological features:	The tumour comprises multilocular cystic spaces and solid nodules with

confluent glandular and papillary architecture and extracellular mucin. The tumour cells are heterogenous in appearances with moderate to marked nuclear atypia (nuclear grade 3). Frequent mitotic activity and necrotic debris are seen. Endometrioid glandular cells, tumour cells with mucinous and serous features are seen. Some tumour cells are squamoid with eosinophilic cytoplasm and distinct cell border. Immunostudy shows wild-type expression for p53 and diffuse positive staining for p16. WT-1 stain is negative. PAX8 and ER stains are positive. Vimentin stain is focally positive.

Ovarian capsule/surface:	No tumour is seen on capsular surface; Capsular opened before submission.
Lymphovascular invasion:	Not identified.
Right fallopian tube:	Uninvolved.

Uterine tumour:	Two separate tumours are found.
Tumour site of tumour 1:	Endometrial cavity
Tumour size:	18 x 15 mm in area
Histologic tumour type:	Endometrioid adenocarcinoma
Histologic FIGO grade:	Grade 3 (6-50% non-squamous solid growth), nuclear grade 3
Histologic features:	The tumour form confluent glandular and cribriform glandular architecture

mingled with solid areas. Mucinous differentiation and focal squamoid appearance are notable. There is frequent mitosis; atypical mitosis, tumour necrosis and and marked nuclear atypia.

Myometrial invasion:	Microinvasion is noted (Block A9 and A10), depth of invasion < 1 mm
	Depth of invasion < 50% thickness of the myometrium

Tumour site of tumour 2:	Posterior uterine wall, separate from the endometrial tumour (Tumour 1), closest distance to tumour 1 is 7 mm.
Tumour size:	18 mm in greatest dimension
Histologic tumour type:	Endometrioid adenocarcinoma
Histologic FIGO grade:	Grade 2 (< 5 % non-squamous solid growth), nuclear grade 3
Histologic features:	The tumour form angulated and branching glands with intraglandular

papillation and bridging. They are surrounded by desmoplastic stroma, involving myometrium and extending to serosa. Marked nuclear atypia is notable. Immunostudy shows weak staining of p53 in tumour cells and p16 staining is patchy. The tumour cells are positive for ER and negative for WT-1.

Lymphovascular invasion:	Peritumoral lymphatic tumour invasion present (3 vessels involved)
Left parametrium:	Involved by endometrioid adenocarcinoma.
Right parametrium:	Uninvolved
Uninvolved endometrium:	Inactive endometrium
Cervix:	Uninvolved; low-grade squamous intraepithelial lesion seen.
Other pathological findings:	Endometriosis is noted near serosa.

Report Time:
24/08/2020 18:23

If there is any inconsistency or ambiguity between the English version and the Chinese version, the English version shall prevail.

晚期宫颈癌康复

司女士因宫颈癌，于2021年1月份做了全子宫切除以及盆腔中器官如双侧输卵管、双侧卵巢等全部切除手术。当时的她65岁，以为经过这样彻底的、大面积的手术切除之后，就不会再有什么问题了。但术后还不到1年，即2021年年底，就出现腹部疼痛不适。急忙去医院做检查，经确诊为肿瘤复发，于是尽快开始化疗和放疗。因为她还有严重的糖尿病、高血压、高血脂病史，加上化疗和放疗导致身体非常虚弱。特别是化疗、放疗后，全身皮肤严重过敏，起了大大小小的水疱非常痛苦，最为严重的是她的臀部，肛门、尿道部位有非常剧烈的疼痛，令她无法忍受。虽然她每日服止痛药，但是即使用吗啡和最强的麻醉止痛药也都没有任何效果，甚至后来把吗啡类止痛药增加至最高剂量，每日服用4次，仍然感到剧烈疼痛。

2022年4月10日，司女士前来就诊，来诊时非常痛苦，疼痛非常严重。她当时每日服用吗啡和其他止痛药有2个多月了，但是疼痛依旧非常严重，不能忍受，无法睡觉，无法休息。根据对她的病症的辨证，我们采取了活血化瘀，驱毒止痛的方法。在治疗1周以后臀部的剧烈疼痛减轻，吗啡类的止痛药由原来的每天服用4次减少到每天2次。双侧髂骨大量肿大的淋巴结明显缩小。用活血化瘀、驱毒止痛的方法再治疗1周，疼痛明显减轻，因为她服用吗啡类止痛药时间过长，有一定的成瘾性，如果晚上不服用就会影响睡眠，所以只需晚上服用 1 次即可。我们又继续努力治疗了 2 周，于 2022 年 5 月上旬疼痛感完全消失。她自己告诉我们已经有 2 周没有服用止痛药了，同时血压、血糖，白细胞指数都已恢复正常。

2022 年 5 月中旬，司女士来就诊时说，已经停用吗啡类止痛药 3 周了，所有止痛药都停了。她本人和我们大家都非常高兴，她的 CEA 癌指数，由 2022 年 4 月 1 日的 188，降到 4 月 26 日的 75，5 月 17 日的 24，在 6 月 12 日再次检查 CEA 癌指数时，降为 12.87。精神也明显好转，继续坚持认真治疗。就这样到了 2022 年的 8 月初，因为疼痛已经没有了，所以想了解肿瘤的大小情况，于是再次做了 PET/CT。检查报告显示，经过生命修复的中医药治疗后，盆腔和阴道的复发肿瘤都已明显缩小。肿瘤的大小为 2.8cm×1.6cm×2.4cm，同时腹腔多发的大量转移肿瘤和双侧髂部淋巴转移病灶均已消失。治疗有明显的效果，大家都非常高兴。但是从 2022 年 9 月中旬以后就没有见到司女士再来就诊治疗，或许是因为工作忙碌。

时间过得很快，转眼 3 个月过去了，2022 年 12 月中旬，司女士又来看病就诊了。这次她来的时候是由家人推着轮椅，而她坐在轮椅上，完全不能行动，并且左右辗转，痛苦呻吟。原来在这 3 个月里，经过其他人的大力推荐，她采用了当前最先进的免疫结合靶向治疗，一共做了 4 个疗程，一心盼望能够彻底消灭肿瘤。但是事与愿违，疼痛再次出现，并且越来越重，甚至完全不能行动，即便是坐着、躺着也会不停地辗转，寻找一个能短暂缓解一下的姿势，否则连几秒钟都不能忍受。同时检查报告还显示肿瘤再次明显增大，SUVmax（最大的标准摄取值）达 22.36，已压迫神经及周围组织。在这种情况下，她又想到了原先用中医药的方法治疗，所以再次前来就诊。

看到她非常痛苦，我们也尽快地给她进行治疗。除了活血化瘀、驱毒消瘤之外，也加用了针灸等方法。这样很快地就能减轻痛苦，减少疼痛。经过一段时间的治疗，她终于可以从站立开始，慢慢迈步行走，到最后可以自己行动了。很快，经过几周的治疗之后，她不再需要坐轮椅了。在这种情况下，她还在进行着化疗。因为有医生告诉她，这个化疗是不能停止的，否则会有非常严重的后果，所以她选择继续化疗。之后又有 1 周没有见到司女士，因担心治疗不到位，所以我们就打电话问她是怎么回事。原来她在化疗之后，突然意识丧失并陷入昏迷，紧急入院进行急诊和抢救。经过 1 周左右的多种措施监测治疗才恢复过来。

司女士身体已经到了不能承受化疗等带来的严重毒副作用，只能选择使用温和传统的天然药物，用生命修复的中医药治疗。经多方检查，明确了造成疼痛的原因是肿瘤生长迅速，严重压迫神经导致。疼痛消失证实肿瘤是在逐渐缩小，使得多处神经解除严重压迫。现在她继续认真治疗，等待在一定时间之后再次做 CT 检查。因为这些放射性的检查是需要在有一定的间隔时间之后才能再次进行。但经过长期化疗，免疫治疗后，在腹股沟处还是有大量成团块状聚集，质地坚硬的肿瘤结节继续生长，而现在经过生命修复的中医药治疗，这些结节逐渐消失了。这是不需要经过 CT 等深层检查，在体表就可以用手触摸到的明证。现在的她身心愉悦，吃得好，睡得香，她高兴地告诉前来就诊的其他患者，中医药不仅没有毒副作用，而且治病救人立竿见影，确实令人信服。

 治疗原则

活血化瘀，祛毒消瘤。

常用中药

1. 蒲公英、野菊花、桃仁、红花、水蛭、土鳖虫、鳖甲、猕猴梨根、威灵仙等。
2. 同时服用祛毒散、消瘤丸。

影像学、病理学检查报告及诊疗记录

1. 2022 年 3 月 24 日 PET/CT 检查报告证实患宫颈癌，于 2021 年 1 月行全子宫及输卵管、卵巢等切除手术。并术后化疗。现阴道有高代谢 4.4cm 肿瘤复发。腹腔有大量肿瘤复发，双侧髂部淋巴结肿大。

2. 经生命修复中医药治疗后，2022 年 8 月 5 日 PET/CT 检查报告显示阴道复发肿瘤缩小，为 2.80cm×1.63cm×2.45cm。腹腔多发转移及双髂部淋巴结均消失。

3. 停用中药转用靶向、免疫等治疗后，2022 年 12 月 14 日 PET/CT 检查报告证实肿瘤再次增大代谢活性增高，为 5.67cm×5.17cm×4.38cm，SUVmax 22.36。

附：患者检查报告

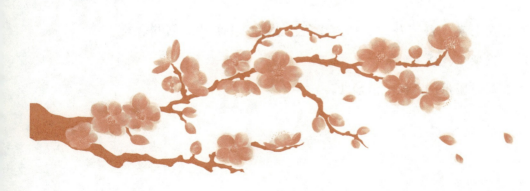

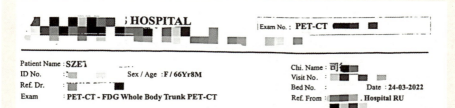

Patient Name : SZE1

ID No. :   Sex / Age : **F / 66Yr8M**

Ref. Dr. :

Exam : **PET-CT - FDG Whole Body Trunk PET-CT**

Chi. Name : 司1

Visit No. :

Bed No. :   Date : **24-03-2022**

Ref. From :   . Hospital RU

No abnormal uptake is noted in the axial skeleton.

(SUV = Standardized Uptake Value.)

Opinion:

Status-post THBSO. Hypermetabolic nodular mass measuring about 4.4 cm is present at the left superior aspect of the vagina vault, most consistent with recurrent tumour. Multiple lesions are also present in the peritoneal cavity, most consistent with recurrent tumours. Mildly active lymph nodes at bilateral iliac areas are worrisome for early recurrent tumours. The supraclavicular fossae are clear. There is no recurrent tumour in the liver and other abdominal visceral organs.

No recurrent tumour is present in the head and neck, lungs and bones.

Thank you for your referral.

(This examination does not include the brain.)

No. of image prints : 22   No. of DVD : 1

Remark :

NGWH

Report No. : 22'

Authorized and Reported on 24-03-2022 @ 13:51 by

.. .. 醫生

DR.

MBBS (HK), FHKCR, FHKAM (Radiology)

Diplomate American Board of Nuclear Medicine   Version No   1

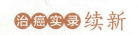

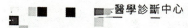

Hong Kong Advanced Imaging – Examination Report

Appointment Time:	05/08/2022 09:30	Patient ID:	
Patient Name:	SZET	Gender:	F
Age:	67	DOB:	07/07/1955
Referring Doctor:	Dr.		

keeping with known tumor recurrence.

Previously noted multiple peritoneal nodules have resolved. No residual hypermetabolic peritoneal lesion is seen. Previously noted mildly active lymph nodes at bilateral iliac regions have also resolved.

Physiologic FDG uptake is seen in the liver, spleen, and bowel. No hypermetabolic lesion is detected in the liver, spleen, adrenal glands and pancreas. The kidneys, ureters and urinary bladder are visualized per normal clearance of the radiotracer. There are no pathologically enlarged or hypermetabolic abdominal, pelvic, or inguinal lymph nodes.

MUSCULOSKELETAL:

Physiologic FDG uptake is seen in the axial and proximal appendicular skeleton. No aggressive osseous lesion is seen on CT.

CONCLUSION:

1. CA cervix status post-THBSO. Previously noted local tumor recurrence at the left vaginal vault shows interval decrease in size with similar uptake (2.80 x 1.63 x 2.45cm, SUVmax 9.82).

2. Previously noted peritoneal metastases and mildly active bilateral iliac lymph nodes have resolved. No other metabolically active lesion is detected elsewhere in the body.

(A whole body CT scan was performed, but was used only for attenuation correction and anatomic correlation. If a comprehensive diagnostic CT is required, the Radiology Department should be consulted for an adjunct CT study.)

Thank you Dr. your referral.

Report Date: 05/08/2022

/at

Dr.
Specialist in Radiology
MBBS (HK), FRCR, FHKCR, FHKAM (Radiology)

Page 2 of 2

258

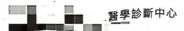

醫學診斷中心

Hong Kong Advanced Imaging – Examination Report

Appointment Time:	14/12/2022 10:30	**Patient ID:**	
		Site:	HKAI
Patient Name:	SZE	**Gender:**	F
Age:	67	**DOB:**	07/07/1955
Referring Doctor:	Dr.		

ABDOMEN AND PELVIS:

Previous THBSO noted. Previously noted hypermetabolic lesion suggestive of local recurrence at the left vaginal vault/ pararectal region shows further increase in size and activity compared to previous CT and PET-CT, now measuring 5.67 x 5.17 x 4.38cm/ SUVmax 22.36 (vs last CT 3.60 x 2.46 x 3.33cm, last PET-CT SUVmax 9.82). It is suggestive of local disease progression. The lesion now shows invasion of the left levator ani muscle. Mild left sided hydronephrosis noted with prominent left ureter. Findings could be due to adhesive effect by the lesion.

No hypermetabolic lesion is detected in the liver, spleen, adrenal glands and pancreas. The right kidney, right ureter and urinary bladder are visualized per normal clearance of the radiotracer. There are no pathologically enlarged or hypermetabolic abdominal, pelvic, or inguinal lymph nodes.

MUSCULOSKELETAL:

Spondylosis noted along the cervical, thoracic and lumbar spine. Relative decrease in bony uptake noted at the lumbosacral region in keeping with post-radiation change. Physiologic FDG uptake is seen in the rest of axial and proximal appendicular skeleton. No aggressive osseous lesion is seen on CT.

CONCLUSION:

1. Previously noted local tumour recurrence at the left vaginal vault/ pararectal region shows further increase in size and activity, now measuring 5.67 x 5.17 x 4.38cm/ SUVmax 22.36. Finding is suggestive of local disease progression. The lesion now shows invasion of the left levator ani muscle.

2. No other metabolically activity lesion is detected elsewhere in the body.

Thank you Dr. for your referral.

Report Date:14/12/2022

/JY

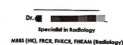

Dr.

Specialist in Radiology

MBBS (HK), FRCR, FHKCR, FHKAM (Radiology)

Page 2 of 2

病案 **39**

晚期甲状腺癌咽喉癌康复

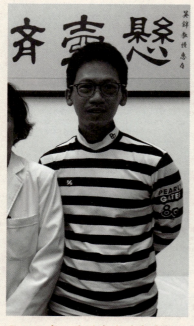

🔊 2024年2月刘先生前来诊治时合影留念

刘先生是一家公司的主管。2005年，31岁的他做了鼻咽癌手术，手术后又进行了33次的放疗。在身体恢复之后，又投身于工作。就这样过了12年，又感到颈部不适，用手可以摸到肿大的包块。他急忙去医院做检查，结果发现患有甲状腺癌。刘先生实在是不想再做手术了，但迫于无奈，拖了一些时间之后，于2019年3月再次做了甲状腺癌的切除手术。手术后的病理报告显示，甲状腺癌已经转移扩散，在鼻咽部、甲状腺旁边的组织中以及气管旁等多处都有癌细胞的转移，还有多数淋巴结转移。手术无法把这些转移的肿瘤切除干净，因为有些肿瘤的部位，如喉部、气管旁等均无法切除。手术之后，他采用放射性碘治疗，但是效果并不理想。

他于2020年4月再次做手术，这已经是他第3次做手术，但仍然不能够完全切除转移性的恶性肿瘤。组织病理报告显示咽喉部位，甲状腺周围，颈部多处部位，以及气管旁等处仍然有肿瘤的存在和转移。手术后他再次接受放射性碘治疗，但效果依旧不明显，仍然有多数转移病灶。并且肿瘤分布在人体最重要的颈部，呼吸、消化等功能均受到破坏。

他在没有其他选择的情况下，于2021年10月前来进行生命修复的中医药治疗。刘先生来时声音非常低弱、说话困难，声音嘶哑，并有吞咽困难，呼吸困难，喉咙干燥，心悸，咳嗽多痰等严重问题。因为颈部做过放疗，整个颈部的肌肉非常僵硬，按之如石。经辨证分析，对他的治疗首先采用祛毒化瘀，之后逐渐加强软坚散结的力量。

刘先生服用中药后病情逐渐好转，影响生活和生命最严重的症状——呼吸困难和吞咽困难也都陆续减轻或好转，其他症状也在慢慢缓解，就这样经过2个月的治疗，刘先生告诉我们现在没有什么特别不舒服的了。我们鼓励他继续治疗，以巩固疗效，所以他现在还在继续认真的治疗中，虽然已经恢复工作，但他说并没有感到工作疲劳，每天都过得非常充实和快乐。

治疗原则

攻毒化瘀，软坚散结。

常用中药

1. 鱼腥草、金银花、皂角刺、杏仁、桃仁、红花、海藻、昆布、田七、牡丹皮等。
2. 同时服用攻毒散、消瘤丸。

影像学、病理学检查报告及诊疗记录

2019 年 3 月 21 日病理检查报告说明：2005 年鼻咽癌手术。右侧甲状腺乳头状癌并甲状腺外浸润，甲状腺旁多发淋巴结，乳头状癌转移。咽喉头部甲状腺乳头癌转移。气管旁淋巴结甲状腺乳头状癌转移。

附：患者检查报告

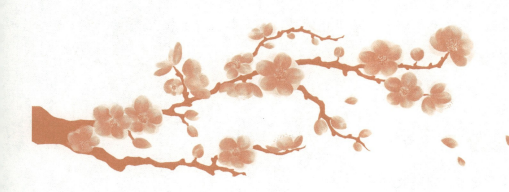

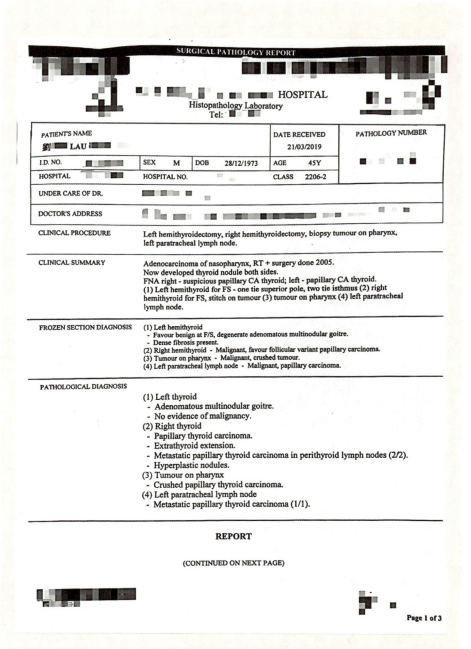

SURGICAL PATHOLOGY REPORT

HOSPITAL
Histopathology Laboratory
Tel:

PATIENT'S NAME				DATE RECEIVED		PATHOLOGY NUMBER
劉 LAU				21/03/2019		
I.D. NO.	SEX M	DOB	28/12/1973	AGE	45Y	
HOSPITAL	HOSPITAL NO.			CLASS	2206-2	

UNDER CARE OF DR.

DOCTOR'S ADDRESS

CLINICAL PROCEDURE
Left hemithyroidectomy, right hemithyroidectomy, biopsy tumour on pharynx, left paratracheal lymph node.

CLINICAL SUMMARY
Adenocarcinoma of nasopharynx, RT + surgery done 2005.
Now developed thyroid nodule both sides.
FNA right - suspicious papillary CA thyroid; left - papillary CA thyroid.
(1) Left hemithyroid for FS - one tie superior pole, two tie isthmus (2) right hemithyroid for FS, stitch on tumour (3) tumour on pharynx (4) left paratracheal lymph node.

FROZEN SECTION DIAGNOSIS
(1) Left hemithyroid
  - Favour benign at F/S, degenerate adenomatous multinodular goitre.
  - Dense fibrosis present.
(2) Right hemithyroid - Malignant, favour follicular variant papillary carcinoma.
(3) Tumour on pharynx - Malignant, crushed tumour.
(4) Left paratracheal lymph node - Malignant, papillary carcinoma.

PATHOLOGICAL DIAGNOSIS

(1) Left thyroid
  - Adenomatous multinodular goitre.
  - No evidence of malignancy.
(2) Right thyroid
  - Papillary thyroid carcinoma.
  - Extrathyroid extension.
  - Metastatic papillary thyroid carcinoma in perithyroid lymph nodes (2/2).
  - Hyperplastic nodules.
(3) Tumour on pharynx
  - Crushed papillary thyroid carcinoma.
(4) Left paratracheal lymph node
  - Metastatic papillary thyroid carcinoma (1/1).

REPORT

(CONTINUED ON NEXT PAGE)

Page 1 of 3

263

病案 **40**

晚期胰腺癌康复

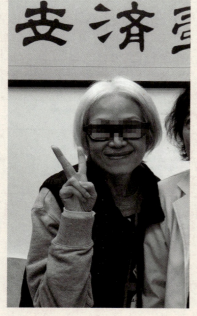

🔊 王太太 2023 年 10 月前来诊治时合影留念

王太太 62 岁，她在 2022 年 7 月感到腹痛、腹胀、消化差，并伴有胃痛。于是在 2022 年 8 月进行抽血化验，结果显示有关胰腺癌的指数 CA19-9 数值很高，达到 280 多。又于 2022 年 8 月 31 日做了 CT 检查，报告显示：①患有胰腺癌。②肝内胆管及大量分支胆管，肝外胆管均明显扩张，并在胰头处有狭窄和压迫、突出。报告指出，应做进一步的检查，以排除肝脏及肝内管道的病变。③胆囊肿大，胆内泥沙样结石和大量胆结石。④肾结石。⑤升结肠憩室。⑥肝门处淋巴结肿大，腔静脉后，主动脉腔静脉，胃周等部位有明显的肿大淋巴结。

医院要求尽快做肿瘤切除手术。王太太非常害怕，她不想做手术，但是医生反复强调胰腺癌是癌中之王，不能耽误时间，家人和亲戚也一直催促，大家都认为她应该做手术。于是王太太于 2022 年 9 月做了肿瘤切除手术，手术使用的是 Whipple 术方法，这是传统的腹腔镜胰、十二指肠切除术。术中切除了胰腺头部及十二指肠、胆囊、胆总管、部分胃及小肠等。但最严重的问题是，手术后的病理检查报告明确指出：手术切口处有肿瘤存在。这也就是说手术并没有将肿瘤完全切除，或者说没有切除干净。这对于已经有多处淋巴转移的胰腺癌患者来说，真是非常不幸，无疑是雪上加霜。王太太的肝也有明显的问题，碱性磷酸酶、丙种谷氨酰转肽酶、谷草转氨酶、谷丙转氨酶等是反映肝脏功能，肝外胆道梗阻、肝内占位性病变的重要指标，而她的这些指数都非常高，存在一些隐患。虽然手术切除的范围已经很大，但是并没有在报告中见到对肝脏做任何进一步的诊治。手术后这些指标仍然居高不下，有关检测指标高于正常值的20倍，甚至70多倍。王太太于2022年10月17日前来诊治。她来的时候是坐在轮椅上由家人推着她的，身体非常虚弱，面色苍白贫血，精神疲惫。腹部胀满，大量的腹水使得腹部严重膨胀隆起，腹大如鼓。最重要的是仍有严重的腹痛、腹胀，无法进食，咳嗽多痰，双下肢严重水肿，失眠盗汗，四肢冰冷等症状。

对王太太的治疗，我们开始是以扶阳补正为主，随着身体状态逐渐好转，逐步将治疗的重点放在扶正祛邪，消除腹水，水肿，消除肿瘤等方面。王太太的肚子慢慢变小，吃东西逐渐增加，精神状态好转，在一天一天中好起来了。因为她的病情非常严重，所以在治疗中增加了穴位治疗、针灸治疗等方法。虽然王太太特别怕痛，每次扎针都会大呼小叫，要求医生轻一点，手下留情。但是即便这样，也并没有影响她继续前来做针灸治疗。经过治疗，她的血液检测指标以及癌指数 CA19-9 等恢复正常。现在她自己就可以步行前来，不需要再坐轮椅了。虽然整个治疗周期不长，只有 2～3 个月的时间，但是因为她的身体恢复是非常好的，证明抗癌的中药治疗是很有效的，所以把她的病例介绍出来，以便鼓励更多的患者。现在王太太仍在积极的治疗中，她自己也能感觉到身体恢复得很好，也更信任生命修复的抗癌治疗。

治疗原则

扶阳补正，抗癌逐水。

常用中药

1. 鹿茸、淫羊藿、黄芪、人参、当归、牵牛子、茯苓、泽漆、蜂房、炙甘草等。
2. 同时服用消瘤丸、扶阳散。

影像学、病理学检查报告及诊疗记录

1. 2022 年 8 月 31 日 CT 检查报告证实患有胰腺癌及胆结石。肝内胆管及大量分支胆管，肝外胆管的扩张并在胰头处狭窄突出压迫，应做进一步的检查以排除肝管道病变。肝门处淋巴结肿大，腔静脉后，主动脉腔静脉胃周等部位有明显淋巴结肿大等。

2. 2022 年 12 月 22 日检查报告显示各项指数及癌指数等均恢复正常。

附：患者检查报告

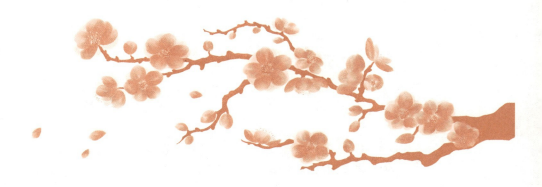

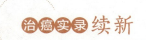

▆▆ Hospital ▆醫院

MEDICAL IMAGING DEPARTMENT

Patient's Name	: WONG ▆▆ ▆ ▆	Unit Record No.	: ▆▆▆▆
Sex	: F	Age	: 61
Examination Date	: 31-AUG-2022	Accession No.	: ▆▆▆▆
Ward / Class	: 635B	Attending Doctor	: ▆▆▆▆

EXAMINATION / PROCEDURE REPORT

COMMENTS:

- A lobulated lesion with mixed microcystic and macrocystic appearance is again seen at the pancreatic head, measuring approximately 1.9 x 2.0 x 2.5 cm (TS x AP x CC). No associated calcifications are seen. The central solid component of the tumour demonstrates predominant delayed contrast enhancement, and may represent scar tissue. Given the lack of significant FDG uptake and lack of visible connection with the main pancreatic duct, findings may represent a serous cystadenoma. Imaging differentials would include other cystic neoplasms, such as an IPMN.

- Dilated central intrahepatic and proximal to mid extrahepatic duct with focal abrupt tapering at level of the pancreatic head is again noted. This could be due to extrinsic compression. ERCP and cytological correlation would be helpful to exclude ductal pathology.

- The gallbladder is distended and contains sludge and stones.

- A few tiny non-obstructive calyceal stones (less than 2 mm) are seen in both kidneys.

- Ascending colonic diverticulosis is noted.

- Mildly enlarged lymph nodes up to 9 mm are seen at the porta hepatis region. Small to mildly prominent lymph nodes are seen at the retrocaval, aortocaval, and perigastric (pericardial) regions. These are non-specific.

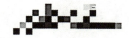

Approved on : 31-AUG-2022 05:05 PM
Page 3 of 3

(Electronically Signed)

Specialist in Radiology
MBBS(HK), M Res (Med) (HK), FRCR, FHKCR, FHKAM(Radiology)

MR-C101

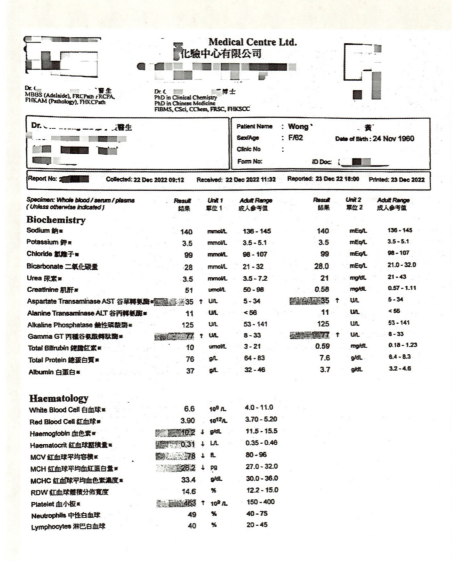

Medical Centre Ltd.
化验中心有限公司

Dr. ( ) 医生
MBBS (Adelaide), FRCPath FRCPA,
FHKAM (Pathology), FHKCPath

Dr. ( ) 博士
PhD in Clinical Chemistry
PhD in Chinese Medicine
FIBMS, CSci, CChem, FRSC, FHKSCC

Dr. 医生		

Patient Name	: Wong 黄
Sex/Age	: F/62
Clinic No	:
Form No:	

Date of Birth : 24 Nov 1960

ID Doc:

Report No:	Collected: 22 Dec 2022 09:12	Received: 22 Dec 2022 11:32	Reported: 23 Dec 22 18:00	Printed: 23 Dec 2022

Specimen: Whole blood / serum / plasma (Unless otherwise indicated)	Result 結果	Unit 1 單位 1	Adult Range 成人參考值	Result 結果	Unit 2 單位 2	Adult Range 成人參考值
Biochemistry						
Sodium 鈉 ▣	140	mmol/L	136 - 145	140	mEq/L	136 - 145
Potassium 鉀 ▣	3.5	mmol/L	3.5 - 5.1	3.5	mEq/L	3.5 - 5.1
Chloride 氯離子 ▣	99	mmol/L	98 - 107	99	mEq/L	98 - 107
Bicarbonate 二氧化碳量	28	mmol/L	21 - 32	28.0	mEq/L	21.0 - 32.0
Urea 尿素 ▣	3.5	mmol/L	3.5 - 7.2	21	mg/dL	21 - 43
Creatinine 肌酐 ▣	51	umol/L	50 - 98	0.58	mg/dL	0.57 - 1.11
Aspartate Transaminase AST 谷草轉氨酶 ▣	35 ↑	U/L	5 - 34	35 ↑	U/L	5 - 34
Alanine Transaminase ALT 谷丙轉氨酶	11	U/L	< 56	11	U/L	< 56
Alkaline Phosphatase 鹼性磷酸酶 ▣	125	U/L	53 - 141	125	U/L	53 - 141
Gamma GT 丙種谷氨酰轉肽酶	77 ↑	U/L	8 - 33	77 ↑	U/L	8 - 33
Total Bilirubin 總膽紅素	10	umol/L	3 - 21	0.59	mg/dL	0.18 - 1.23
Total Protein 總蛋白質 ▣	76	g/L	64 - 83	7.6	g/dL	6.4 - 8.3
Albumin 白蛋白 ▣	37	g/L	32 - 46	3.7	g/dL	3.2 - 4.6
Haematology						
White Blood Cell 白血球 ▣	6.6	10⁹ /L	4.0 - 11.0			
Red Blood Cell 紅血球 ▣	3.90	10¹² /L	3.70 - 5.20			
Haemoglobin 血色素 ▣	10.2 ↓	g/dL	11.5 - 15.5			
Haematocrit 紅血球壓積量 ▣	0.31 ↓	L/L	0.35 - 0.46			
MCV 紅血球平均容積 ▣	78 ↓	fL	80 - 96			
MCH 紅血球平均血紅蛋白量 ▣	26.2 ↓	pg	27.0 - 32.0			
MCHC 紅血球平均血色素濃度 ▣	33.4	g/dL	30.0 - 36.0			
RDW 紅血球體積分佈寬度 ▣	14.6	%	12.2 - 15.0			
Platelet 血小板 ▣	463 ↑	10⁹ /L	150 - 400			
Neutrophils 中性白血球	49	%	40 - 75			
Lymphocytes 淋巴白血球	40	%	20 - 45			

Page 1 of 2

269

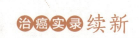

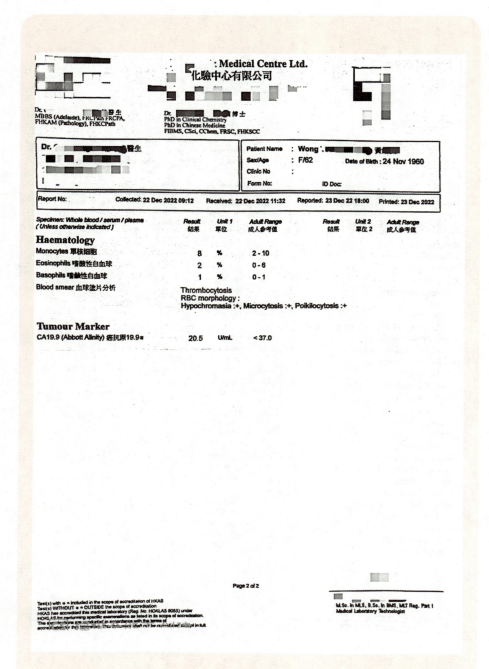

: Medical Centre Ltd.
化驗中心有限公司

Dr.
MBBS (Adelaide), FRCPath FRCPA,
FHKAM (Pathology), FHKCPath

Dr. 博士
PhD in Clinical Chemistry
PhD in Chinese Medicine
FIBMS, CSci, CChem, FRSC, FHKSCC

Dr. 醫生

Patient Name	: Wong 黃
Sex/Age	: F/62 Date of Birth : 24 Nov 1960
Clinic No	:
Form No:	ID Doc:

Report No: Collected: 22 Dec 2022 09:12 Received: 22 Dec 2022 11:32 Reported: 23 Dec 22 18:00 Printed: 23 Dec 2022

Specimen: Whole blood / serum / plasma
(Unless otherwise indicated)

	Result 結果	Unit 1 單位	Adult Range 成人參考值	Result 結果	Unit 2 單位 2	Adult Range 成人參考值
Haematology						
Monocytes 單核細胞	8	%	2 - 10			
Eosinophils 嗜酸性白血球	2	%	0 - 6			
Basophils 嗜鹼性白血球	1	%	0 - 1			
Blood smear 血球塗片分析	Thrombocytosis					
	RBC morphology :					
	Hypochromasia :+, Microcytosis :+, Poikilocytosis :+					
Tumour Marker						
CA19.9 (Abbott Alinity) 癌抗原19.9≡	20.5	U/mL	< 37.0			

Page 2 of 2

M.Sc. in MLS, B.Sc. in BMS, MLT Reg. Part I
Medical Laboratory Technologist

病案 41

晚期卵巢癌多发肝、腹腔、胸膜等转移康复

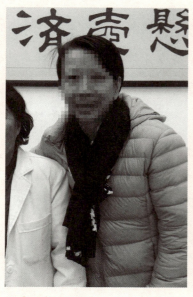

🎧 郭女士 2023 年 6 月前来诊治时合影留念

郭女士在 2021 年，48 岁的时候患了卵巢癌，当时经过检查发现卵巢肿瘤的体积很大，达到了 11cm。于是她在 2021 年 7 月做肿瘤切除手术。手术后的病理报告证实为卵巢透明细胞癌，并且有淋巴和血管的侵入。手术中除了子宫全部切除之外，双侧输卵管也被切除了，同时还切除了腹腔网膜，双侧盆腔的转移性淋巴结。手术之后身体稍有恢复后，就于 8 月开始进行化疗。从 8 月到 12 月共进行了 6 个疗程的化疗，但是化疗结束不到 2 个月肿瘤又再次复发。后来郭女士得知在手术过程中，腹腔的肿瘤被切破了，导致整个腹腔都充满了破损肿瘤中出来的各种物质。也就是说，肿瘤细胞满布于整个腹腔。手术后 1 个多月，在接受化疗和靶向治疗过程中就已经复发。当时的癌指数为 200 多，于是入院抽腹水，后又有肺部塌陷，又连续抽胸腔积液 1 个多星期。2022 年 3 月，郭女士又感染上了 COVID-19，病情再次加重。当

时的癌指数 CA125 高达 276。以后又多次连续抽取肺的胸腔积液，她也一直在坚持做化疗和靶向治疗，但是病情并没有得到缓解。因为病情严重，其家人和她本人都考虑配合一些其他自然疗法，以减少长期严重的毒性作用。

她于 2022 年 8 月底前来进行诊治。当时她是在继续化疗和靶向治疗的过程中，前来求助是想减少化疗和靶向治疗带来的毒副作用。郭女士当时身体非常瘦弱，精神状态很差，气短胸闷，呼吸困难，腹部高高隆起，胸、腹部大量胸、腹水，面色萎黄，精神不振，腹痛严重，双侧胸部疼痛，腹部可以摸到多个肿块。郭女士来治疗的同时，仍然在接受化疗和靶向治疗，同时也在断断续续地做抽胸腔积液、腹水等治疗。即使化疗中发生口腔溃烂，流鼻血，完全不能进食，呕吐，脱发等严重副作用，她也还是按照医生的要求坚持了下来。2022 年 9 月经过血液检查，癌指数等指标与上个月一样，还是很高，CA125 达89.6。她说 2021 年的下半年做了 6 个疗程的化疗，2022 年的上半年使用药力更强、毒性更强的药物进行了 4 个疗程的化疗，2022 年的 7 月至 10 月又做了 8 个疗程的靶向治疗。现在身体非常疲惫，全身都因为化疗和靶向治疗而变的黢黑，双手十指伸出来，就好像是刚扒过煤炭的颜色。做了这么多次的化疗和靶向治疗，就是期盼着能有一个好的结果。

她于 2022 年 10 月 5 日再次做 PET/CT 检查。结果显示以前的多发性腹腔转移病灶增多增大，并且有新的转移病灶，腹水也大量增加。肝脏在原有转移灶的基础上又有了新的肝转移病灶。甚至胸腔积液，甲状腺肿瘤，乳腺也有病变。检查报告的结论与上次检查报告相比较，病情明显加重。郭女士感到十分的灰心丧气。这段时间里，她也看到了很多患者使用生命修复的中药治疗的情况。医生要求他继续做化疗和靶向，她问还要做多少次，什么时候停止？得到的答复是没有停止的时间，要一直不停地做下去。但是问到有什么结果，病会好吗？答案是非常不明确和令人沮丧的。郭女士于 2022 年 10 月 24 日做了一个重大的决定，就是她不再做化疗和靶向了。因为身体太虚弱了，副作用太大了，她已经无法承受这些治疗带来的副作用了。

于是郭女士停止了化疗和靶向治疗，转为每周都来我们的中心，单纯进行生命修复的中医药治疗。时至今日，停止化疗和靶向治疗已有 2～3 个月的时间，郭女士之前化疗和靶向带来的许多严重的副作用在逐渐减少或消失，煤炭一样的黑色慢慢褪去，皮肤的颜色逐渐恢复到正常。颈部等多处肿大的淋巴结也摸不到了，腹腔中大大小小的肿瘤也逐渐消失了。腹水逐渐减少，她感到全身温暖舒适，不像以前那样全身冰冷。虽然治疗的时间还比较短，郭女士也需要进一步加强治疗，但是她感觉自己的身体已经有了明显的好转和改善。这几天郭女士到医院里复查，回来后告诉我们，给她治病的医生和长期给她打针的护士见到她后都感到非常的惊奇，问她为什么现在看起来这么好了，郭女士说是在用生命修复中医药治疗。医生告诉她，既然效果这样好就继续治疗吧。郭女士充满信心，继续中医药的抗癌治疗。

治疗原则

软坚消瘤，通经攻癌。

常用中药

1. 柴胡、山慈菇、丹参、大黄、玄明粉、三棱、莪术、夏枯草、人参、附子、熟地黄等。
2. 同时服用消瘤丸、散结丸。

影像学、病理学检查报告及诊疗记录

1. 2021 年 7 月 7 日手术后病理报告证实为卵巢细胞癌，并有淋巴血管侵入，手术子宫切除，双附件双侧输卵管切除，网膜切除，双侧盆腔淋巴结切除。

2. 2022 年 10 月 5 日 PET/CT 检查报告证实：以前的多发性腹腔转移增大，并在横膈膜、肾周、胸膜、盆腔等部位有新的转移病灶。腹水大量增加。有新的肝转移病灶。右胸腔积液。左甲状腺结节，左乳房病变。与 2022 年 5 月 30 日检查报告比较，病情明显加重。

附：患者检查报告

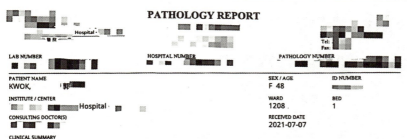

PATHOLOGY REPORT

Hospital

Tel:
Fax:

LAB NUMBER ▓ ▓ ▓

HOSPITAL NUMBER

PATHOLOGY NUMBER

PATIENT NAME
KWOK, 郭▓

SEX / AGE
F 48

ID NUMBER

INSTITUTE / CENTER
▓▓▓ Hospital ▓

WARD
1208

BED
1

CONSULTING DOCTOR(S)

RECEIVED DATE
2021-07-07

CLINICAL SUMMARY
Large pelvic mass. PET-CT: ? Malignant ovarian tumor. Right ovarian cyst content for frozen section - Carcinoma of ovary. Large fibroid. Laparotomy, total hysterectomy + bilateral salpingo-oophorectomy + omentectomy + pelvic lymphadenectomy.

FROZEN SECTION DIAGNOSIS
1) Carcinoma, favor clear cell.

DIAGNOSIS
1-6) Uterus with bilateral adnexa, total hysterectomy and bilateral salpingo-oophorectomy + omentectomy + bilateral pelvic lymph nodes sampling
- Clear cell adenocarcinoma (透明細胞腺癌) of right ovary
- Lymphovascular permeation present
- Clear margins
- Adenomyosis (子宮腺肌症)
- Leiomyoma (肌瘤)
- Benign hemorrhagic cyst (良性出血性囊腫) of left ovary
- No metastasis in bilateral pelvic lymph nodes

NATURE OF SPECIMEN
1) Right ovarian cyst content. Follow-up specimens: 2) Uterus + right ovary and tube. 3) Left ovary and tube. 4) Omentum. 5) Right pelvic lymph node. 6) Left pelvic lymph node.

MACROSCOPIC EXAMINATION

1) Right ovarian cyst content. The specimen is submitted in multiple fragments consisting of pale yellow to tan-colored solid nodules measuring from 0.8 cm to 3.2 cm. Sectioning shows fleshy tumor with focal hemorrhage. There is no necrosis. Cassette (1) 3 tissue blocks for frozen section. Cassette (2) to (4) Multiple additional tumor blocks. Figure 1 shows the submitted specimen.

2) Uterus and right ovary and tube. Received is a uterus with attached right adnexa weighing 886 g. There is marked congestion and hemorrhage over the right adnexal region. The right fallopian tube measures 8 cm long and 0.7 cm in diameter. The right ovary is enlarged to a cyst measuring up to 11 cm. It is ruptured on submission. The ovarian capsule is up to 1.2 cm thick. There are abundant degenerated blood inside and focal hemorrhagic solid nodules are identified. The nodules measure up to 3.8 cm. The uterus measures 17 cm from fundus to cervical os, 13 cm from cornu to cornu and 8 cm anteroposteriorly. The endometrium and myometrium measure 0.2 cm and 5 cm. There are a few foci of adenomyosis in the thickened myometrium. Two fibroid masses measure 6 cm and 11 cm with white whorled cut surface are also found near the fundus. There is no hemorrhage or necrosis of the fibroid. Cassette (1) Right fallopian tube and parametrium, 2 tissue blocks. Fibroids, 2 tissue blocks. Cassette (2) Left parametrium, 1 tissue block. Cervical margin, 1 tissue block. Cervix, 2 tissue blocks. Cassettes (3) & (4) Multiple tissue blocks from right ovarian cyst. Cassette (5) Endometrium and myometrium, 2 tissue blocks. Figure 2 shows the submitted specimen. Figure 3 shows cut surface of right ovary. Figure 4 shows cut surface of uterus.

3) Left ovary and tube. Received is a fallopian tube and ovary. The fallopian tube measures 5 cm long and 1 cm in diameter. The ovary measures 4 cm. Sectioning shows a 2 cm hemorrhagic cyst. Ovary, 2 tissue blocks. Fallopian tube, 1 tissue block. Figure 5 shows the submitted specimen. Figure 6 shows cut surface.

REPORT READ BY DOCTOR FAXED ON _____ (DATE/TIME)

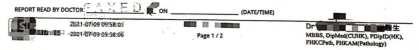

Page 1 / 2

Dr ▓▓▓▓ 醫生
MBBS, DipMed(CUHK), PDipID(HK),
FHKCPath, FHKAM(Pathology)

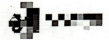

放射部 **Radiology Department**
電話 Tel: ▮▮▮▮▮▮▮   傳真 Fax: ▮▮▮ ▮▮

Hosp Patient ID: ▮▮▮ ▮   Exam Date: 05.10.2022
Name: KWOK,▮▮▮▮   Sex: F   DOB: 08.12.1972
Referrer: ▮▮▮▮   Location: PET-CT01
Section: PET-CT   Document No.: ▮▮▮▮▮
Case ID: ▮▮▮▮▮▮▮▮▮   HIS Order Number: ▮▮▮▮▮
Exam No: ▮ ▮ ▮▮▮▮

---

level are seen, being largely stable. Compressive atelectasis over basal right lung is noted. No hypermetabolic lung mass or nodule is detected. No left pleural or pericardial effusion is noted. No hypermetabolic lymphadenopathy in bilateral hila, mediastinum, internal mammary chains, supraclavicular fossa and bilateral cervical regions. A non-FDG-avid left lobe thyroid nodule (1.7 x 1.3 x 1.0cm) is noted. Orbits, paranasal sinuses and nasopharynx are unremarkable. Pharyngeal lymphoid activity is within physiological limit. An oval non-FDG-avid hypodense lesion (1.3 x 0.8cm) at medial left breast is noted. No hypermetabolic lesion is detected in both breasts. Axillae are clear.

SKELETAL SYSTEM
No hypermetabolic or aggressive lytic-sclerotic bone lesion in the visualized skeleton is noted.

Summary of representative lesions are tabulated as below:
(Reference liver background has SUVmax of 2.7)
(The measurement of SUV values may vary in different imaging centres and direct comparison should be made with caution.)

Location	Size (cm)	SUVmax
R pleural deposits	2.7 x 0.9 x 1.3	3.8
	1.7 x 0.9 x 1.1	3.8
Gastrohepatic peritoneal lesions	2.0 x 1.6 x 1.1	6.1
	1.2 x 1.0	4.7
L abdominal peritoneal lesion	6.5 x 3.4 x 5.1	6.7
L omentum peritoneal lesion	4.7 x 1.6 x 3.4	6.8
Para-splenic peritoneal lesion	1.2 x 0.8 x 2.0	4.7
R mesenteric peritoneal lesion	1.1 x 1.1 x 0.9	4.5
L mesenteric peritoneal lesion	1.3 x 1.0 x 0.9	5.3
Peritoneal lesion abutting R diaphragmatic crux	1.1 x 0.5	4.5
Peritoneal lesion at R Gerota's fascia	1.0 x 0.9	4.4
Pelvic peritoneal lesion	0.6 x 0.6	5.3
R lobe liver lesion	1.2 x 1.4	8.8

Thank you for the courtesy of this referral
Electronically Signed

Approved Date: 06.10.2022 16:55

SPECIALIST IN RADIOLOGY
MBChB(CUHK) FRCR FHKCR FHKAM(RADIOLOGY)

Page 2 of 3

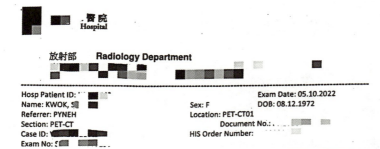

晋院 Hospital

放射部 **Radiology Department**

Hosp Patient ID: Exam Date: 05.10.2022
Name: KWOK, S   Sex: F   DOB: 08.12.1972
Referrer: PYNEH   Location: PET-CT01
Section: PET-CT   Document No.:
Case ID: HIS Order Number:
Exam No:

IMPRESSIONS:

Note is made to history of CA ovary with TAHBSO, omentectomy and pelvic lymph node dissection performed.

- Previous multiple peritoneal metastases show overall mild increase in extent, with new small active deposits noted abutting right diaphragmatic crux, right Gerota's fascia and pelvic region. Gross ascites, showing significant interval increase in amount.
- A new hypermetabolic liver lesion at inferior right hepatic lobe is noted, suspicious of new liver metastasis.
- Previous right pleural deposits at mid thoracic level are largely stable. Moderate right pleural effusion.
- Other incidental findings including non-FDG-avid left thyroid nodule and medial left breast lesion are seen.
- Overall, the disease shows progression when compare to previous PET/CT study dated 30-May-2022.

Thank you for your referral.

SUV = Standardised Uptake Value which is a quantification of glucose metabolic rate

Thank you for the courtesy of this referral
Electronically Signed

DR
SPECIALIST IN RADIOLOGY
MBChB(CUHK) FRCR FHKCR FHKAM(RADIOLOGY)

Approved Date: 06.10.2022 16:55

Typed By:

Page 3 of 3

病案42

晚期乳腺癌多发脑、骨转移康复

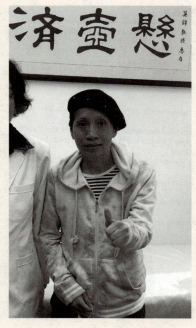

🎧 梁女士2024年1月前来诊治时合影留念

梁女士是一位中学教师，工作勤奋，认真负责，检查学生的作业一丝不苟，教书育人非常有耐心，讲课和教导学生时，表达能力也非常好。但是在2011年年末突然发现了乳腺的包块，她急忙去医院就诊。经过一系列的检查，得到的诊断，是她万万没有想到的乳腺癌，并已有局部的侵入扩散。她于2012年1月到医院去做手术，切除有癌症的乳腺肿瘤以及扩散的部分。自感以后不会再有问题了，期间也常服用一些保健品。但是在2014年10月，经过检查，发现仅仅过了2年，就又有局部乳腺癌的扩散和淋巴转移。她急忙在医院里做各种现代化治疗，并长期坚持，以对抗癌症。2021年2月经过检查，发现乳腺癌不仅是局部的复发和淋巴转移，还发生了多发性双肺转移，甚至连胰腺也发生了转移。2022年6月，又发现了全身多发性骨转移和多发性脑转移。脑部的癌肿非常大也非常多，其中最大的肿瘤达到了 5.4cm，梁女士非常瘦弱，整个头部的体积也没有多大，却被这么多这样大的肿瘤占据了颅脑的最重要的部分，同时脊椎的肿瘤向硬脊膜扩散。她一直使用最先进的靶向治癌药物，发现脑的多发转移之后，又增加了类固醇激素治疗。尽管不停地使用各种先进的治疗方法，但病情越来越重，最后完全不能活动，瘫痪在床。脑部的多发和巨大肿瘤以及脊椎的肿瘤都是造成她瘫痪的重要原因。大脑越来越糊涂，不能说话，无法用语言表达，思维混乱。医院明确表示因为病情已经到了无药可医，无法治疗的阶段，他们也没有什么好的治疗方法了。

梁女士于 2022 年 9 月 25 日前来就诊，开始用生命修复的中医药来治疗癌症。她来看病时属于全身瘫痪的状态，由家人协助抬入诊所。她当时骨瘦如柴，奄奄一息，生活完全不能自理，吞咽困难，只能吃流食。失去语言功能，头痛，全身瘫痪，全身无力还做噩梦，时常有幻觉，咳嗽多痰，气短、呼吸困难，腹胀腹痛。

治疗原则采用扶助正气，祛除癌毒。因为身体过分虚弱，所以开始时用了大量补助阴阳气血的中药，待稍有改善以后，陆续增加抗癌中药。在治疗 1 周之后，梁女士前来看病时精神好转，自诉全身的瘫痪状况有所改善，并且自己能够扶住桌椅站立一会儿。可是就在治疗的第 2 周，出现了发热，严重头痛，尿道感染，尿痛的症状，其主要原因是靶向、化疗的副作用造

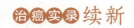

成，只好住院治疗。医院给她减少了靶向药物的治疗剂量，期间有 10 多天住院中，无法服用中药。待症状缓解后，梁女士又前来看诊。经服用中药，她说头晕头痛的情况已经有所改善，并且在 11 月上旬，能够自己走路了，右侧的上臂可以活动一些，但下肢仍有不适。她非常高兴的告诉我们，现在语言表达能力恢复的很明显。11 月中旬，她的精神状态和活动能力继续好转，可以自己去上厕所，不需要人帮助了。乳腺部位伤口的癌肿明显缩小，流出的分泌物减少。12 月上旬，病情继续好转，精神也有明显好转，胃口恢复，语言流利，已经与正常人讲话没有两样。听到她用手机给朋友打电话安排教学事宜，吐字清楚，表达准确，用词恰当，有非常好的语言才华，并且还用英文给大家唱歌，赢得了掌声和欢迎。12 月中旬发现乳腺的癌肿伤口明显缩小，液体渗出明显减少，接近痊愈和封口。梁女士现在信心百倍，继续认真的使用生命修复中医药治疗。

燮理阴阳，补助正气，消瘤抗癌。

常用中药

1. 人参、鹿角胶、龟胶、黄芪、黄精、淫羊藿、半枝莲、猕猴桃根、乌梢蛇、蜈蚣、猫爪草等。
2. 同时服用消瘤丸、散结丸。

影像学、病理学检查报告及诊疗记录

1. 2022 年 9 月 6 日癌症中心的病情介绍：2012 年 1 月患乳腺癌并局部侵入。2014 年 10 月局部和淋巴转移复发。2021 年 2 月多发肺转移和胰腺。2022 年 6 月多发骨和脑转移。

2. 2022 年 8 月 2 日脑 MRI 检查结果显示：大脑有大量转移病灶，最大的位于脑顶叶——枕叶部位有 4.8cm×3.8cm×5.4cm 肿瘤。

3. 2022 年 8 月 4 日 PET/CT 检查报告显示：乳腺癌手术之后，右胸部有很大的蘑菇状肿瘤显示肿瘤复发。双侧肺转移，右肺胸膜转移。右胸部腋下纵隔等大量淋巴转移。胰腺体部有很大的高代谢强度的肿瘤提示第二个原发胰腺癌，建议可进一步检查。左第五右第八肋骨和腰四椎骨骨转移，并向邻近软组织和硬脊膜扩散，应进一步检查脊椎和神经根状态。

附：患者检查报告

281

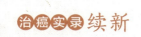
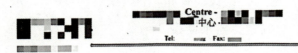

Centre - 中心 -

Tel: ▬▬ Fax: ▬

Date: 06 September, 2022

To whom it may concern

       Re: LEUNG ▬ ▬ ▬ *(梁▬)*, ▪ ▪ ▪ ▪ *Female/56Y*

The abovenamed patient is suffering from CA right breast papillary with foci of invasion (HR+ve, HER2-ve) (Jan 2012)
Local and nodal recurrence (ER+ve, HER2-ve) (Oct 2014)
Multiple lung metastases and ?BRCA1/2 related pancreatic mass IDC Grade II (ER+ve, PR-ve, HER2-ve with Ki-67=35%) (Feb 2021)
Bone and brain metastases (June 2022)
I've recommended as followings:

1) MR-Brain(P+C) asap
2) Continue Palbociclib 125mg daily(3/4 weeks) + Letrozole 2.5mg daily (PALOMA2) to until intolerable toxicities or disease progression, whichever happens earlier
3) Assess tumour response after C2-Palbociclib
4) Assays for gBRCA1/BRCA2 mutations asap
5) Consider Temozolomide or SRT if brain metastases deterioration

Thank you very much for your kind attention.

Yours faithfully,

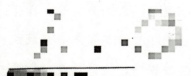

MD, MBBS(HK), FRCR, FHKCR, FHKAM (Radiology), DMRT(UK)

Hospital

DEPT. OF CLINICAL ONCOLOGY
Tel: ▓▓▓▓
23/09/2022
Case no: RW ▓▓▓

To: Whom it may concern

Dear Sir/Madam,

Re: LEUNG, ▓▓ ▓ ▓ ▓ 梁▓ ▓ ▓ ▓

This letter is to certify the patient latest MRI brain result in 2/8/2022 and PET-CT reuslt 4/8/2022 for medical purpose with patient consent.

MRI brain 2/8/2022
There are multiple enhancing metastatic deposits in the cerebral and cerebellar hemispheres as follow:
- Dominant lesion at the right parieto-occipital region measuring 4.8x3.8x5.4cm, with eccentric heterogeneous enhancing component. Dependent haemosiderin layering is suggestive of previous haemorrhage.
- Left lateral cerebellar hemisphere, measuring 1.7cm.
- Right medial occipital lobe, measuring 10mm.
- Along right superior frontal sulcus, measuring 7mm.
- There is resultant mass effect from the dominant left parieto-occipital metastasis with effacement of the occipital horn and trigone of left lateral ventricle.
- No hydrocephalus.
- No acute infarct or microhaemorrhage in rest of the brain.

PET CT 4/8/2022
1. CA right breast status surgery with large fungating masses along the right chest wall, suggestive of
local tumour recurrence.
2. Bilateral pulmonary metastases and pleural-based metastasis along the right middle lobe.
3. Metastatic nodes along the right pectoral and level I and II right axillary region. Smaller nodes in the
mediastinum could represent additional metastatic nodes.
4. Large hypermetabolic cystic lesion at the pancreatic body with internal solid component could represent a second primary pancreatic tumour (mucinous cystadenoma/cystadenocarcinoma). Correlation with old film +/- dedicated MR pancreas is recommended for further evaluation if there are clinical needs.
5. Bone metastases at left 5th rib, right 8th rib and L4 with adjacent soft tissue & epidural extension. The spinal canal is narrowed at this site. Suggest correlation with neurological examination +/- MR spine if there are concerns about the nerve root status.
6. Hypodense lesion in included left occipital lobe of the brain is suspicious of brain metastasis (not completely included in the current examination). Suggest correlation with MR/CT brain for complete intracranial disease status.

Thank you for your attention.

Printed on 23/09/2022 17:40   Printed by: ▓▓▓▓   Page 1 of 2

病案 43

晚期肺癌多发脑转移康复

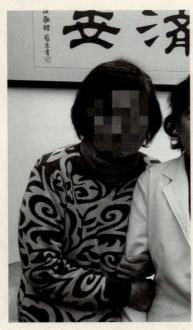

曾太太 2022 年 12 月前来诊治时合影留念

曾太太在 1999 年时患了肺癌，她当时 50 岁，在医院做手术切除了肿瘤和左侧部分肺。之后多年身体状况一直良好，没有发现什么大的问题。2020 年，因为咳嗽、气短到医院去做检查，6 月经组织学检查，确诊为肺腺癌。她当时经朋友介绍吃了一些营养产品，也服用过一些中草药。到 2021 年 10 月的时候，她的身体状况非常差，整个人非常疲倦和虚弱，走路失去平衡，不能站稳，整天卧床，进食越来越差。直至后来完全不能走路，瘫痪在床。因为她的病情越来越严重，于是在 2021 年 11 月 1 日住进了医院，经过多方面的检查，确诊为肺癌多发性脑转移。她在医院住了 1 个多月，服用靶向药物，并注射类固醇进行治疗，但是病情仍然非常严重。当时的 CEA 癌指数达到 681（正常值为小于 5），数值非常之高，病情危重。她不仅感觉疲倦，活动困难，还出现双下肢水肿，睡眠差，进食差，头痛，双手震颤。2021年11月中旬，在曾太太住院期间，她的女儿前来咨询，并预约出院之后前来治疗的日期。2021年12月曾太太出院之后就直接到我们的生命修复研究中心进行就诊和治疗。当时她的病情非常严重，完全不能行动，坐轮椅由家人推着她前来就诊。她身体很虚弱，全身无力，双腿双足严重水肿，不能睡觉，需要依靠安眠药。有时神志不清，并且咳嗽严重，多痰气喘，大便秘结。经过治疗之后，慢慢地曾太太一天天的好转起来。咳嗽逐渐减少，痰液减少，气短胸闷减轻，胃口好转，她也可以慢慢地尝试着站起来几分钟，然后再坐在轮椅上。能够迈步后，开始像幼儿一样慢慢地学习迈步和走路。2022年2月23日，曾太太的CEA癌指数降为5.4。2022年8月再次复查时，她的CEA癌指数已经为2.9，完全恢复正常。曾太太依旧坚持着治疗和练习，就这样过了1~2个月，她可以比较正常地行走了。以后她慢慢地一边活动，一边在家里做行走的练习。她自己计算，从开始能走几步，慢慢地增加到十几步，二十几步，三十几步。大约治疗4~5个月，曾太太就完全恢复正常的行走。以前每次前来看诊都需要乘坐出租车或者找人开车带她过来，现在她说可以正常的上街去买东西，在家操持家务，做饭，打扫卫生。她告诉我们今天走了几千步，再往后她可以自己前来，还高兴地告诉我们，现在是自己乘坐公交车前来的，这在以前是根本不可能办到的。在过年之前的复诊中，她流着眼泪回想说，上一年过年时瘫痪在床，全家一片哀愁。这一次她提前打扫房间，给孩子们准备喜爱的礼物，给全家制作好吃的年糕。虽然曾太太已经73岁了，但依然充满活力，她的生活已经完全恢复正常。

治疗原则

补中祛毒，化痰消癌。

常用中药

1. 黄芪、白术、人参、礞石、海浮石、胆南星、半夏、厚朴、重楼等。
2. 同时服用消瘤丸、散结丸。

影像学、病理学检查报告及诊疗记录

1. 2021年11月24日PET/CT检查报告显示肺癌双肺转移，肺塌陷，多侧肾上腺转移。多淋巴转移，考虑双侧肾上腺转移。

2. 2022年4月1日脑部MRI检查证实有多发脑转移，慢性脑血管缺血等病变。

附：患者检查报告

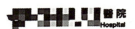 醫院 Hospital

Tel: ▮▮▮ Fax: ▮▮▮

PET-CT

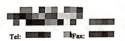

Name:	LEE ▮▮▮ 李▮▮		**Referral Doctor:**	▮▮ ▮ ▮▮▮
Sex/Age:	F / 72Y	**DOB:** 15.01.1949	**Ordering Doctor:**	▮ ▮▮ ▮▮
HN No.:	▮▮ ▮	**ID:** ▮ ▮ ▮	**Exam Date:**	24.11.2021
Epi No.:	▮▮		**Clinic /Ward Bed:**	▮▮▮ ▮▮ ▮ ▮

COMMENT:

1. Status treated pulmonary malignancy post left lower lobectomy. The known hypermetabolic left suprahilar lung mass has slightly decreased in FDG uptake. New segmental left upper lobe lung collapse distal to the mass with mild patchy FDG uptake could be inflammatory, with or without neoplastic infiltration.

2. Multiple new inactive solid nodules in right lung, some of them cavitary, are highly suggestive of intrapulmonary metastases.

3. Loculated left apical pleural effusion with subtle FDG uptake, and trace inactive free left pleural fluid.

4. The known hypermetabolic mediastinal and right axillary lymph nodes have generally improved in size and/or FDG uptake, except for a previously inactive aortopulmonary window lymph node which is now mildly FDG-avid.
   A prominent FDG-avid left level IV cervical lymph node has slightly worsened. Other previously noted bilateral lower cervical lymph nodes have improved or normalized.

5. Mildly increased bilateral adrenal glands FDG uptake is non-specific but would deserve follow-up imaging to exclude early adrenal metastasis.

6. No other metabolic evidence of distant metastasis is demonstrated.

Thank you for your kind referral.

SUV = Standard Uptake Value which is a quantification of glucose metabolic rate

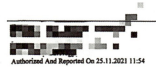

Authorized And Reported On 25.11.2021 11:54

Page 3 of 3

287

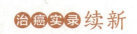

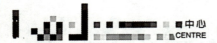 中心
CENTRE

	REPORT DATE : 01 APR 2022
	EXAM DATE : 01 APR 2022
Hospital	**OUR REF NO** : ▓▓ ▓▓▓ ▓▓
(▓▓▓▓醫院)	
NAME : LEE ▓▓▓▓	**YOUR REF NO** : ▓▓▓
HKID : ▓▓▓	
SEX/AGE : F/73 **DOB : 15 JAN 1949**	**ACCESSION NO** : ▓▓▓▓▓▓▓▓▓

MRI BRAIN (CONTRAST)

FINDINGS:

Mild background chronic microvascular ischaemic changes.

There is a nodular enhancing lesion seen over the left occipital lobe measuring 0.6 x 0.5 cm in size. There is also a nodular enhancing lesion measuring 0.7 x 0.5 cm just posterior to the posterior horn of the right lateral ventricle in the occipital lobe, in keeping with metastatic focus. Comparison is not possible with previous CT brain plain scan. Another tiny 3 mm nodular enhancing focus over right cerebellum may represent a metastatic focus as well.

The ventricles are not dilated. No midline shift. No focal mass effect. Sulcal spaces are normal.
The gray and white matters differentiation appears normal. No abnormal signal intensity identified otherwise.
No evidence of acute cerebral infarction is identified on the diffusion weighted sequence.
There is no intracranial haemorrhage seen.
Pituitary gland is not enlarged.
No abnormal leptomeningeal enhancement noted.

IMPRESSION:
1. Bilateral occipital lobe and right cerebellar metastases as described. Comparison with previous plain CT brain is not possible and not accurate.
2. Mild background chronic microvascular ischaemic changes noted.
3. No extra-axial fluid collection.
4. No midline shift and hydrocephalus.

MBBS(HK), FRCR
FHKCR, FHKAM(Radiology)

CY

病案44

三次癌症手术后康复

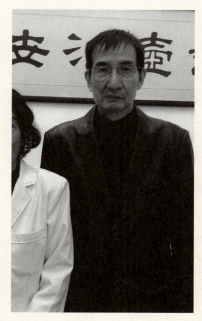

叶先生 70 岁了，他在 2020 年至 2021 年的 15 个月的时间里连续做了 3 次癌症切除的手术。叶先生是位有拼搏精神，努力工作的企业家，但是他从小患有乙型肝炎，并有肝硬化病史多年。在 2020 年中期的时候，他很不幸的发现患了肝癌。于 2020 年 7 月手术切除了肝右叶的恶性肿瘤。手术后身体刚刚恢复不久，又感到肝区不适，再次去做检查，发现肝的另外部分也有肿瘤。于是在 2021 年 8 月，不得已再次做了肝癌肿瘤的切除手术，这次是肝左叶的癌肿。手术后才 2 个月，刚刚松口气，就因吃饭进食的时候有吞咽困难并感到疼痛，于是在 2021 年 10 月到医院再次检查，结果确诊他患了口腔癌，伴有淋巴转移，已是第 Ⅳ 期，又接着做了口腔癌的切除手术。第 3 次手术之后，医院要求叶先生尽快做放疗，否则病情非常严重，非常危险。连续 3 次的手术，使得叶先生

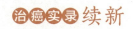

长期遭受痛苦。他感觉自己再也不能承受这样严重地打击了，所以他拒绝了医生尽快做放疗的要求，转向求治于生命修复的中医药治疗。

　　叶先生刚来时精神状态很差，手术后的口腔、牙槽都会疼痛，颈部疼痛，耳朵听不到，吞咽困难，说话困难，腹部的手术伤口也在疼痛，站立不稳，感觉每天的日子都非常难熬。叶先生的太太鼓励他，并且每次都陪他一起前来诊治。逐渐的，叶先生的身体慢慢好起来了，肝区疼痛从减轻到消失，口腔内疼痛逐步减少。吃东西慢慢地变得自然，吞咽困难逐渐改善。这样治疗了3个月后，再次检查身体。乙肝病毒的指数降到最低0，肝癌的指数甲胎蛋白降到1.8，在正常值以下，其他各项指标均在正常范围内。叶先生和他太太都非常高兴，决定认真服用中药坚持治疗。现在叶先生早就恢复了他的工作，虽然每天忙忙碌碌，但还在坚持服用中药巩固治疗。叶先生通过自身疾病的治疗过程，增强了对中医药的了解和信任，他决定用生命修复的中医药作为长期养生、调理身体的优选方法。

攻毒祛邪，扶正抗癌。

常用中药

1. 白花蛇舌草、海藻、夏枯草、半枝莲、全蝎、蜈蚣、鳖甲、山豆根、鸡骨草等。
2. 同时服用消瘤丸、攻毒丸。

影像学、病理学检查报告及诊疗记录

1. 2020 年 7 月 28 日手术后病理报告为肝细胞癌。

2. 2021 年 8 月 3 日肝脏再次手术后病理报告为肝细胞癌。

3. 2021 年 10 月 22 日 PET/CT 检查显示口腔上腭骨癌肿，有淋巴转移，手术后病理报告确诊为鳞状细胞癌 PT_4a（第 Ⅳ 期）。

附：患者检查报告

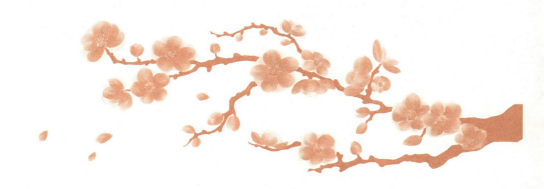

HOSPITAL 醫院
HISTOPATHOLOGY LABORATORY
組織病理化驗室

Tel :
Fax :

Path. No. :
Record status : C
Patient's name : YIP ▉▉ ▉ 葉▉▉　　　　　　　　　　　　ID# : ◀▉ ▉▉ ▉
Hospital no.: ▉▉▉▉▉ ▉▉▉▉▉　Room : M5A　　Bed : 506-5　　Sex : M　　Age : 67Yr1▉
Under the service of : ▉▉▉▉ ▉▉▉▉▉
Clinical history :　Segment 5/8 HCC.
Surgical procedure :　Segment 5/8 subsegmentectomy.
Nature of specimen :　Segment 5/8 subsegmentectomy specimen.
Frozen section diagnosis (if any) :　　　　　　　　　　　　Date received :　28/07/202▉

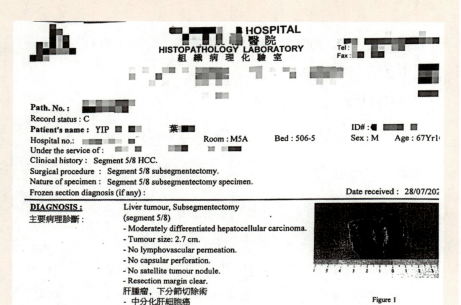

DIAGNOSIS :
主要病理診斷 :

Liver tumour, Subsegmentectomy
(segment 5/8)
- Moderately differentiated hepatocellular carcinoma.
- Tumour size: 2.7 cm.
- No lymphovascular permeation.
- No capsular perforation.
- No satellite tumour nodule.
- Resection margin clear.
肝腫瘤，下分節切除術
- 中分化肝細胞癌

Figure 1

MACROSCOPIC EXAMINATION:

(KCH, jc)
Segment 5/8 liver tissue. Submitted is a wedge of liver tissue weighing 48 gm and measuring 5 x 5 x 4.5 cm. It has be▉
partially cut opened on receipt showing a yellowish lobulated tumour mass measuring 2.7 x 1.9 x 1.5 cm. It is located
0.9 cm from the nearest liver resection margin. The tumour is located at the subcapsular region with no definite tumou▉
infiltration into the capsule. It shows lobulated appearance with friable consistency. No necrosis is seen. Cut surface
the other parts of the liver parenchyma shows vaguely nodular appearance but there is no cirrhotic nodule identified.
There is no satellite tumour nodule. (A) 1 tissue block from liver resection margin. 1 random tissue block from the ot▉
parts of the liver parenchyma. (B)to(E) 4 tissue blocks from tumour. Figure 1 shows the submitted specimen.

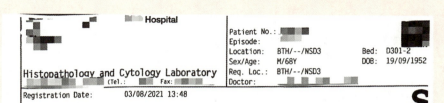

Hospital

Patient No.:	
Episode:	
Location: BTH/--/NSD3	Bed: D301-2
Sex/Age: M/68Y	DOB: 19/09/1952
Req. Loc.: BTH/--/NSD3	
Doctor:	

Histopathology and Cytology Laboratory
(Tel.:   Fax:)

Registration Date: 03/08/2021 13:48   **S**

Final Report

Specimen :
Segment 3 hepatectomy specimen

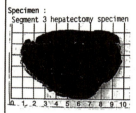

Clinical Summary :
Segment 3 HCC

Gross Description :
Specimen designated 'segment 3 hepatectomy specimen' received in formalin. It consists of a piece of brownish liver tissue, weighing 92 gm. The liver tissue measures 80 x 60 x 45 mm in size. The specimen is received cut opened at multiple areas before submission. The liver tissue is also received partially disrupted. A stitch is identified which connects the partially disrupted liver tissue. A plastic clip is detected inside the liver tissue clipping the bile duct. Serial cut section of the liver tissue shows a roundish tumour nodule located underneath the liver capsule. The tumour measures 11 x 8 mm in size. The tumour shows tan whitish coloured cut surface. The liver resection margin is clear with minimal clearance grossly measuring 25 mm. The liver capsule shows no tumour perforation. The rest of the liver parenchyma appears mildly cirrhotic. Representative sections are submitted as follows:
Block (A) The clipped bile duct margin.
Block (B) Liver resection margin.
Blocks (C & D) Liver tumour.
Block (E) Random sampling of liver tissue. (LKC)

Microscopic Description :
Sections of the liver show a moderately-differentiated hepatocellular carcinoma. The tumor is composed of proliferation of polygonal tumor cells arranged in thick trabeculae with sinusoidal pattern. The tumor cells show enlarged nuclei, moderate nuclear pleomorphism and hyperchromasia, prominent nucleoli and abundant eosinophilic cytoplasm. The tumor cells contain eosinophilic globules and occasional bile pigments. Mitotic figures are readily seen. Bile duct is inconspicuous in the tumor. Histochemical stain (reticulin) shows decreased staining inside the tumor and highlights the thick trabecular pattern of the tumor. Immunohistochemically, the tumor cells are positive for Hep-Par1 (hepatocyte marker) and focally positive for glypican-3. They are negative for CK19. The overall features of the liver tumor are consistent with hepatocellular carcinoma. Lymphovascular permeation is not seen in the section. The tumor shows no perforation of the visceral peritoneum (liver

---

Report Date & Time: 04/08/2021 19:02   Generated on: 04/08/2021 20:05
Report Destination: BTH/--/NSD3 - D3   Page No.: 1/2

HISTOPATHOLOGY REPORT

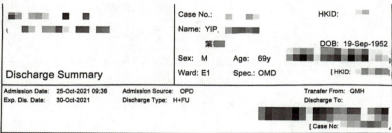

Case No.:		HKID:	
Name: YIP,			
葉			DOB: 19-Sep-1952
Sex: M	Age: 69y		
Ward: E1	Spec.: OMD		[HKID:

Discharge Summary

Admission Date:	25-Oct-2021 09:36	Admission Source:	OPD	Transfer From:	QMH
Exp. Dis. Date:	30-Oct-2021	Discharge Type:	H+FU	Discharge To:	
				[Case No:	

Discharge Note:

non-specific, could indicate dysplastic nodule or early HCC. Follow up for progress is recommended.

CT 10/06/2021
- Liver cirrhosis.
- Known focus of hyperenhancement on arterial phase at S3 has interval increase in size (0.7cm). Features are non-specific, could indicate dysplastic nodule or early HCC. Follow up for progress is recommended.

XR meeting: plan for USG guided biopsy of the S3 lesion. if lesion could not be identified by USG, consider arrange primovist MRI for characterize the lesion.

FNAC refused by pt in view of possible risk of bleeding and seedling of tumour

Pt has already attended private Dr. Yeung YP
Laparoscopic segment 3 resection performed on 3/8/21
Pathol:
Segment 3 hepatectomy specimen
Hepatocellular carcinoma, moderately differntiated
The tumour measures 11mm in maximal dimension
No lymphovascular permeation seen
Tumour shows no perforation of the visceral peritoneum
All resection margins clear

MRI appt 22/04/2022
FU OGD 30/03/2022

Ix:
1. Incisional biopsy tumor at maxilla 22/10/21
- SQUAMOPROLIFERATIVE LESION suggestive of DYSPLASIA;
- CANDIDA organisms present on surface;
- Superficial biopsy only, SUBOPTIMAL for assessment of invasive carcinoma.

2. PET-CT 22/10/2021
- A hypermetabolic soft tissue lesion is noted at right maxilla region. Malignancy cannot be excluded. Infection/inflammation is possible differential. Please kindly correlate histologically.
- A few shotty hypermetabolic right cervical level Ib and level IIa lymph nodes are seen. Nodal metastasis has to be considered.
- Non-FDG avid calcified granulomata are seen at left lower lobe.
- A few shotty mildly hypermetabolic mediastinal lymph nodes are seen at subcarinal, right hilum and right interlobar region. These are likely reactive nodes.
- Status post-segment VII/VIII hepatectomy. Focal subcapsular hypermetabolic soft tissue mass is noted at segment III. It could represent known hepatocellular carcinoma. Please kindly correlate.

DISCHARGE SUMMARY

QM9601/DS

病案 **45**

晚期肺癌双肺转移骨转移康复

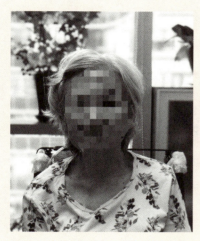

李太太 2022 年 10 月前来诊治时合影留念

李太太在 2020 年 6 月确诊了肺癌。当时她 64 岁，在相当一段时间内，咳嗽、胸闷、气短的症状越来越严重。当时是尽快做的化疗和放疗，但经检查发现病情加重。她原先是右肺有肿瘤，大小约 5.3cm×5.1cm×4.9cm，并且有气管、右肺门等多处的淋巴转移，经过化疗和放疗后再次检查，报告指出除了原来的肿瘤，双肺满布多发新的肿瘤，并有多处转移病灶，还在右侧的第一和第二肋骨发现了新的骨转移病灶。在这种情况下，李太太只好放弃化疗和放疗，前来求助于生命修复的中医药治疗。李太太来到我们的治疗中心时病情非常严重，是坐着轮椅，带着氧气罐持续吸氧的。虽然她在不停地吸着氧气，但是仍然有非常严重的气喘，呼吸困难。痰非常多，上气不接下气。她介绍说，一直在反复的住院吸痰，长期使用吗啡和抗生素。并在 2021 年 7 月的时候，因为上不来气，在医院里做了支气管支架的手术，用于暂时缓解呼吸困难的症状，但病情仍然发展较快，

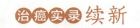

并出现了胸腔积液，在医院里做抽胸腔积液的治疗。所有的症状都显示，李太太的病情是非常严重的。即使给予增加氧气，还是咳嗽，气短，出汗，呼吸困难。经过辨证，我们尽快给李太太用中医药治疗，因为痰液太多，严重气喘，开始只能急则治其标，消炎解毒，化痰定喘。以后逐渐增加消除肿瘤的治疗。虽然病情很严重，但是李太太每次由家人带来时都充满信心，积极配合治疗。病情逐渐好转。2022年10月5日，李太太的复查报告出来了，显示出双肺的肿瘤已经完全消失，已有的2处骨转移也一并消失，并且没有见到新的转移病灶。虽然治疗的时间并不是太长，但是李太太取得了非常好的治疗效果。

她原本肺癌肿瘤大并有淋巴转移，已经是非常严重的病情。经过现代医学治疗后检查又发现了双肺转移、骨转移，属于到了最晚期的阶段。根据医学统计，晚期肺癌骨转移的中位存活期仅为3个月。在这种情况下，李太太只好放弃了常规的化疗等治疗方法，而选择用生命修复的中医药，并取得了良好的效果。肺部肿瘤全部消失，多处骨转移也已经消失，非常值得庆幸。

开胸散结化痰，祛邪扶正消瘤。

常用中药

1. 人参、半夏、瓜蒌、薤白、葶苈子、杏仁、半枝莲、重楼、百部等。

2. 同时服用散结丸、消痰丸。

影像学、病理学检查报告及诊疗记录

1. 2021年6月15日PET/CT检查报告肺癌，右肺中叶肿瘤5.3cm×5.1cm×4.9cm，并有多处气管旁肺门等淋巴转移，骨转移。

2. 2021年10月11日检查报告显示，肺癌多发双肺转移，淋巴转移骨转移。

3. 2022年10月5日PET/CT检查报告证实肺部肿瘤已完全消失，骨转移消失，没有见到转移病灶。

附：患者检查报告

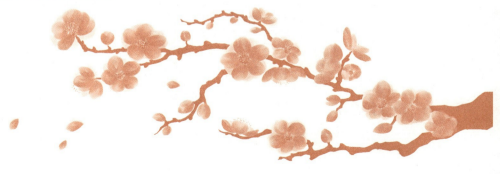

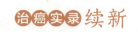

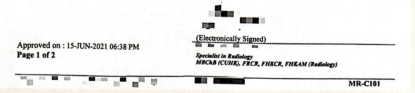

MEDICAL IMAGING DEPARTMENT

Patient's Name	: LEE,	**Unit Record No.**	:	
Sex	: F	**Age**	: 64	
Examination Date	: 15-JUN-2021	**Accession No.**	:	
Ward / Class	: 631B	**Attending Doctor**	:	

EXAMINATION / PROCEDURE REPORT

^{18}F-FDG PET/CT SCAN WHOLE BODY AND BRAIN (PLAIN)

CLINICAL INFORMATION:

Ca lung

TECHNIQUE:

Attenuation corrected PET scans of 4mm thickness were obtained from vertex to pelvis 1 hour after 6.96 mCi (body weight 61 kg) of ^{18}F-FDG was injected via right hand vein. Whole body volumetric CT Scan was performed for the same region. CT-PET fused images were subsequently obtained. Blood glucose level prior to injection of FDG was 5.5 mmol/l.

FINDINGS :

Liver tissue normal reference uptake has SUVmax of 2.9.

NECK AND THORAX

An irregular hypermetabolic mass with central photopenic area suggesting necrosis is noted in the lateral segment of right middle lobe lung. It shows disease extension across the right minor fissure invading into the inferior part of right upper lobe. Adjacent pleural tagging is also noted. No direct mediastinal or diaphragmatic invasion is noted. Multiple bulky hypermetabolic lymphadenopathies at right upper and lower paratracheal, right hilar and subcarinal region are seen. Tiny calcified granuloma in the left lung lingular segment is noted. No pleural or pericardial effusion is noted. No hypermetabolic lymphadenopathy in left hilum, left mediastinum, bilateral supraclavicular fossa and along bilateral jugular lymphatics. Thyroid gland and nasopharynx are unremarkable. No hypermetabolic lesion is detected in both breasts. Axillae are clear.

ABDOMEN AND PELVIS

There is normal size and metabolism of liver, spleen, adrenal glands and pancreas. No hyperdense gallstone. Kidney configuration is normal. Stomach and bowel activities are physiological. Colonic diverticula are seen. Focal bulging (2.3cm) with calcification at the anterior uterine wall, likely due to fibroid, is noted. No hypermetabolic mass in the pelvis is noted. There is no hypermetabolic lymphadenopathy in abdomen, pelvis or inguinal regions. No ascites.

(Electronically Signed)

Approved on : 15-JUN-2021 06:38 PM
Page 1 of 2

Specialist in Radiology
MBChB (CUHK), FRCR, FHKCR, FHKAM (Radiology)

MR-C101

Hospital ■ 醫院
MEDICAL IMAGING DEPARTMENT

Patient's Name	: LEE	Unit Record No.	:	
Sex	: F	Age	:	64
Examination Date	: 15-JUN-2021	Accession No.	:	
Ward / Class	: 631B	Attending Doctor	:	

EXAMINATION / PROCEDURE REPORT

BRAIN

There is normal intense tracer uptake in the cerebral cortex and basal ganglia. No discrete hypermetabolic intracranial lesion is noted. Please be aware that FDG PET/CT has a limited sensitivity for detection of cerebral metastasis. No acute intracranial hemorrhage or midline shift is noted.

SKELETAL SYSTEM

No hypermetabolic focal marrow lesion in the axial and proximal appendicular skeleton is noted. Focal mild uptake (SUVmax 4.3) at left L4/5 facet joint is likely due to inflammatory/degenerative activity. Grade 1 L3/4 spondylolisthesis and degenerative changes in the skeleton are seen.

IMPRESSION:

- The irregular mass in right middle lobe lateral segment with transfissural invasion of inferior part of right upper lobe is highly suspicious of malignant lung tumour. Histological correlation is suggested. No direct mediastinal or diaphragmatic invasion is noted.
- Multiple bulky hypermetabolic lymphadenopathies at right upper and lower paratracheal, right hilar and subcarinal region are suggestive of regional nodal metastases.
- Incidental findings of colonic diverticula and uterine fibroid.
- No focal FDG-avid distant metastasis is demonstrated in the rest of current study.

Selected measurements are tabulated as below:

Location	Size (cm)	SUVmax
R middle lobe lung mass	5.3 x 5.1 x 4.9	21.7
R upper paratracheal LN	1.7	19.1
R lower paratracheal LN	0.7	16.0
R hilar LN	1.4	3.4
Subcarinal LN	3.0	19.5

Thank you for your referral.

SUV = Standardised Uptake Value which is a quantification of glucose metabolic rate

(Electronically Signed)

Approved on : 15-JUN-2021 06:38 PM
Page 2 of 2

Specialist in Radiology
MBChB (CUHK), FRCR, FHKCR, FHKAM (Radiology)

MR-C101

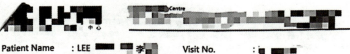

Patient Name : LEE ▮▮▮ 李▮	Visit No. : ▮ ▮▮
Patient ID : ▮▮▮▮	Client No. : ▮▮ ▮▮
Sex/Age, DOB : F/64, ▮▮ ▮ ▮▮	Accession No. : ▮▮▮▮ ▮
Exam Date : 11/10/2021	Referring Doctor : ▮▮ ▮▮
Reporting Date : 12/10/2021	Your Reference : 210125CM

PET-CT WHOLE BODY (PLAIN)

No ascites or loculated intraabdominal collection. No hypermetabolic intra-abdominal or retroperitoneal lymphadenopathy.

Bones

A new hypermetabolic segment is seen near anterior end of right 1st rib (SUVmax 5.8). Another new hypermetabolic short segment is seen in the anterolateral part of right 2nd rib (SUVmax 4.6). No other focally hypermetabolic body lesion is seen.

There is increased FDG uptake in the left L4/5 facet joint (SUVmax 3.9), likely inflammatory change.

CONCLUSION

- The previously shown hypermetabolic RML/RUL tumor has shown significant interval improvement.
- Multiple new hypermetabolic lesions are seen scattered in both lungs. Most of the lesions are ill-defined patchy infiltrates or ground glass densities, which are likely active inflammatory / infective change. One of the lesions in RLL appears as a solid nodule, which raises suspicion of metastasis, but could otherwise be part of the same multifocal inflammatory/infective change. Please correlate with clinical finding. Interval imaging follow up could also be helpful.
- Hypermetabolic lymph nodes seen in right side of mediastinum have shown interval improvement.
- New hypermetabolic segments in right 1st and 2nd ribs are suspicious of new metastasis.
- No metabolic evidence of other new distant metastasis.

Thank you for your referral.

Authorized and Reported: 12/10/2021 04:11:35 PM
Printed: 18/10/2021 08:16:59 AM
▮▮ ▮▮

(Electronic signature)
▮▮ ▮▮▮
Consultant Radiologist
MBChB, FRCR, FHKCR,
FHKAM(Radiology)

Page 3 of 3

300

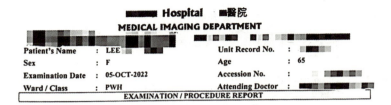

■■ Hospital ■醫院

MEDICAL IMAGING DEPARTMENT

Patient's Name	: LEE	Unit Record No.	:	■■
Sex	: F	Age	:	65
Examination Date	: 05-OCT-2022	Accession No.	:	■■■
Ward / Class	: PWH	Attending Doctor	:	■■■

EXAMINATION / PROCEDURE REPORT

PET/CT SCAN WHOLE BODY WITH BRAIN (CONTRAST)

CLINICAL INFORMATION

CA lung on immunotherapy.   Pneumonitis noted in previous study.
For follow up.

TECHNIQUE

Attenuation corrected PET scans of 4mm thickness were obtained from vertex
to pelvis 1 hour after 5.2 mCi (body weight 45 kg) of F18 -FDG was injected
via left arm vein. Whole body volumetric CT Scan with brain was performed
for the same region.   CT-PET fused images were subsequently obtained.
Blood glucose level prior to injection of FDG was 6.5 mmol/l.

Liver reference SUVmax/mean: 2.4/1.8

REPORT

Comparison is made with the previous PET/CT study done on 12/03/2022.

HEAD AND NECK

Post contrast CT scan shows no mass lesion in the brain and neck.   No
lymphadenopathy detected.   The thyroid gland is not enlarged.

THORAX

There is no hypermetabolic mass lesion detected in both lungs.   Right lung
volume is decreased.   Multiple areas of fibrosis, atelectasis and traction
bronchiectasis are still noted in both lungs with mild uptake (SUVmax up to
2.5, previous up to 3.3).   No significant progression.   The previous noted
right apical pneumothorax has resolved.   There is no pleural effusion.

Approved on : 08-OCT-2022 04:42 PM
Page 1 of 2

(Electronically Signed)

Consultant in Radiology
MBBS(HK), DMRD, FRCR, FHKCR, FHKAM(Radiology)

MR-C101

301

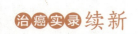

■■ Hospital ■■醫院
MEDICAL IMAGING DEPARTMENT

Patient's Name	: LEE ■■ ■ ■	Unit Record No.	:
Sex	: F	Age	: 65
Examination Date	: 05-OCT-2022	Accession No.	:
Ward / Class	: PWH	Attending Doctor	:

EXAMINATION / PROCEDURE REPORT

ABDOMEN AND PELVIS

The liver, spleen, pancreas and adrenal glands are unremarkable. There is no mass lesion detected. The kidneys are normal. There is no paraaortic lymphadenopathy or ascites. Bowel pattern is normal.

The small uterine fibroid with calcifications is unchanged.

AXIAL SKELETON

Focal uptake is noted at left fourth, fifth and sixth ribs with SUVmax up to 4.3. These are suggestive of healing crack fractures. No skeleton metastasis.

COMMENT

The primary lesion in right lung cannot be identified, no evidence of tumour recurrence. The right apical pneumothorax has resolved. Multiple areas of fibrosis, atelectasis and traction bronchiectasis in right lung due to previous infection. No pleural effusion.

No evidence of metastasis detected in the body and skeleton.

Some healing crack fractures at left fourth to sixth ribs.

Small uterine fibroid.

Thank you for your referral.

SUV = Standardised Uptake Value which is a quantification of glucose metabolic rate

/kk

(Electronically Signed)

Approved on : 08-OCT-2022 04:42 PM

Page 2 of 2

Consultant in Radiology
MBBS(HK), DMRD, FRCR, FHKCR, FHKAM(Radiology)

MR-C101

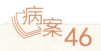

晚期肺癌多发肝、肾上腺、骨、卵巢等转移康复

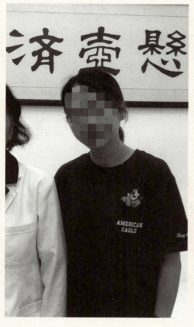

🔹 刘女士 2022 年 11 月前来诊治时合影留念

刘女士于 2022 年 4 月 17 日前来就诊，当时她 45 岁。自诉已经确诊为第 IV 期晚期肺癌，就诊时面色灰暗，疲倦无力，神情黯淡，不断呻吟。她说现在有严重的咳嗽，咯血，血痰症状。肝区疼痛非常严重，晚上痛得不能睡觉，或被痛醒，无法睡觉，吃止痛药也没有效果。在此之前已经咳嗽了半年多，在 2 周之前开始发生严重疼痛。咳嗽严重，血丝、血块很多。她带来了 2022 年 4 月 6 日和 2022 年 4 月 9 日在医院做的 PET/CT 检查报告。看了刘女士的检查报告，发现肿瘤的严重程度让人非常吃惊。在报告上明确写着：①肺脏有不规则的大肿瘤，肿瘤的大小有 5.4cm×4.3cm×3.7cm，SUV 值 15.6。同时肿瘤紧接左侧心脏的边缘和左肺门位置，邻近的肺组织已经有部分的塌陷。②纵隔部位有大量高代谢的弥漫性的转移性肿大淋巴结，沿着气管

303

旁、肺动脉窗、主动脉旁等位置分布，双侧颈部转移性淋巴结肿大。③肝脏肿瘤大的体积有 4.7cm×5.7cm×6.3cm，SUV 值 16.9。肿瘤可能是原发性的，也可能是转移来的。还有一些比较小的高代谢的肿瘤在肝右叶分布。④肝门处有肿大的高代谢的转移性淋巴结分布。⑤肾上腺有转移性的肿瘤，大小体积是 2.2cm×1.8cm×3.3cm，SUV 值 13.2。⑥右侧卵巢高代谢增强，有肿瘤分布。⑦脊椎有高代谢的转移性的骨质破坏，在脊椎胸九和腰四有骨转移，胸九的骨转移有向椎管内侵犯的表现。刘女士还做了有关的，在超声引导下器官取材的活组织检查，经过检测证明，肝脏的肿瘤是从肺脏，肺腺癌转移而来，明确了原发病灶在肺脏。在给她进行身体检查时，我们发现肝脏的肿瘤非常巨大。肿瘤在平肚脐以上的位置都是质地坚硬的大肿块，压痛明显不可触碰，全身有散在瘀斑。经过辨证施方，我们用中医药进行积极的治疗，同时因为疼痛严重也增加了穴位针灸治疗等多种方法。

刘女士对治疗的反应非常好，几天之后肝区的疼痛就有所减轻，告诉我们晚上可以睡觉了，也不用吃原本就不起作用，没有效果的止痛药了。治疗 2 周之后肝区已经没有疼痛了。以后医院给开了靶向药，并做了放疗。医生听说疼痛已经没有了，效果很快很好，也说道如果单纯只靠现代医学的治疗，是达不到这种效果的。又过了 2 周，刘女士恢复胃口，吃饭好，睡觉好。之后我们就把重点放在治疗咳嗽，多痰，咯血等问题上面。

2022 年 6 月 17 日的 CT 检查报告显示，肺部的肿瘤已经明显缩小，现在的大小是 2.5cm×2.6cm×1.4cm。大量的转移性的淋巴结明显缩小或消失。双侧颈部转移性肿大淋巴结完全消失，肝脏最大的肿瘤明显缩小，现在的大小是 2.6cm×2.7cm×3cm，SUV15.6。而肝脏的其他比较小的一些肿瘤已经全部消失。肾上腺的肿瘤也消失了，剩下残余的 SUV 值 2.9。肝门处肿大的转移性淋巴结完全消失。胸九的骨转移缩小，活性和大小都有所减少。脊椎腰四的骨转移已经消失。

到 2022 年 8 月 17 日，也就是她前来治疗整整 4 个月时，经医院检查肺部肿瘤已经消失。全家甚感欣慰，刘女士的丈夫更是去掉了笼罩多时的满面愁云。刘女士一直都有很好的心态，她一直用积极、乐观的态度去治疗癌症，这也是她能够卓有成效的战胜癌症的强大力量。

当前刘女士仍在认真的治疗过程中。虽然整个治疗的疗程时间还不够长，但我认为还是应该将这个治疗过程发布出来，以鼓励更多的重症患者。

治疗原则

燮理阴阳，扶正祛邪。

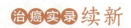

常用中药

1. 人参、淫羊藿、肉苁蓉、大黄、红花、杏仁、牡蛎、桃仁、牵牛子等。

2. 同时服用消瘤丸、散结丸。

影像学、病理学检查报告及诊疗记录

1. 2022年4月9日PET/CT检查报告显示全身多个器官有大量肿瘤及转移性肿瘤。其中肺脏大的肿瘤为5.4cm×4.3cm×3.7cm，肝脏大的肿瘤有4.7cm×5.7cm×6.3cm，另外纵隔、肝门、颈部等多发淋巴转移，肾上腺、脊椎、卵巢等转移。

2. 2022年4月7日病理组织学检查报告确定肝脏肿瘤为转移性肺腺癌。

3. 2022年6月17日PET/CT检查报告显示，全身多器官多发肿瘤明显减少或消失。

4. 2022年4月25日X线片显示肺部大的肿瘤。

5. 2022年8月17日X线片显示肺部肿瘤全部消失。

附：患者检查报告

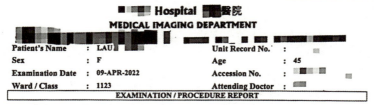

Hospital 醫院
MEDICAL IMAGING DEPARTMENT

Patient's Name	: LAU	Unit Record No.	:	
Sex	: F	Age	: 45	
Examination Date	: 09-APR-2022	Accession No.	:	
Ward / Class	: 1123	Attending Doctor	:	

EXAMINATION / PROCEDURE REPORT

PET/CT SCAN OF WHOLE BODY (PLAIN)

TECHNIQUE:

Attenuation corrected PET scans of 4mm thickness were obtained from skull base to pelvis 1 hour after 5.23 mCi (body weight 49.2 kg) of F18 -FDG was injected via left wrist vein. Whole body volumetric CT Scan was performed for the same region. CT-PET fused images were subsequently obtained. Blood glucose level prior to injection of FDG was 4.8 mmol/l.

FINDINGS:

NECK

Normal pharyngeal and tonsillar tracer uptake is noted.

Mildly enlarged and hypermetabolic bilateral lower neck lymph nodes are seen, in particular at right supraclavicular region, with size measuring up to 0.8 x 0.9 cm and activity up to SUVmax 10.8, compatible with metastatic lymph nodes.

No other abnormal tracer uptake is demonstrated in the neck region.

No other significant cervical or supraclavicular lymphadenopathy is seen.

THORAX

A large and irregular, heterogeneous and hypermetabolic left lung upper lobe anterior segment tumour (size = 5.4 x 4.3 x 3.7 cm, SUVmax 15.6) is seen, compatible with malignant lung tumour. It is also partly involving the left lung lingular segment. Medially, the tumour is in close contact with the left heart border and left anterior hilar region. Adjacent lung mild partial collapse is also seen.

Multiple and diffuse, enlarged and hypermetabolic mediastinal lymph nodes are seen along paratracheal, precarinal, subcarinal, aortopulmonary window regions, periaortic region. They

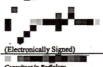

(Electronically Signed)

Approved on : 09-APR-2022 01:10 PM
Page 1 of 5

Consultant in Radiology
MBBS(HK), FRCR, FHKCR, FHKAM(RADIOLOGY)

MR-C101

307

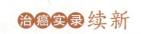

Hospital 醫院

MEDICAL IMAGING DEPARTMENT

Patient's Name	: LAU	Unit Record No.	:
Sex	: F	Age	: 45
Examination Date	: 09-APR-2022	Accession No.	:
Ward / Class	: 1123	Attending Doctor	:

EXAMINATION / PROCEDURE REPORT

have size measuring up to 0.9 x 2.1 cm and activity up to SUVmax 13.6, compatible with diffuse metastatic lymph nodes.

No pleural effusion or pericardial effusion is seen.

The oesophagus appears unremarkable.

ABDOMEN & PELVIS

A large and partly necrotic, hypermetabolic liver tumour (size = 4.7 x 5.7 x 6.3 cm, SUVmax 16.9) is seen at segment 5 of liver. It could either represent primary or secondary tumour.

Several other smaller size and hypermetabolic lesions (up to 1.6 cm, SUVmax 15.2) are seen at right hepatic lobe.

Enlarged and hypermetabolic porta hepatis lymph node (size = 1.8 x 2.5 x 2.2 cm, SUVmax 13.2) is seen, compatible with metastatic lymph node.

The spleen, pancreas and both kidneys appear unremarkable. Right adrenal is unremarkable.

Hypermetabolic left adrenal mass (size = 2.2 x 1.8 x 3.3 cm, SUVmax 13.2) is seen, compatible with adrenal metastasis.

Trace amount of lower pelvis fluid is noted, likely physiological in nature.

Uterus is unremarkable. Minimal endometrial uptake is seen. Right ovary shows increased uptake (SUVmax 8.6) is seen, could be due to physiological uptake or underlying ovarian lesion/ tumour.

Tiny right renal stone (0.2 cm) is seen.

No abnormal bowel pattern, bowel wall thickening or bowel dilatation is seen. No abnormal increased uptake is seen along the bowel and stomach.

(Electronically Signed)

Approved on : 09-APR-2022 01:10 PM
Page 2 of 5

Consultant in Radiology
MBBS(HK), FRCR, FHKCR, FHKAM(RADIOLOGY)

MR-C101

Hospital 醫院

MEDICAL IMAGING DEPARTMENT

Patient's Name	: LAU	Unit Record No.	:	
Sex	: F	Age	:	45
Examination Date	: 09-APR-2022	Accession No.	:	
Ward / Class	: 1123	Attending Doctor	:	

EXAMINATION / PROCEDURE REPORT

SKELETON

Hypermetabolic bony erosion at T9 and L4 vertebra (SUVmax up to 13.1) is seen, compatible with bony metastases. The T9 metastasis shows suspicious mild intraspinal extension. Mild degeneration is seen along the spine.

COMMENTS:

1. A large and irregular, heterogeneous and hypermetabolic left lung upper lobe anterior segment tumour (size = 5.4 x 4.3 x 3.7 cm, SUVmax 15.6) is seen, compatible with malignant lung tumour. It is also partly involving the left lung lingular segment. Medially, the tumour is in close contact with the left heart border and the left anterior hilar region. Adjacent lung mild partial collapse is also seen.

2. Multiple and diffuse, enlarged and hypermetabolic mediastinal lymph nodes are seen along paratracheal, precarinal, subcarinal, aortopulmonary window regions, periaortic region. They have size measuring up to 0.9 x 2.1 cm and activity up to SUVmax 13.6, compatible with diffuse metastatic lymph nodes.

3. A large and partly necrotic, hypermetabolic liver tumour (size = 4.7 x 5.7 x 6.3 cm, SUVmax 16.9) is seen at segment 5 of liver. It could either represent primary or secondary tumour. Several other smaller sized and hypermetabolic lesions (up to 1.6 cm, SUVmax 15.2) are seen at right hepatic lobe.

4. Enlarged and hypermetabolic porta hepatis lymph node (size = 1.8 x 2.5 x 2.2 cm, SUVmax 13.2) is seen, compatible with metastatic lymph node.

5. Hypermetabolic left adrenal mass (size = 2.2 x 1.8 x 3.3 cm, SUVmax 13.2) is seen, compatible with adrenal metastasis.

6. Right ovary shows increased uptake (SUVmax 8.6) is seen, could be due to physiological uptake or underlying ovarian lesion/ tumour.

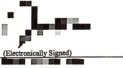

(Electronically Signed)

Consultant in Radiology
MBBS(HK), FRCR, FHKCR, FHKAM(RADIOLOGY)

Approved on : 09-APR-2022 01:10 PM
Page 3 of 5

MR-C101

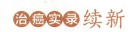

Hospital 醫院

MEDICAL IMAGING DEPARTMENT

Patient's Name	: LAU		Unit Record No.	:
Sex	: F		Age	: 45
Examination Date	: 09-APR-2022		Accession No.	:
Ward / Class	: 1123		Attending Doctor	:

EXAMINATION / PROCEDURE REPORT

7. Hypermetabolic bony erosion at T9 and L4 vertebra (SUVmax up to 13.1) is seen, compatible with bony metastases. The T9 metastasis shows suspicious mild intraspinal extension.

/dw

Location	Size (cm)	Max SUV
Right lower cervical LN	0.9x0.8	10.8
Left SCF LN	0.6	3.1
LUL Mass	5.4x4.3x3.7	15.6
Adjacent lung collapse	--	3.8
Left hilar LN	1.5x1.2	13.6
Thoracic inlet LN	0.8x0.7	7.0
Right paratracheal LN	1.4x1.0	7.2
Precarinal LN	1.3x1.0	13.6
AP window LN	1.5x0.8	8.9
Subcarinal LN	2.1x0.9	9.8
Periaortic LN	1.2x1.0	11.1
Liver lesions	Up to 5.7x4.7x6.3	Up to 16.9
Left adrenal	2.2x1.8x3.3	13.2
Porta hepatis LN	2.5x1.8x2.2	13.2
Right ovary	--	8.6

(Electronically Signed)

Approved on : 09-APR-2022 01:10 PM

Page 4 of 5

Consultant in Radiology
MBBS(HK), FRCR, FHKCR, FHKAM(RADIOLOGY)

MR-C101

Hospital 醫院
MEDICAL IMAGING DEPARTMENT

Patient's Name	: LAU	Unit Record No.	:
Sex	: F	Age	: 45
Examination Date	: 09-APR-2022	Accession No.	:
Ward / Class	: 1123	Attending Doctor	:

EXAMINATION / PROCEDURE REPORT

Uterus	--	4.4
GS	--	--
Right renal stone	0.2	--
T9	--	13.1
L4	--	6.6

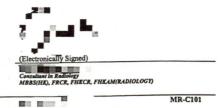

(Electronically Signed)

Consultant in Radiology
MBBS(HK), FRCR, FHKCR, FHKAM(RADIOLOGY)

Approved on : 09-APR-2022 01:10 PM
Page 5 of 5

MR-C101

311

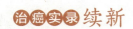

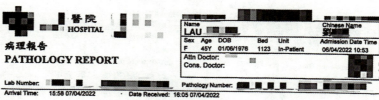

病理報告
PATHOLOGY REPORT

Name		Chinese Name
LAU		
Sex Age DOB Bed Unit		Admission Date Time
F 45Y 01/06/1976 1123 In-Patient		06/04/2022 10:53
Attn Doctor:		
Cons. Doctor:		

Lab Number: Pathology Number:

Arrival Time: 15:58 07/04/2022   •   Date Received: 16:05 07/04/2022

Pathology Report

SPECIMEN TYPE
Ultrasound guided biopsy liver lesion.

CLINICAL DETAILS
Abdominal pain. No fever.
CT shows 4 cm liver mass with central non-enhancing component.
? liquefying liver abscess. ? tumour with central necrosis. For ultrasound guided biopsy performed.

MACROSCOPIC EXAMINATION
Specimen labeled as ultrasound guided biopsy liver lesion, submitted in formalin with patient's particulars. It consists of multiple cores of tan tissue, ranging from 0.2 cm to 0.5 cm long. Specimen is all embedded in 2 blocks.

MICROSCOPIC EXAMINATION
The section shows cores of tumor tissue covered by infiltrative clusters of polygonal malignant cells with moderate nuclear pleomorphism and hyperchromasia, rare nucleoli, as well as modest amphophilic and rarely vacuolated cytoplasm. Poorly formed gland is noted. Squamous differentiation is absent. There is no spindle cell component. Tumor necrosis is discerned. Immunohistochemically, the tumor cells are immunoreactive towards CK7, CK19 and TTF-1. Stain for ER, CK20 or CDX2 is negative. The overall features are those of metastatic pulmonary adenocarcinoma.

DIAGNOSIS
Liver lesion, ultrasound guided biopsy - Metastatic pulmonary adenocarcinoma.

Reported by:

Report Time: 13:35 09/04/2022

MBBS (HK), FRCPA, FHKCPath,
******** End of Report ********   FHKAM (Path), Grad Dip (Derm) NUS

Effective Date Since 01-01-2022   Page 1 of 1

■■Hospital ■■醫院
MEDICAL IMAGING DEPARTMENT

Patient's Name	: LAU ■■	Unit Record No.	: ■■
Sex	: F	Age	: 46
Examination Date	: 17-JUN-2022	Accession No.	: ■■
Ward / Class	: 1128	Attending Doctor	: ■■

EXAMINATION / PROCEDURE REPORT

Clinical Information: metastatic lung cancer

PET/CT SCAN OF WHOLE BODY

TECHNIQUE:

Attenuation corrected PET scans of 4mm thickness were obtained from skull base to pelvis 1 hour after 4.3 mCi (body weight 48.6 kg) of F18 -FDG was injected via right hand vein.

Whole body volumetric CT Scan was performed for the same region. CT-PET fused images were subsequently obtained. Blood glucose level prior to injection of FDG was 4.9 mmol/l.

CORRELATIVE STUDIES: previous PET-CT scan dated 9/4/2022

FINDINGS:

NECK

Normal pharyngeal and tonsillar tracer uptake is noted.

Previously noted metastatic bilateral neck lymph nodes are resolved in this study.

No other abnormal tracer uptake is demonstrated in the neck region.

No other significant cervical or supraclavicular lymphadenopathy is seen.

THORAX

Previously noted large left lung upper lobe anterior segment malignant tumour shows significant interval decrease in size and activity in this study, with the residual tumour measuring (size=2.5 x 2.6 x 1.4cm, SUVmax 16.0), compatible with significant disease response to treatment.

Previously noted multiple and extensive, metastatic mediastinal lymph nodes also show significant interval decrease in size and activity in this study. There are only several residual lymph nodes seen, with the most prominent one seen at the left hilar region (size=0.7 x1cm, SUVmax 2.9), compatible with significant disease response to treatment.

Fibrotic changes are seen in the rest of both sides of lung, in particular at bilateral lung bases.

Left lung lingular segment atelectasis and mild consolidation changes are seen.

No pleural effusion or pericardial effusion is seen. The oesophagus appears unremarkable.

(Electronically Signed)

Approved on : 17-JUN-2022 04:10 PM
Page 1 of 4

■■
Consultant in Radiology
MBBS(HK), FRCR, FHKCR, FHKAM(RADIOLOGY)

MR-C101

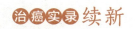

Hospital ■■醫院

MEDICAL IMAGING DEPARTMENT

Patient's Name	: LAU ███	Unit Record No.	: ███
Sex	: F	Age	: 46
Examination Date	: 17-JUN-2022	Accession No.	: ███
Ward / Class	: 1128	Attending Doctor	: ███

EXAMINATION / PROCEDURE REPORT

ABDOMEN & PELVIS

Previously noted large and necrotic right hepatic lobe metastasis shows significant decrease in size and activity in this study, now measuring about (size=2.6x2.7x3cm, SUVmax 5.6), compatible with significant disease response to treatment. Rest of the previously noted liver metastases are resolved.

Previously noted left adrenal metastasis is also mostly resolved, with minimal residual activity (SUVmax 2.9).

Previously noted metastatic lymph node at the porta hepatis is also resolved.

Minimal uptake along the uterus endometrium (SUVmax 3.0) is seen, likely physiological uptake. No abnormal adnexal mass lesion is seen. Both ovaries are unremarkable.

Right adrenal is unremarkable.

The spleen, pancreas and both kidneys appear unremarkable except for tiny right renal stone (0.2cm).

No significant abdominal or pelvic lymphadenopathy is noted.

No ascites is noted.

No abnormal bowel pattern, bowel wall thickening or bowel dilatation is seen. No abnormal increased uptake is seen along the bowel and stomach.

SKELETON

Previously noted T9 bony metastasis shows decrease in size and activity in this study, with residual uptake (SUVmax 6.9). Previously noted left L4 vertebra metastasis appears resolved in this study. No other abnormal tracer uptake is seen. No other significant focal bony abnormality is seen.

(Electronically Signed)
███
Consultant in Radiology
MBBS(HK), FRCR, FHKCR, FHKAM(RADIOLOGY)

Approved on : 17-JUN-2022 04:10 PM
Page 2 of 4

MR-C101

▆▆ Hospital ▆▆醫院
MEDICAL IMAGING DEPARTMENT

Patient's Name	: LAU ▆	Unit Record No.	: ▆▆ ▆
Sex	: F	Age	: 46
Examination Date	: 17-JUN-2022	Accession No.	: ▆▆▆▆
Ward / Class	: 1128	Attending Doctor	: ▆ ▆ ▆▆▆▆

EXAMINATION / PROCEDURE REPORT

COMMENTS:

1. Previously noted large left lung upper lobe anterior segment malignant tumour shows significant interval decrease in size and activity in this study, with the residual tumour measuring (size=2.5 x 2.6 x 1.4cm, SUVmax 16.0), compatible with significant disease response to treatment.

2. Previously noted multiple and extensive, metastatic mediastinal lymph nodes also show significant interval decrease in size and activity in this study. There are only several residual lymph nodes seen, with the most prominent one seen at the left hilar region (size=0.7 x1cm, SUVmax 2.9), compatible with significant disease response to treatment.

3. Fibrotic changes are seen in the rest of both sides of lung, in particular at bilateral lung bases. Left lung lingular segment atelectasis and mild consolidation changes are seen.

4. Previously noted metastatic bilateral neck lymph nodes are resolved in this study.

5. Previously noted large and necrotic right hepatic lobe metastasis shows significant decrease in size and activity in this study, now measuring about (size=2.6x2.7x3cm, SUVmax 5.6), compatible with significant disease response to treatment. Rest of the previously noted liver metastases are resolved.

6. Previously noted left adrenal metastasis is also mostly resolved, with minimal residual activity (SUVmax 2.9).

7. Previously noted metastatic lymph node at the porta hepatis is also resolved.

8. Previously noted T9 bony metastasis shows decrease in size and activity in this study, with residual uptake (SUVmax 6.9). Previously noted left L4 vertebra metastasis appears resolved in this study.

9. Overall, the disease is showing significant response to treatment. /ll

(Electronically Signed)
▆▆▆▆
Consultant in Radiology
MBBS(HK), FRCR, FHKCR, FHKAM(RADIOLOGY)

Approved on : 17-JUN-2022 04:10 PM
Page 3 of 4

MR-C101

315

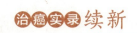

Hospital 醫院
MEDICAL IMAGING DEPARTMENT

Patient's Name	: LAU	Unit Record No.	:
Sex	: F	Age	: 46
Examination Date	: 17-JUN-2022	Accession No.	:
Ward / Class	: 1128	Attending Doctor	:

EXAMINATION / PROCEDURE REPORT

Location	Size (cm)		Max SUV	
	Present study	Previous study	Present study	Previous study
right lower cervical LN	--	0.9x0.8	--	10.8
left SCF LN	-	0.7	--	3.1
LUL mass	2.6x2.5x1.4	5.4x4.3x3.7	6.0	15.6
left hilar LN	1.0x0.7	1.5x1.2	2.9	13.6
thoracic inlet LN	--	0.8x0.7	--	7.0
R paratracheal LN	--	1.4x1.0	--	7.2
precarinal LN	--	1.3x1.0	--	13.6
AP window LN	--	1.5x0.8	--	8.9
subcarinal LN	--	2.1x0.9	--	9.8
periaortic LN	--	1.2x1.0	--	11.1
liver lesions	up to 2.7x2.6x3.0	up to 5.7x4.7x6.3	up to 5.6	up to 16.9
left adrenal	--	2.2x1.8x3.3	2.9	13.2
periaortic LN	--	2.5x1.8x2.2	--	13.2
right ovary	--	--	--	8.6
uterus	--	--	3.0	4.4
GS	--	--	--	--
right renal stone	0.2	0.2	--	--
T9	--	--	6.9	13.1
L4	--	--	--	6.6

(Electronically Signed)

Approved on : 17-JUN-2022 04:10 PM
Page 4 of 4

Consultant in Radiology
MBBS(HK), FRCR, FHKCR, FHKAM(RADIOLOGY)

MR-C101

316

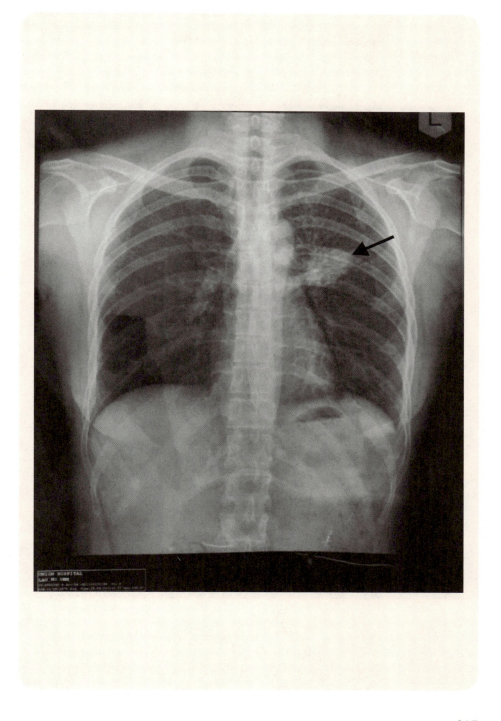

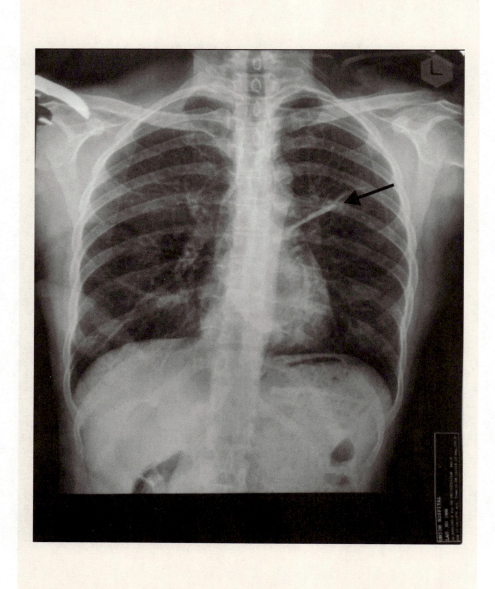

病案**47**

卵巢癌康复 15 年

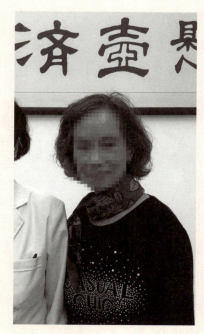

🔊 李女士 2024 年 1 月前来诊治时合影留念

在 2009 年李女士 54 岁的时候，有一段时间内经常感到腹部不舒服，消化不良，胃口不好，她以为就是消化不良，起初没有过于在意。后来又发展为腹部隐隐作痛，并且晚上睡觉时腹胀的感觉越来越重，整晚都难以入睡。后来在洗澡的时候摸到肚子里有肿块，她急忙到医院里去检查，结果诊断她患的是卵巢癌，并有腹腔淋巴转移。李女士非常紧张，因为她丈夫也是患了癌症，在不久前去世的。她想一定要治好自己的疾病，如果她也走了，这个家就完了，两个孩子要怎么办呢？都还需要她操劳。于是在 2009 年 5 月，李女士在医院做了手术，切除了子宫、卵巢、输卵管等腹部的所有生殖器官。手术后医生告诉她要尽快地进行化疗和放疗。但因为有丈夫以前治疗的经历，所以李女士决定走另外一条治病的路。

她在手术之后的第 21 天前来看诊治疗。当时她腹部疼痛不能触摸，大便秘结，食欲很差，在相当一段时间内除了腹痛之外，胸部疼痛也很严重，并且伴有咳嗽多痰，气短胸闷的症状。医生怀疑她发生了肺部的转移，并且在 2009 年 11 月的 CT 检查报告中被证实，腹腔中还有多个肿大淋巴结存在，医生要求尽快做化疗和放疗，否则后果不堪设想。李女士对于丈夫患癌症的治疗经过历历在目，其丈夫受尽各种化疗、放疗的痛苦，最后人还是没有了。所以她决定坚持中医药治疗，不去做化疗和放疗等治疗，也不去医院做检查。以后的 2~3 年时间内，她认真服用中药，坚持治疗，在之后断续前来看病，断续服用中药。她的身体逐渐恢复正常，咳嗽多痰症状逐渐减轻到最后消失，体重逐渐增加，胃口逐渐变好，感到全身力气也恢复了。她返回工作，操劳家务，照顾子女，生活完全恢复正常。在以后的时间内，她也曾断断续续的前来，但大多数是因为关节痛、肩痛等方面的问题。如今 15 年过去了，李女士仍一直在做她喜爱的司机工作。她开的是货车，除了开车之外，还要兼顾卸货。虽然工作忙累，但是她却精力充沛，不感到疲乏。只是有时会有腰痛、腿酸等问题前来调理一下。她常说，现在的身体非常健康，非常的快乐，并经常对人说起是中医药帮助她战胜了癌症。

卵巢癌是女性生殖系统恶性肿瘤，早期症状不明显，常被误认为胃肠道不适，消化不良等。虽然患卵巢癌的人数没有子宫颈癌多，但近年来却是死亡率上升最快的癌症，原因就在于大多数的患者都是早期没有被发现。尽管近年来现代医学在不断发展，但通过标靶、化疗，Ⅲ期的患者平均五年存活率也并不高。因此进一步发展中医药长久疗效的治疗非常必要。

治疗原则

活血化瘀，扶助正气，软坚消瘤。

常用中药

1. 人参、黄芪、鹿角胶、黄精、肉苁蓉、三七、土鳖虫、三棱、乌梢蛇等。
2. 同时服用消瘤丸、化瘀丸。

影像学、病理学检查报告及诊疗记录

2009 年 5 月 18 日手术病理报告证实为卵巢癌。

附：患者检查报告

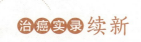

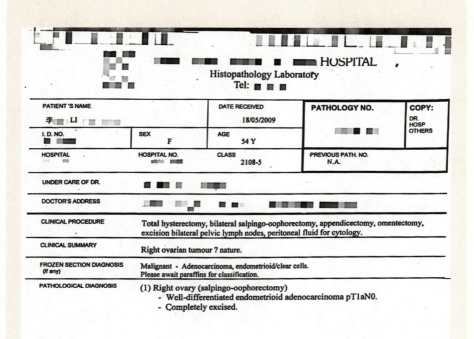

HOSPITAL

Histopathology Laboratory
Tel: ■ ■ ■

PATIENT'S NAME		DATE RECEIVED		PATHOLOGY NO.		COPY:
李 ■ LI ■ ■		18/05/2009		■ ■ ■		DR. HOSP OTHERS
I. D. NO. ■ ■ ■	SEX F	AGE 54 Y				
HOSPITAL ■	HOSPITAL NO. ■ ■	CLASS 2108-5		PREVIOUS PATH. NO. N.A.		

UNDER CARE OF DR.	■ ■ ■ ■
DOCTOR'S ADDRESS	■ ■ ■ ■ ■ ■
CLINICAL PROCEDURE	Total hysterectomy, bilateral salpingo-oophorectomy, appendicectomy, omentectomy, excision bilateral pelvic lymph nodes, peritoneal fluid for cytology.
CLINICAL SUMMARY	Right ovarian tumour ? nature.
FROZEN SECTION DIAGNOSIS (if any)	Malignant - Adenocarcinoma, endometrioid/clear cells. Please await paraffins for classification.
PATHOLOGICAL DIAGNOSIS	(1) Right ovary (salpingo-oophorectomy) - Well-differentiated endometrioid adenocarcinoma pT1aN0. - Completely excised.

REPORT

Macroscopic examination:

(1) "Right ovarian tumour" - Smooth-surfaced ovarian mass 23.6 grams in weight, 3.6 x 3 x 2.7 cm. with fallopian tube 6 cm. long, 1 cm. in diameter. Cut surfaces showed internal mucoid nodules, fairly well-circumscribed upto 2.5 x 2.2 x 2 cm. No macroscopic capsular invasion was found.

(2) "Peritoneal washings" - Approximately 200 ml. of brownish turbid fluid.

(3) "Uterus, both fallopian tubes and left ovary" - Uterus and left fallopian tube and ovary, 69 grams in weight, uterine corpus measured bicornual 3.5 cm., anterior-posterior 3.2 cm., fundus to cervical os 7.4 cm., endocervical cavity 2.4 cm. long, uterine cavity 3.5 cm. long, uterine wall 1.2 to 1.7 cm. thick, endometrium was paper-thin less than 0.1 cm. thick. No fibroids were found. The cervix was moderately eroded and focally congested and vaginal cuff measured 1.2 x 0.4 cm. in area, 0.2 cm. thick. Left ovary measured 2 x 2 x 0.8 cm. with two opened cysts 1.2 x 1.2 x 0.5 cm. and 1 x 0.7 x 0.4 cm. Left fallopian tube measured 5.5 cm. long, 0.5 cm. in diameter, twisted and normal, adhered to the ovary.

Blocks: (A, B) cervix, (C) endometrium, (D) left ovary and fallopian tube, (E) left, (F) right parametrium.

(4) "Left pelvic LN" - A yellowish fatty mass 4.8 x 2.4 x 1.5 cm. with five lymph nodes, largest 1.3 x 0.8 x 0.5 cm. and smallest 0.5 x 0.3 x 0.2 cm.

(CONTINUED ON NEXT PAGE)

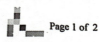 Page 1 of 2

病案 48

恶性脂肪肉瘤康复

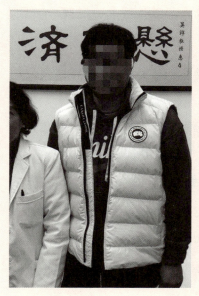

林先生 2023 年 1 月前来诊治时合影留念

　　林先生，在 1990 年 50 岁的时候就做过一个大手术。他当时患了生殖细胞肿瘤，并且胸腹部都有转移，于是他做了肿瘤切除手术，随即也进行了手术后的化疗和放疗，以后一直平安无事。但是到了 2019 年，常感觉腹部不适，隐隐腹痛。以后又有进食减少，消瘦等症状。于是他在 2019 年 5 月去做身体检查。自以为就是消化不良的问题，并没有什么其他太大的问题，只是做个常规的身体检查，所以一直拖着没有去取回检查报告。一直到 2020 年 5 月他才得知，原来他的肚子里面长了一个非常大的肿瘤。肿瘤的大小，大概有 7.0cm×8.6cm×15.3cm，他急忙去找医生。医生说他这么大的肿瘤，需要尽快做手术切除，于是林先生在 2020 年 7 月做了切除腹部肿瘤手术。手术后的病理报告，又使他大吃一惊，原来他患的是脂肪肉瘤。脂肪肉瘤是一种非常恶性的软组织肿瘤，在手术后1个月林先生就开始做放疗。在放疗中了解到，这种肿瘤是非常容易复发的，于是他急忙在放疗的同时前来接受生命修复的中医药治疗。

当时他非常疲累，身体状况很差，无法进食，腹痛、腹胀，全身出皮疹，胃胀气，全身疼痛，感觉快坚持不下去了。经过我们的辨证分析，在放疗的同时加用了中药以后，他的精神状态慢慢好转，各种疼痛慢慢消失。他的身体恢复得很快，开始锻炼身体，经常做爬山、打球、慢跑等运动。他感觉身体已经完全恢复了，没有什么不舒服了，但是查到的资料以及朋友、医生都告诫他，说这种病是非常容易复发的，要千万小心，所以他坚持服用中药。现在4年多了，经过身体检查，肿瘤并没有复发。我们告诉他，还需要继续坚持治疗一段时间，所以尽管他的工作很忙碌，需要经常出差，也经常带着全家到国外去旅游，他也没有停止服用中药。

脂肪肉瘤是一种由脂肪细胞在深层软组织异常增生导致的癌症，是一种比较少见的发生于软组织的恶性肿瘤。其可以发生在身体任何部位的脂肪细胞中，但大多数病例发生在四肢或腹部肌肉。可发生于任何年龄，老年人比较多见。

目前现代医学对于这种恶性软组织肿瘤的治疗，存在的主要问题：手术后高复发率，大部分肉瘤并无有效的化疗药物，大多数脂肪肉瘤对化疗和放疗并不敏感。所以开拓有效的治疗方法，发挥传统医药学的优势，是治疗这些疑难病症的新途径。

治疗原则

解毒化瘀，活血攻癌。

常用中药

1. 白花蛇舌草、半枝莲、红花、桃仁、当归、田七、贝母、海藻等。
2. 同时服用消瘤丸。

影像学、病理学检查报告及诊疗记录

1. 2020 年 6 月 19 日 CT 检查报告证实为腹膜后有巨大肿瘤 7.0cm×8.6cm×15.3cm。

2. 2020 年 7 月 11 日手术后病理报告证实为脂肪肉瘤。

3. 2021 年 3 月 15 日检查报告证实无肿瘤复发。

附：患者检查报告

■ ■ ■ ■ ■   ▲   ■ ■ . . 2

Imaging Department
Radiological Report

Name:	LIN■ ■	In-Hospital No.:	■ ■ ■
Sex / DOB:	M/■ ■	Exam No.:	■ ■ ■
Ref Dr.:	■ ■	Ward:	■ ■ ■
Exam Type:	CT	Date of Exam:	19 June 2020

CT ABDOMEN & PELVIS (PLAIN & CONTRAST) P.2 of 2
Impression:
1. A large predominantly fat-containing mass at left retroperitoneum abutting the lateral aspect of the left psoas muscle. It measures 7.0x8.6x15.3cm (TD x AP x CC) in size. Multiple internal thin septa are noted. Small enhancing solid components are seen at the medial aspect (~1.2cm) and inferior aspect (~0.9cm) of the mass. Overall features are suggestive of a retroperitoneal lipomatous tumor e.g. a liposarcoma. Further management is suggested.

2. The lumbar veins, hemiazygos veins, superficial veins in the anterior abdominal subcutaneous layers, veins in right anterior and right lateral abdominal wall are dilated. There is no evidence of obstruction from the IVC to the right atrium. No evidence of portal hypertension. Superior vena cava obstruction has to be considered. Further investigation with CT thorax with contrast is suggested.

3. No focal mass or significant fatty infiltration at S4b of liver.

Reported on 19 June 2020

MBChB (CUHK), FRCR,
FHKCR, FHKAM (Radiology)

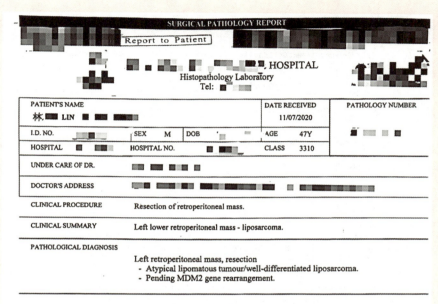

SURGICAL PATHOLOGY REPORT

Report to Patient

■ HOSPITAL

Histopathology Laboratory
Tel: ■ ■

PATIENT'S NAME				DATE RECEIVED	PATHOLOGY NUMBER
林■ LIN ■ ■ ■				11/07/2020	■ ■ ■ ■
I.D. NO. ■	SEX M	DOB '■	AGE 47Y		
HOSPITAL ■	HOSPITAL NO. ■ ■		CLASS 3310		

UNDER CARE OF DR.	■ ■ ■ ■ ■ ■
DOCTOR'S ADDRESS	■ ■ ■ ■ ■ ■ ■
CLINICAL PROCEDURE	Resection of retroperitoneal mass.
CLINICAL SUMMARY	Left lower retroperitoneal mass - liposarcoma.

PATHOLOGICAL DIAGNOSIS

Left retroperitoneal mass, resection
- Atypical lipomatous tumour/well-differentiated liposarcoma.
- Pending MDM2 gene rearrangement.

REPORT

Macroscopic examination:

"Retroperitoneal liposarcoma" - A tan to yellow fairly well-circumscribed fatty mass with focal lining of muscle externally 620 g in weight, 15.5 x 9.5 x 7.5 cm. Cut surfaces showed yellow fat-like tissue with scattered pale fibrous septa.
Blocks: (A) to (J) Two pieces each random from one end to the other; (K) to (U) Further blocks random.

Microscopic examination:

Sections show a lipomatous tumour with predominant mature adipose connective tissue. Scattered foci of mildly atypical stromal cells are seen within fibrous septa, with very occasional lipoblast-like cells. Immunohistochemical studies show scattered expression of MDM2 and CDK4 with very low Ki67 proliferation index (less than 1%). The appearances are consistent with atypical lipomatous tumour /well-differentiated liposarcoma, but a further report will follow FISH analysis for MDM2 gene rearrangement. There is infiltration into peripheral skeletal muscle bundles. No features of de-differentiation are found in multiple blocks examined. Excision appears narrowly clear, but the lesion merges with normal adipose tissue.

Date Reported: 16/07/2020

■ ■ ■

Reported and
Authorized by: _

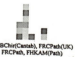

MBBChir(Cantab), FRCPath(UK)
FRCPath, FHKAM(Path)

Page 1 of

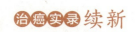

醫院 | 診斷及介入放射部
Hospital | Department of Diagnostic & Interventional Radiology

Tel :

Name:	LIN,	ID:
Sex / DOB:	M /	Ward / Dept: Liver Surgery & Transplant Centre
Ref. Dr.:		Hosp No.:
Exam ID(s):		Date of Exam: 15-MAR-2021

MRI SCAN OF ABDOMEN AND PELVIS WITH AND WITHOUT CONTRAST

Clinical data:

Liposarcoma, resected.

Technique:

Abdomen:
Pre-contrast:
Axial T1, T2, T2 fat sat, T1 fat saturation
Coronal T2 weighted

Post-contrast (Gadolinium):
Axial T1 fat saturation
Coronal T1 fat saturation

Pelvis:
Pre-contrast:
Axial T1, T2, T1 fat saturation
Coronal T2 weighted
Sagittal T2 weighted

Post-contrast (Gadolinium):
Axial T1 fat saturation
Coronal T1 fat saturation
Sagittal T1 fat saturation

Findings:

Correlation made with previous MRI in December 2020.

Liver is not enlarged.   Stable lesion is noted at right lobe of liver, could be a hemangioma. It measures 1.1 x 1.2 cm.
No other enhancing is seen in rest of the liver.
Biliary tree is not dilated.   Main portal vein is opacified.
No sizeable gallbladder stone is seen.
Spleen is not enlarged.
No gross pancreatic or adrenal mass is seen.
Kidneys are comparable in size and contrast enhancement.
Small right renal cysts are noted.
Bilateral renal collecting systems are not dilated.

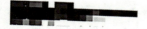 Page 1 of 2

扁桃体癌和舌癌康复

陈先生于 2012 年 4 月发现颈部有多个包块，当时他不怎么在意，也没有当回事。但是包块越长越大，于是在 2013 年 4 月去做了检查，经组织化验确诊为扁桃体的恶性肿瘤。于是在当月做了手术切除癌变的扁桃体，随即于 2013 年 5 月前来进行生命修复的中医药治疗。那时他 53 岁，刚做完扁桃体的切除手术，身体虚弱，头晕，味觉丧失，呕吐，不能进食，喉咙非常痛，就连喝一点水都困难。

我们根据他的病情，给他进行了积极的中医药治疗。清热解毒，化痰软坚。经过 3 个多月的中药治疗，他的情况恢复得很好。喉咙不痛了，能够正常进食，气色不错，吞咽困难没有了，味觉也恢复了正常，手术的创伤也恢复了。这时医院里要求他做进一步治疗，于是陈先生就去做了放疗和化疗。就这样过了一段时间，完成了所有放疗和化疗。他觉得现代医学最先进的治疗方法如手术、放疗、化疗都已经完成了，应该没有问题了，他就不用再来做治疗了。我们曾经提醒他根本性抗癌的治疗只用了 3 个月是不够的，还应该再坚持一些时日才更加彻底。但是他认为现代医学的所有手段，他已经全部使用并且完成治疗了，应该是不会有问题了。以后也就没有他的消息了。

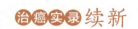

　　但是在近8年没有过联系之后，陈先生又来找我们了。原来他因吞咽困难去做检查，发现了原先患癌邻近的舌头部位的癌症。于是在2021年2月再次做了舌的切除手术。手术后的化验报告，证实为恶性鳞状细胞癌。这次他吸取教训，尽早前来做治疗，吃中药。由于他的颈部经过之前的放疗已变得非常僵硬，医生告诉他不适合再做放疗，化疗也有困难，且他的这种癌细胞对于药物和射线还有相当强的抗药性和耐受性。主诊医生告诉他，这种情况再次复发的可能性是非常大的。但因为是在口腔这个特殊的部位，也很难再做更大范围的手术切除。如果不大面积切除，那么复发的可能性就很大。在这种治疗困难的情况下，陈先生只有选择生命修复的中医药治疗，用天然的中草药、穴位等方法治疗。他当时吞咽困难，腹部疼痛、胀满，头痛，便秘，身体非常虚弱，但是这次他认真治疗后就没有再停下来。他的医生朋友很担心，让他去做检查。于是2022年11月他再去做了一次全面的身体检查，全身各处显示正常，没有发现转移的情况。从患癌症至今已经11年过去了，陈先生的治疗经过使他深深地体会到癌症的破坏性、顽固性和中医药生命修复治疗的优越性。

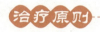

　　解毒化浊，散结消瘤。

常用中药

1. 鱼腥草、败酱草、夏枯草、蜂房、皂角刺、猕猴桃根、山慈菇、贝母等。
2. 同时服用散结丸。

影像学、病理学检查报告及诊疗记录

1. 2013年4月27日手术后病理报告证实为扁桃体低分化鳞状细胞癌。

2. 2021年2月17日舌的手术切除后病理报告为鳞状细胞癌，有淋巴和血管侵入。

3. 2022年11月21日MRI检查结果显示，没有癌症复发和转移迹象。

附：患者检查报告

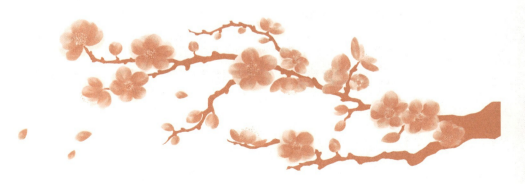

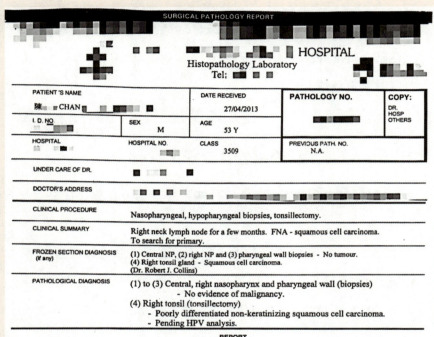

SURGICAL PATHOLOGY REPORT

HOSPITAL

Histopathology Laboratory
Tel:

PATIENT'S NAME 陳 CHAN		DATE RECEIVED 27/04/2013	PATHOLOGY NO.	COPY: DR. HOSP OTHERS
I.D. NO.	SEX M	AGE 53 Y		
HOSPITAL	HOSPITAL NO.	CLASS 3509	PREVIOUS PATH. NO. N.A.	

UNDER CARE OF DR.

DOCTOR'S ADDRESS

CLINICAL PROCEDURE: Nasopharyngeal, hypopharyngeal biopsies, tonsillectomy.

CLINICAL SUMMARY: Right neck lymph node for a few months. FNA - squamous cell carcinoma. To search for primary.

FROZEN SECTION DIAGNOSIS (if any): (1) Central NP, (2) right NP and (3) pharyngeal wall biopsies - No tumour. (4) Right tonsil gland - Squamous cell carcinoma. (Dr. Robert J. Collins)

PATHOLOGICAL DIAGNOSIS:
(1) to (3) Central, right nasopharynx and pharyngeal wall (biopsies)
- No evidence of malignancy.
(4) Right tonsil (tonsillectomy)
- Poorly differentiated non-keratinizing squamous cell carcinoma.
- Pending HPV analysis.

REPORT

Macroscopic examination:

(1) "Central NP biopsy" - Two tan-coloured pieces 5 x 4 x 2 mm. and 4 x 2 x 2 mm.
(2) "Right NP biopsy" - Two tan-coloured pieces, each 3 x 3 x 2 mm.
(3) "Pharyngeal wall biopsy" - Eight tan-coloured pieces, largest 2 x 2 x 1 mm. and smallest 1 mm. in diameter.
(4) "Right tonsil gland" - Tan-coloured mucosal tonsillar mass 3 x 1.5 x 0.7 cm., 1.2 grams in weight.

Microscopic examination:

(1) & (2) Paraffin sections of both specimens confirm the frozen section appearances and show nasopharyngeal mucosa without atypia or malignancy.

(3) Paraffin sections confirm the frozen section appearances and show squamous mucosa with patchy haemorrhage but no dysplasia or malignancy is seen.

(CONTINUED ON NEXT PAGE)

Page 1 of 2

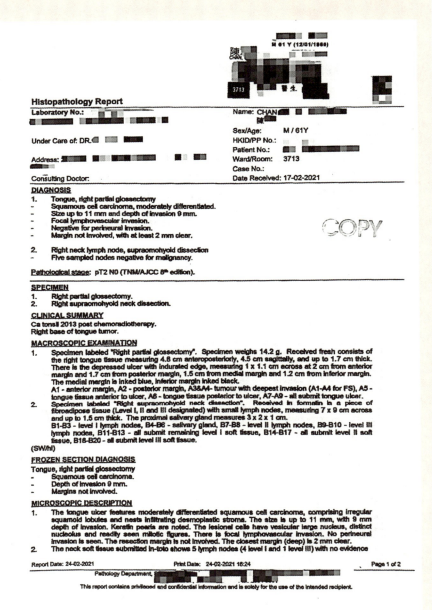

Histopathology Report

Laboratory No.:	Name: CHAN 陳
	Sex/Age: **M / 61Y**
Under Care of: DR.	HKID/PP No.:
	Patient No.:
Address:	Ward/Room: **3713**
	Case No.:
Consulting Doctor:	Date Received: 17-02-2021

M 61 Y (12/01/1960)

3713

COPY

DIAGNOSIS

1. Tongue, right partial glossectomy
- Squamous cell carcinoma, moderately differentiated.
- Size up to 11 mm and depth of invasion 9 mm.
- Focal lymphovascular invasion.
- Negative for perineural invasion.
- Margin not involved, with at least 2 mm clear.

2. Right neck lymph node, supraomohyoid dissection
- Five sampled nodes negative for malignancy.

Pathological stage: pT2 N0 (TNM/AJCC 8th edition).

SPECIMEN

1. Right partial glossectomy.
2. Right supraomohyoid neck dissection.

CLINICAL SUMMARY

Ca tonsil 2013 post chemoradiotherapy.
Right base of tongue tumor.

MACROSCOPIC EXAMINATION

1. Specimen labeled "Right partial glossectomy". Specimen weighs 14.2 g. Received fresh consists of the right tongue tissue measuring 4.8 cm anteroposteriorly, 4.5 cm sagittally, and up to 1.7 cm thick. There is the depressed ulcer with indurated edge, measuring 1 x 1.1 cm across at 2 cm from anterior margin and 1.7 cm from posterior margin, 1.5 cm from medial margin and 1.2 cm from inferior margin. The medial margin is inked blue, inferior margin inked black.
   A1 - anterior margin, A2 - posterior margin, A3&A4- tumour with deepest invasion (A1-A4 for FS), A5 - tongue tissue anterior to ulcer, A6 - tongue tissue posterior to ulcer, A7-A9 - all submit tongue ulcer.
2. Specimen labeled "Right supraomohyoid neck dissection". Received in formalin is a piece of fibroadipose tissue (Level I, II and III designated) with small lymph nodes, measuring 7 x 9 cm across and up to 1.5 cm thick. The proximal salivary gland measures 3 x 2 x 1 cm.
   B1-B3 - level I lymph nodes, B4-B6 - salivary gland, B7-B8 - level II lymph nodes, B9-B10 - level III lymph nodes, B11-B13 - all submit remaining level I soft tissue, B14-B17 - all submit level II soft tissue, B18-B20 - all submit level III soft tissue.

(SW/hl)

FROZEN SECTION DIAGNOSIS

Tongue, right partial glossectomy
- Squamous cell carcinoma.
- Depth of invasion 9 mm.
- Margins not involved.

MICROSCOPIC DESCRIPTION

1. The tongue ulcer features moderately differentiated squamous cell carcinoma, comprising irregular squamoid lobules and nests infiltrating desmoplastic stroma. The size is up to 11 mm, with 9 mm depth of invasion. Keratin pearls are noted. The lesional cells have vesicular large nucleus, distinct nucleolus and readily seen mitotic figures. There is focal lymphovascular invasion. No perineural invasion is seen. The resection margin is not involved. The closest margin (deep) is 2 mm clear.
2. The neck soft tissue submitted in-toto shows 5 lymph nodes (4 level I and 1 level III) with no evidence

Report Date: 24-02-2021	Print Date: 24-02-2021 16:24	Page 1 of 2

Pathology Department,

This report contains privileged and confidential information and is solely for the use of the intended recipient.

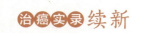

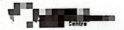 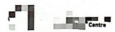

RADIOLOGY REPORT

Ref. / To	:		
Patient	: CHAN, ▮▮▮		
Attending Dr.	: Referring Doctor		
Sex / Age	: Male / 62Y 10M	ID	: ▮▮
Exam. Date	: 21-Nov-2022 14:19	PRN	: ▮▮
		DOB	: 12-Jan-1960

MRI NASOPHARYNX (PLAIN AND CONTRAST)

CLINICAL INFORMATION: CA right back of tongue resected in 1.2021. For surveillance.

TECHNIQUE:

Axial: T1 SE, T2 FS PROPELLER, T2 PROPELLER (brain stem), T2 STIR (neck), DWI (b0, 1000), T1 FS SE + C
Coronal: T2 PROPELLER, T1 IDEAL + C
Sagittal: T1 FSE, T1 3D BRAVO + C

COMPARATIVE STUDIES:
Contrast MRI pharynx and neck on 12.7.2022, 11.1.2022, 25.8.2021 & 17.05.2021, and MRI neck angiogram on 25.08.2021 (HKIDIC).
FDG PET-CT WB on 03.02.2021 (HKIDIC).

FINDINGS:
There is evidence of partial glossectomy and flap reconstruction for prior right back of tongue cancer.
There is no abnormal enhancing mass in the oral cavity and oropharynx.
Bilateral pterygopalatine fossae and the pterygo-maxillary fissures are clear.
The sphenoid floor is intact. There is post-sellar pneumatization of sphenoid sinus.

There is no enlarged lymph node detected on both sides of the retropharyngeal, cervical and supraclavicular regions.
There is no obliteration of the fossae of Rosenmüller.
Mild retention change is noted in left maxillary sinus. Bilateral mastoids and paranasal sinuses are otherwise clear.

The included brain is unremarkable. No sellar or parasellar mass is seen. Cavernous sinuses on both sides are normal.
Alignment of cervical spine is normal. No abnormal thickening of prevertebral soft tissue. No destructive bone lesion.

CONCLUSION:

1. There is no significant interval change compared with previous MRI studies. History of right tongue base cancer with resection and flap reconstruction. There is no MRI evidence of local recurrence or metastasis in scan range.

Consultant Radiologist
MBChB (CUHK) FRCR (UK) FHKCR FHKAM (Radiology)

Tel電話 ▮▮▮
Fax傳真 ▮▮▮

334

晚期肝癌康复

　　李女士在国外工作，非常忙碌。2022年年初，她因为母亲病故，料理后事而返回香港家中。母亲因癌症去世使李女士非常伤心，她很后悔自己为了工作疏忽了对父母的照顾。父亲一直在照顾病重的母亲，无暇顾及自己的起居饮食，导致看起来身体瘦弱，腹部胀大，全身发黄，腿脚也都非常肿胀。李女士急忙处理完后事准备返回工作地，但看到父亲腹部胀大，下肢水肿严重，就带父亲去做了身体检查。结果使人大吃一惊，原来她的父亲已经患了晚期肝癌。但是父亲并不知道他得了这么严重的病，因为李女士的母亲刚刚因为癌症去世，她的父亲无法再承受更大的打击，于是李女士对父亲隐瞒了病情。

　　她带着父亲的检查报告前来求医问药。检查报告上显示肝癌指数 AFP 高达 2000 多，其他肝功能转氨酶胆红素也都明显增高，于是她要求我们给她父亲治疗。开始只能根据他的症状进行辨证分析，辨证用药。以后李先生也都不知道自己的真实病情，他只知道是因为肚子膨胀，双腿严重水肿，每天吃几次中药即可。同时他还有严重的痛风，面色萎黄等问题都需要治疗。经过几个月的治疗之后，他的病情有所好转，水肿和黄疸逐渐减少到消失。就这样在患者完全不知情的情况下经过治疗使得病情一步步好转。患者本人因为完全不了解病情反而没有任何精神压力。他自己说，现在能吃能睡，痛风也没有发作了，身体非常好。

肝癌是严重危害着人们健康的重大疾病，病死率高，症状隐匿，发现时多已是晚期。作为中华文化的瑰宝，采用博大精深的生命修复中医药治疗包括肝癌的多种癌症，都取得了成功，确实值得进一步研究和发扬。

大多数肝癌患者在确诊时已属晚期，所能采用的现代综合治疗方法常限制在放、化疗和免疫治疗上，但治疗的毒副反应大，疗效也并不理想。而中医药没有毒副作用，对癌症的预防和治疗都有着明确的作用，无疑可以发扬中西医学的优势。

李先生确诊已属晚期，加上高龄，手术、TACE（肝动脉插管化疗栓塞）、射频消融术等均不适合，故此首选生命修复中医治疗，以扶正祛邪，先稳定病情，并逐步深入治疗。

肝癌在中医古代文献的记载中，包括了黄疸、鼓胀、肝积等范畴。发病多由正气亏虚，不能抵御外邪，加上感受邪毒、情志抑郁、饮食损伤，以致肝气郁结，气滞血瘀，肿块因而产生。肝癌患者常见症状有胁痛、上腹肿块、腹胀、食欲不振、消瘦、甚至黄疸、腹水等，虽然临床症状复杂，但在治疗上仍以辨证论治为原则。具有中医学特色的为"三肝症"，如患者李先生可见到的，有红丝赤缕（蜘蛛痣）、朱砂掌（肝掌）、肝瘿线，即舌体两侧边缘呈青紫色的条纹状或斑状瘀点。他表现出肝郁脾虚证，常伴有疲倦乏力，纳少便溏，舌胖大或齿印，苔白，脉弦细等，治疗时以疏肝散结、益气健脾为主。

治疗原则

扶正祛邪，疏肝散结，化瘀健脾。

常用中药

1. 人参、黄芪、山药、枳实、郁金、鳖甲、土鳖虫、白花蛇舌草、八月炸、夏枯草等。
2. 同时服用消瘤丸、化瘀丸。

影像学、病理学检查报告及诊疗记录

1. 2022 年 4 月 12 日检查报告显示肝酶、胆红素等多项指数显著异常。

2. 2022 年 4 月 20 日检查报告显示肝脏有 4.1cm×3.7cm×4.8cm 肿瘤，考虑肝癌。

3. 2022 年 4 月 20 日肝癌指数甲胎蛋白 AFP 显著升高达 2214ng/ml。

4. 2023 年 1 月 5 日检查报告显示肝酶指数等多项指标明显好转，已达正常。

附：患者检查报告

體檢診斷中心有限公司
Healthcheck & Diagnostic Centre Limited

Print Date : 2022/04/13

Send To 送呈　　　：DR.

Date 日期：**2022/04/12**

Name 姓名　　　：LEE

Age 年齡：-　　　　Sex 性別：M

Sample ID 檢驗編號：

Patient ID：

#	TEST 項目	RESULT 結果	NORMAL RANGE 正常值
	Biochemistry 生化檢驗		
1	Urea 尿素	7.01 mmol/l	M: 3.2-7.4 F: 2.5-6.7
2	Creatinine 肌酸酐	91.4 umol/l	Child (0-13 yrs) : 1.8-6.0
			Female : 50.4-98.1
			Male : 63.6-110.5
3	Sodium 鈉	139.8 mmol/l	135-150
4	Potassium 鉀	4.68 mmol/l	3.5-5.0
5	Chloride 氯	100.7 mmol/l	98-110
6	Uric Acid 尿酸	↑ 508 umol/l	M:210-420 F:150-350
7	Protein Total 總蛋白	61.4 g/l	60-80
8	Albumin 白蛋白	↓ 30.6 g/l	35-50
9	Globulin 球蛋白	30.8 g/l	22-35
10	A/G Ratio 白蛋白球蛋白比	↓ 0.99	1.0-2.27
11	Total Bilirubin 總膽紅素	↑ 39.1 umol/l	3.4-20.5
12	Direct Bilirubin 直接膽紅素	↑ 24.7 umol/l	0-8.6
13	Alk.phosphatase 鹼性磷酸酶	↑ 304 U/l	Ad: 40-150 Ch: <750
14	SGOT/AST 谷草轉氨酶	↑ 307 IU/l	5-40
15	SGPT/ALT 谷丙轉氨酶	↑ 251 IU/l	0-55

Remark:　Icteric +

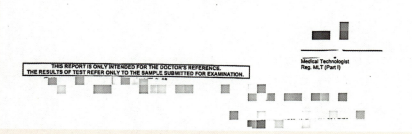

Medical Technologist
Reg. MLT (Part I)

體檢診斷中心有限公司
Healthcheck & Diagnostic Centre Limited

To Dr. :

Name LEE :   **Date** 20 Apr. 2022

Sex M   **Age** 71   **Exam. No.**

Examination(s): Ultrasound of the Upper Abdomen

Report :-

Ultrasound Upper Abdomen:

The liver size is enlarged. There is generalised accentuation of hepatic echogenicity with preserved architecture, compatible with fatty change. A 4.1 x 3.7 x 4.8cm hypoechogenic area is seen in segment 7 ?HCC. The intrahepatic biliary ducts are not dilated. The common bile duct is normal. The portal vein is not dilated. Gallbladder is normally distended. No gallbladder wall thickening or filling defect. There is no gallstone.

The spleen is not enlarged. No focal abnormality is seen.

Both kidneys are of normal size and smooth outline. There is normal cortico-medullary differentiation. No mass lesion is seen. No abnormal renal sinus echogenicity.

No dilated calyces. No evidence of hydronephrosis.   The perinephric areas are clear.

Pancreas outlines normally. There is preservation of the peri-pancreatic tissue plane. No mass lesion is noted.

Aorta is normal in calibre. No aneurysm is seen.

Comment:

Mild fatty liver.
Hepatomegaly.
Hepatic hypoechogenic area ?HCC. CT liver suggested.

Dr   醫生

339

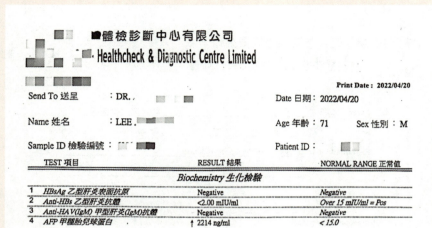

體檢診斷中心有限公司
Healthcheck & Diagnostic Centre Limited

Print Date : 2022/04/20

Send To 送呈 ：DR.

Date 日期：2022/04/20

Name 姓名 ：LEE

Age 年齡：71　　Sex 性別：M

Sample ID 檢驗編號：

Patient ID：

	TEST 項目	RESULT 結果	NORMAL RANGE 正常值
	Biochemistry 生化檢驗		
1	HBsAg 乙型肝炎表面抗原	Negative	Negative
2	Anti-HBs 乙型肝炎抗體	<2.00 mIU/ml	Over 15 mIU/ml = Pos
3	Anti-HAV(IgM) 甲型肝炎(IgM)抗體	Negative	Negative
4	AFP 甲種胎兒球蛋白	↑ 2214 ng/ml	< 15.0

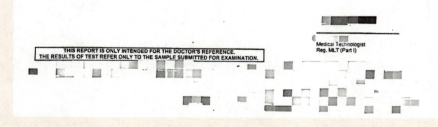

THIS REPORT IS ONLY INTENDED FOR THE DOCTOR'S REFERENCE.
THE RESULTS OF TEST REFER ONLY TO THE SAMPLE SUBMITTED FOR EXAMINATION.

Medical Technologist
Reg. MLT (Part I)

體檢診斷中心有限公司
Healthcheck & Diagnostic Centre Limited

Print Date : 2023/01/05

Send To 送呈　　　：DR.

Date 日期：2023/01/05

Name 姓名　　　：LEE ■

Age 年齡：-　　　Sex 性別：M

Sample ID 檢驗編號：■ ■

Patient ID：■

	TEST 項目	RESULT 結果	NORMAL RANGE 正常值
	Biochemistry 生化檢驗		
1	Protein Total 總蛋白	75.5 g/l	60-80
2	Albumin 白蛋白	42.4 g/l	35-50
3	Globulin 球蛋白	33.1 g/l	22-35
4	A/G Ratio 白蛋白球蛋白比	1.28	1.0-2.27
5	Total Bilirubin 總膽紅素	18.4 umol/l	3.4-20.5
6	Direct Bilirubin 直接膽紅素	6.53 umol/l	0-8.6
7	Alk.phosphatase 鹼性磷酸酶	↑ 174 U/l	Ad: 40-150　Ch: <750
8	SGOT/AST 谷草轉氨酶	29.9 IU/l	5-40
9	SGPT/ALT 谷丙轉氨酶	15.7 IU/l	0-55

Medical Technologist
Reg. MLT (Part I)

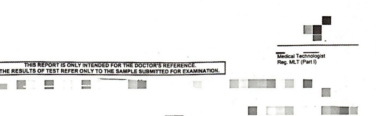

341

病案51

老年人晚期胆管癌同获良效

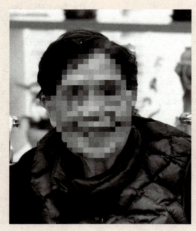

胡老太 84 岁了，身体瘦弱，患有多种慢性疾病，高血压、高血脂、糖尿病病史 30 多年，长期服用治疗三高类疾病的药物也有 30 多年了。平时身体弱不经风，并伴有慢性肾功能衰竭，经过检查肾功能只有常人的 1/3，还有慢性胃病等多种疾病缠身。2022 年 4 月，她的胃痛症状加

○ 胡老太近照

重，并且经常呕吐，以为是老毛病，也没有及时去医院。直到 2022 年 10 月，胃痛越来越重，去医院检查发现患了肝脏肿瘤，有 5cm×7cm 大小。12 月中旬再去检查时发现肿瘤生长很快，已经有 11.6cm×8.1cm 大小。反映胆管癌的癌指数 CA19-9 高达 203.3，反映肝脏癌变的 AFP 指数高达 1071.3。确诊为胆管癌，多发肝脏、气管旁、腹腔、主动脉旁等转移，并有乳腺肿瘤等。因为她的岁数很大了，身体又非常差，儿女们都担心她不能承受化疗、手术等治疗的风险，并且医院已经告知晚期胆管癌是癌中之王。经过家人一起商量，决定不做手术也不做化疗了。这种情况只能前来进行中医药治疗。

　　她刚来时身体非常瘦弱，疼痛严重，不能直起腰身。同时已多日不能进食，腹痛严重，10多天没有大便。根据她的情况，我们给予扶正抗邪为主，进行有效的中医药治疗。服药治疗后，从第2周开始，她的精神面貌大为改观，满面笑容。诉说吃了中药感觉很舒服，没有疼痛，大小便也通畅了，胃口好转。但正当积极治疗之际，胡老太再次来诊的时候又出现精神很差，呻吟不止的情况。详细询问病情，原来老人家不小心突然摔倒，严重摔伤，双手和全身都有很多大的瘀斑，全身疼痛，不能活动，呕吐、腹痛再度加重。根据这种严重情况，再给予辅助正气调理，化瘀、止痛、抗癌、消瘤等多方面的治疗。渐渐地老人家又慢慢恢复起来了。在胡老太有严重疾病的情况下，加上严重摔伤，对一般人来说都是难以承受的，对一位重病缠身的老年人来说，更是非常严重，非常危险的情况。但是生命修复的中医药治疗仍然是非常有效的。老人家现在又恢复了，精神状态良好，胃口不错，每天能正常饮食。全身的疼痛也已经消失，她自己和她的家人们都很有信心进行下一步的抗癌治疗。

　　生命修复中医药治疗年老体弱多病的癌症患者有强大的优势。老年癌症患者全身器官退化，老化，衰竭，生理功能下降，全身正气严重不足，多种疾病并存，同时肿瘤生长迅速，如没有及时正确的治疗，易于短期内严重恶化。

　　生命修复的中医药治疗没有毒副作用，年老体弱者同样从中受益良多。我们重视从整体出发和个体化治疗，对患者的治疗从全身出发，对不能接受手术、放化疗的癌症患者治疗效果也同样显著，能使患者最大程度的受益，进一步战胜癌症，及早恢复正常的生活，使生命之树长青。

治疗原则

扶正祛邪，化瘀消瘤。

常用中药

1. 鹿茸、人参、龟胶、三七、柴胡、红花、山药、赤芍、贝母、八月炸等。
2. 同时服用消瘤丸、化瘀丸。

影像学、病理学检查报告及诊疗记录

1. 2022 年 11 月 10 日 PET/CT 检查报告证实肝脏有 5.44cm×7.42cm 的肿瘤，考虑为胆管癌。

2. 2022 年 12 月 16 日 PET/CT 检查报告证实肝脏肿瘤增大到 11.64cm×8.13cm，并有肝内转移、肝门、腹主动脉旁、气管旁等多处淋巴转移。

附：患者检查报告

▪▪ MRI & Diagnostic Centre
磁力共振及诊断中心

REF. / TO	: DR. ▪ ▪ ▪			
PT's NAME	: Wu, ▪	**PT's ID**	:	▪
中文名	: 胡▪▪	**D.O.B.**	: 28/04/1940	
SEX / AGE	: F / 82Y	**REF. NO.**	:	
EXAM. DATE	: 10/11/2022	**CASE NO.**	: EM▪	

REPORT BY	: DR. ▪ ▪	**MAGNETIC RESONANCE IMAGING REPORT**

COMMENTS

- The intrahepatic ducts appear dilated.
- A mass lesion *(5.44 x 7.42cm)* is noted in the left lobe of the liver involving both medial and lateral segment. Associated dilatation of the left intrahepatic ducts are noted. Medially, this mass has extended to the upper end of the common duct. The right intrahepatic ducts are also dilated. Overall feature is suspicious of a tumour, and a cholangiocarcinoma has to be considered. Infective change and liver abscess is less likely in this case. Further evaluation +/- histology correlation will be needed.
- The left portal vein is not seen, can suggest tumour compression / thrombosis.
- No focal mass of pancreas is seen.
- There are bilateral renal cysts.
- There is no abnormal pelvic mass or fluid collection.

Thank you for your referral.

Dr. ▪▪ ▪
Specialist in Radiology
MBChB (CUHK) FRCR FHKCR FHKAM (Radiology)

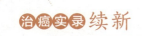

PET 00114650

醫院 同 位 素 及 正 電 子 掃 描 部
Department of Nuclear Medicine & Positron Emission Tomography
HOSPITAL
Tel:
Fax:

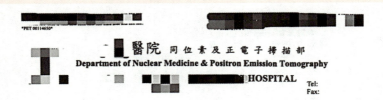

Above the diaphragm, there are multiple primarily ^{11}C-acetate lymph nodes at the right cardiophrenic, right internal mammary, bilateral prevascular and right paratracheal regions. The lymph nodes only demonstrates background to minimal ^{18}F-FDG uptake. In the thorax, there is normal size and metabolism of lung segments. No pleural or pericardial effusion is seen. Thyroid gland is prominent with heterogeneous density, suggestive of benign nodules. Nasopharynx is unremarkable. Bilateral paranasal sinuses are patent. There is a small ^{18}F-FDG-avid focus at the most lateral border of right breast 10 o'clock position. The left breast shows no hypermetabolic intramammary lesion. No hypermetabolic lymphadenopathy is found at bilateral axillae.

Skeletal survey shows scoliosis of thoracolumbar spine with degenerative change. No focal hypermetabolic marrow lesion is detected in axial or proximal appendicular skeleton.

Functional parameters of these lesions are tabulated as below:

WU,			C-11 ACT		F-18 FDG	
	in mm		Standard	Delayed	Standard	Delayed
Site	LD	PD	SUVmax	SUVmax	SUVmax	SUVmax
Large primarily FDG-avid mass at L lobe of liver	116.4	81.3	5.7	5.0	14.2	17.2
Small FDG-avid lesion at subcapsular segment IVa of liver	10.5	9.8	-	-	7.7	-
R internal mammary node	8.9	7.7	4.9	-	1.5	-
R paratracheal node	9.9	9.4	4.2	-	2.0	-
R cardiophrenic node	14.3	10.4	6.2	5.8	1.9	1.9
Aortocaval node	10.5	9.4	4.1	4.3	1.4	1.5
L para-aortic node	10.5	9.9	5.8	5.4	2.0	1.9
L para-aortic node 2	13.0	7.6	4.8	4.5	1.4	1.6
FDG activity at ileocecal junction	23.7	16.0	-	-	6.7	-
Small focus at most lateral border of R breast 10H position	7.2	6.8	-	-	1.7	-

Note: LD=longest diameter; PD=diameter perpendicular to LD

<u>Impression:</u>

1. There is a large and markedly ^{18}F-FDG-avid mass involving the most of left lobe of liver with only mild ^{11}C-acetate activity and significant central necrosis, associated with dilated left intrahepatic ducts. The overall feature are highly suggestive of cholangiocarcinoma or cholangioHCC.
2. A small pure ^{18}F-FDG-avid lesion at the subcapsular region of segment IVa of liver is suggestive of intrahepatic metastasis.
3. There are multiple prominent lymph nodes at the portal, left para-aortic and aortocaval regions, as well as across the diaphragm to right cardiophrenic, right internal mammary, bilateral prevascular and right paratracheal regions. However, these lymph nodes demonstrate different metabolic

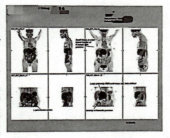

行之有效的养生康复方法

明代《正统道藏洞神部》说："呬主肺，肺连五脏，受风即鼻塞，有疾作呬吐纳治之。呵字，呵主心，心连舌，心热舌干，有疾作呵吐纳治之。呼字，呼主脾，脾连唇，脾火热即唇焦，有疾作呼吐纳治之。嘘字，嘘主肝，肝连目，论云肝火盛则目赤，有疾作嘘吐纳治之。嘻字，嘻主三焦，有疾作嘻吐纳治之。"明代医学专著《寿世保元》说："不炼金丹，且吞玉液，呼出脏腑之毒，吸入天地之清。"又说："五脏六腑之气，因五味熏灼不知，又六欲七情，积久生病，内伤脏腑，外攻九窍，以致百骸受病，轻则痼癖，甚则盲废，又重则伤亡，故太上悯之，以六字诀治五脏六腑之病。其法以呼字而自泻去脏腑之毒气，以吸气而自采天地之清气补气。当日小验，旬日大验，年后百病不生，延年益寿，卫生之宝，非人勿传，呼有六曰：嘘、呵、呼、呬、吹、嘻也，吸则一而已。呼有六者，以呵字治心气，以呼字治脾气，以呬字治肺气，以嘘字治肝气，以吹字治肾气，以嘻字治胆气。此六字诀，分主五脏六腑也。"

六字诀对于人体的益处在于通过呼吸、动作、意念进行导引，天人合一，使人体能够吸地阴之精气上升，吸天阳之轻气。六字诀养生法，是中国古代流传下来的一种养生方法，有悠久的历史渊源，是以自然界春夏秋冬五运六气的变化，结合五行的生克制化与五脏六腑的属性，以五音作为发音，进行的有深邃内涵的健身方法。六字诀传至唐代，著名医药学家孙思邈进一步发扬光大。并按五行相生之顺序，配合四时之季节，进一步完善。

《吕氏春秋》中说："筋骨瑟缩不达，故作为舞以宣导之。"《庄子》中说："吹呴呼吸，吐故纳新，熊径鸟伸，为寿而已矣。"在西汉时期《王褒传》一书中，也有"呵嘘呼吸如矫松"的记载。在《养性延命录》一书中说："凡行气，以鼻纳气，以口吐气，微而行之名曰长息，纳气有一，吐气有六。纳气一者谓吸也，吐气六者谓吹、呼、嘻、呵、嘘、呬，皆为长息吐气之法。时寒可吹，时温可呼，委曲治病，吹以去风，呼以去热，嘻以去烦，呵以下气，嘘以散滞，呬以解极。"隋代天台高僧智顗大法师，在他所著的《修习止观坐禅法要》一书中，也提出了六字诀治病方法。他谈道：但观心想，用六种气治病者，即是观能治病，何谓六种气，一吹、二呼、三嘻、四呵、五嘘、六呬，此六种息皆于唇口中，想心方便，转侧而坐，绵微而用。颂曰：心配属呵肾属吹，脾呼肺呬圣皆知，肝脏热来嘘字治，三焦壅处但言嘻。

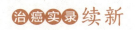
六字诀的功法

◇ 预备式

练习预备式时，可采用从头到脚各部位默念松静二字，逐步放松进而以意领气达到入静。

其中"放松"是最重要的精髓。放松要求精神和肢体均高度放松。精神放松是指大脑神经处于飘然清爽舒松的状态；肢体放松应舒适自然，动作要柔和舒展，切勿僵持。

练习以松静站立为基本方法，具体如下。

1. 松静站立，头要中正，顶要虚悬。头顶如悬，好似在百会穴（在头顶之正中点）处有绳子吊起之意。

2. 含胸拔背，就是胸部微微放松内含，背部撑圆。

3. 沉肩坠肘、松腰塌胯及双腿微屈：如稍下坐姿式；虚腋，就是腋窝处放松留空，两臂自然放松在身体两侧。

预备式姿势的要点就是"头顶如悬"和"松腰塌胯"。

"头顶如悬"时注意下腭内收，颈部垂直，则"含胸拔背""松腰塌胯"及"双腿微屈"就相应的容易做出来。

◇ 顺式腹呼吸法

六字诀是以吐音，呼吸为主的吐纳法。

随呼气吐出脏腑之浊，随吸气吸进天地之清，是以鼻吸口呼的顺式腹呼吸作为练习的方法。呼吸要纯任自然，不疾不徐。呼气时同时作收腹提肛缩肾；吸气时小腹放松，口唇微闭，舌抵上腭，这就叫顺式腹呼吸。

六字诀要求呼有意，吸无意，腹腔内之浊气随读字吐出，大自然界之清气由鼻腔吸进，不必用力下沉而小腹自然隆起。"提肛"随着收腹把肛门逐渐收缩起来。臀部两侧大约环跳穴部位向中间收缩，会阴穴处也同时收缩。"小腹放松"就是随吸气自然慢慢隆起。

◇ 动作配合法

根据养生古籍记载，六字诀还可用动作配合法如下。

肝若嘘时目瞪睛，肺和呬气手双擎；
心呵顶上连叉手，肾吹抱取膝头平；
脾病呼时须撮口，三焦客热卧嘻宁。

下降，吐出五脏六腑之浊毒之气，培补真元，疏通经络，调和脏腑，促进免疫功能，以强身、养生、治病。

锻炼中把预备式要点有机地糅合在一起，以舒松自然为度，形成舒展外延之势，达到"形正势圆"的要求，进入"体松气顺"之境界。

◇ 六字诀发音方法

六字诀有三种发音方法，一是震动声带，即念出声来的发音法；二是以锻炼气息的调控为主，以送出气流为主的发音法；三是不发出声音的锻炼方法。在养生古籍《修龄要指》中特意提出"六字诀，以口吐鼻吸，耳不闻声，乃妙。"

故笔者认为应先重点练习不出声的锻炼方法。根据个人喜好和习惯，也可以后进行出声的六字诀练习，自己作为对比练习。

◇ 六字吐音与功效

嘘（发音 xū），作用于肝。肝为将军之官，肝气与春季相应，可养护肝胆和治疗肝胆疾病。例如胸胁胀满，头目眩晕，急躁易怒，眼目疾病等。

呵（发音 hē），作用于心。心主神明，为五脏六腑之主，心气与夏季相应，念呵可养护心脏，治疗心病。如心神烦躁，失眠健忘，口舌生疮，心悸失眠等症。

呼（发音 hū），作用于脾。脾为后天之本，气血生化之源，念呼可补益脾气，治疗脾病如腹胀腹泻，疲乏无力，食欲不振，肠道疾病，痰湿水肿等症。

呬（发音 sì）作用于肺。肺主一身之气，秋季与肺相应，可养护肺脏，治疗肺病如咳嗽，气短鼻塞，痰喘等症。

吹（发音 chuī）作用于肾。肾为先天之本，冬季与肾相应，念吹可养护肾脏，治疗肾脏疾病如腰痛，阳痿，月经不调，妇科疾病，腰膝无力等症。

嘻（发音 xī）作用于三焦。三焦是六腑之一，是上焦、中焦、下焦的统称，三焦的功能是通调水道，保持上中下三焦气血运行的通畅。念嘻字可养护三焦，对于上、中、下三焦不畅之症，均有调理作用，如眩晕，耳鸣，胸腹胀闷，小便不利等。

以上这六个字，每个字都作用于相应的脏腑，吐音时拖长音，持续于整个呼气的过程。每个字念 6 次为 1 遍，一般念 6～36 遍。

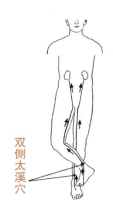
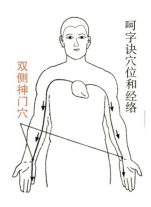
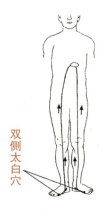

吹字诀穴位和经络　双侧太溪穴

呵字诀穴位和经络　双侧神门穴

呼字诀穴位和经络　双侧太白穴

图 1　六字诀

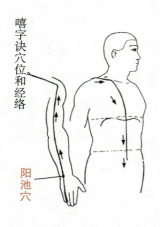

嘻字诀穴位和经络

阳池穴

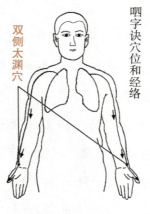

双侧太渊穴

呬字诀穴位和经络

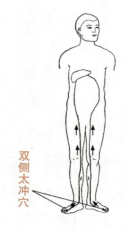

嘘字诀穴位和经络

双侧太冲穴

图1（续）　六字诀

◇　五行相生练习法

五行相生的顺序是木生火、火生土、土生金、金生水、水生木，按照这个次序，六字诀的排列顺序是：嘘、呵、呼、呬、吹、嘻。

按五行相生顺序练习是常规的练习方法。因为肝属木，木生火，肝气可扶助心气，肝藏血可济生心血。心属火，火生土，心气可以生脾胃之土气，心之阳气可化生脾胃之阳，使消化吸收功能健全。脾属土，土生金，可使肺功能健全。金生水，肺气健全生肾气，肾气虚者可补肺气。水生木，肾为肝之母。滋水涵木可使肝气健全。

◇ 五行相克练习法

某脏腑之气血过旺，可用克法。

例如，用金克木的方法，如肝阳太盛，形成肝阳上亢的头痛眩晕时，肝属木，肺属金，可用肺金克肝木。念呬字强健肺气，因肺气足可以平肝、滋水、潜阳，以抑制肝阳上亢，治疗头痛。

◇ 母子同练法

母病及子或子病及母，而成为母子皆病者，则母子同练。母之脏病累及子脏或子之脏病累及母脏而选择练习者，需母子二脏之音都要练。

要辨别分清母脏和子脏的虚实，以做正确练习。如心病，心火旺而致不思饮食，腹胀，便秘，为心脾同病，母子同病。如心脾均为实证，则念呼字和呬字，为泻心之子与泻脾之子的练习。

◇ 季节练习法

根据不同季节与五脏的关系，和六字诀与不同季节的相应而练习。如春季练嘘字，夏季练呵字，秋季练呬字，冬季练吹字。

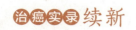

◇ **针对性练习法**

可以针对具体的情况，单练一个字或两个字。如生气时可念嘘字，口舌生疮可念呵字，腹胀腹泻可念呼字，感冒咳嗽可念呬字，肾虚及腰膝疼痛可念吹字，一般念 6～36 遍。

◇ **补虚法**

主要锻炼属于虚损的五脏，为子虚补其母法。

如肾有虚证而致腰膝疲软、失眠、多梦、健忘等症状，可练习和念呬字，因为呬属肺，肺为金，肾为水，补金生水之意，补养肺金以济肾水。以此类推。如肝病练吹字法，心病练嘘字法，脾病练呵字法，肺病练呼字法。

锻炼补虚法之时，一定要注意，先进行辨证分析，确实了解到本脏是属于虚损状态的，才可以用补虚法练习。

◇ **泻实法**

如母病属实证，可用泻其子之法来治疗。

如肝容易患急躁易怒，胸肋痛，头痛目赤，小便黄，大便干等症候，可选用心之音呵字，平心气以泻肝火，以此类推。如心病练呼字法，脾病练呬字法，肺病练吹字法，肾病练嘘字法。

锻炼泻实法之时，一定要注意，先进行辨证分析，确定了解到本脏是属于旺，实状态的，才可以用泻实法练习。

◇ 六字诀经脉循行路线

经络循行练习法有两种方法。

1. 在开始学习和练习时间不长，不够熟练时，在念不同的字诀和呼气时，可意想此经络中指定的一对左右相同的穴位。

2. 练习时间长了，熟悉该条经络循行路线之后，在呼气同时，意念随双侧经络从起端至末端。经络在一定部位发生阻隔时，都会由于经气运行不畅，气滞血瘀而引起疾患。因此在念六字诀时以意导引气血，使之在经络管道中通畅地运行，达到导滞、通瘀的作用。六字诀治病的机制，旨在于此。此即"以意领气"，需要在熟练地掌握吐音、动作、呼吸，了解有关脏器的经脉走向，在松静达到一定程度以后进行。

呼气时意想相应的经络循行，或意念本经原穴，如以下各经练习所述，都能起到很好的疏经活络作用。开始练习可不加意想，在呼气读音时，用心体会每个字气血循经路线，然后逐渐加入意想练习，久而久之水到渠成，自然就能做到意到气到，气到血行的目的。具体练习方法如下。

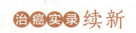

"嘘"字诀

1. 在呼气时同时意想双侧太冲穴。

2. 经络循行：意想呼气时经气从双足部大趾内侧（靠小趾侧）起，沿下肢内侧中线上行，经小腹入肝。

"呵"字诀

1. 呼气时同时意想双侧神门穴。

2. 经络循行：呼气时意想经气从双腋下沿双臂内侧行至小指端。

"吹"字诀

1. 呼气时同时意想双侧足部太溪穴。

2. 经络循行：呼气时意想经气由双足心起，经内踝，沿腿内侧后缘上行，经小腹入两肾。

"呼"字诀

1. 呼气时同时意想双足部太白穴。

2. 经络循行：呼气时意想经气从足部内侧脾经太白穴，沿小腿、大腿内侧中线上行，经小腹入脾。

"呬"字诀

1. 呼气时同时意想双侧太渊穴。

2. 经络循行：呼气时意想经气从胸前体上方沿手臂内侧前缘到大指端外侧。

"嘻"字诀

1. 呼气时同时意想双手腕部阳池穴。

2. 经络循行：呼气时意想经气从双手无名指的外侧起，沿手背向上，在双肩处，至大椎，再向前，入缺盆部，从胸至腹入上、中、下三焦。

六字诀练习需要循序渐进，不能急于求成。其中"经脉循行练习法"比较复杂或不易记住，可先不练习，只有掌握前面简单易学易练的方法，循序渐进，才能收到很好的效果。

◇ 六字诀功法的特点

一、有病无病都可练

对于各种不同疾病，包括癌症患者和不同疑难病症患者，都可起到养生调理，减少病痛，无病养生，增强体质的良好作用。

二、简易实用

六字诀的发声和口型简单，易记。小腹起伏，与大多数人在安静时或睡眠时的呼吸是一致的，都是腹式呼吸。导引的动作也很简单，儿童、少年、青年、成人、老年人均可练习，一般 1～3 个月有显著效果。

三、按需选练

六字诀运用灵活，可以按顺序练习，也可以有针对性地练1个或2个字；既可以长期坚持连续练习六字诀，也可以根据不同情况单独练某1个字；还可根据个人身体条件和病情疾患的虚实需要进行补泻练习。

四、不出偏差

只要按照要求练习，注意松静自然，毫不用力，不要紧张，全身各个部位都完全放松。轻松呼吸、轻松意念，一步一步地进行操练，循序渐进，就不会出现偏差。希望大家都能取得理想的效果。

养生静坐功

在几千年前的中医宝典《素问·上古天真论》中就提到了"提挈天地，把握阴阳，呼吸精气，独立守神，肌肉若一"，就是用运筹阴阳的呼吸锻炼，以及全身肢体，肌肉的协调配合来养生和治疗疾病。

静坐和站桩养生，就是这样的流传千年的养生方法。在当代更被世界各地的科学研究证实是有益健康、康复疾病的方法，也是对健康人和癌症等疑难病症患者的良好健身方法。

静坐应以坐式为准，如果年老体衰，身体过分虚弱，可采取卧式，也是很好的锻炼方法。

一、卧式

卧式分仰卧和侧卧两种。

1.仰卧式

自然平卧。仰面朝天躺着，下肢自然伸直。脚跟靠拢或稍分开，足尖自然分开放松。上肢自然伸直，置于体侧。十指松展，掌心向内或向下，或两掌叠放于腹部。枕的高低要适宜，以身体舒适和有利于放松为限。要保持呼吸流畅，躯干正直。双目微闭，微露一线之光。口轻闭，以鼻吸鼻呼或鼻吸口呼为主。

2.侧卧式

侧身卧于床上，左、右侧卧均可。一般采用右侧卧。头微前俯。头之高低由枕头调节，以舒适和放松为宜。口唇轻闭，躯干微屈。腰宜稍弯，略呈弓形，显现出含胸拔背之势。右侧卧时，右上肢自然弯曲。五指舒松，掌心向上，置于枕上靠头脸部。左上肢自然伸直，五指松开，掌心向下，放于同侧髋部。右下肢自然伸直，或略微弯曲。左下肢膝关节弯曲约120°，轻放于右下肢膝部。

二、坐式

坐式分平坐、自然盘坐、单盘坐和双盘坐四种。

1.平坐

以臀部前半部或前1/3部端坐于硬方凳或椅子上。上身自然端正，头要正直，下颌微收，含胸松肩，放松肘臂。十指舒松略屈，掌心向下，放于大腿膝部，或两手掌交叠放于下腹部。两足平行分开，两膝与肩同宽。两小腿与大腿弯曲的角度约为100°～120°，口眼轻闭。

平坐为坐式中最普遍、最常用的姿势，适合各种年龄与各种体质的静坐者。年老体弱者习练静坐，可将坐式与卧式交替进行。两足以舒适、平展、松弛为宜。

2. 自然盘坐

上半身与平坐式相同。唯两小腿交叉，足掌向后向外，臀部着垫。两手互相轻握，置于腹前或分放于大腿上。

3. 单盘坐

上体与手的位置同自然盘坐。唯将左足置于右腿上，或右足置于左腿上。

4. 双盘坐

上体与手的位置同自然盘坐。将左足置于右腿上，同时将右足置于左腿上。两足心向上朝天。双盘坐有一定难度，可逐步锻炼，不需强求。盘坐有助于思想入静，上身及头部的紧张状态易于解除。练习者可根据自身条件和体质从四种坐姿中选择一种。

三、静坐要点

1.静坐时，首先要全身放松，肌肉不要有任何紧张。感受身体变得轻松安静，并将这种轻松和安静传遍全身。

2.开始练习时，可能无法集中放松，各种想法很多，无法安静下来。这时不要急躁，注意将各种念头拉回自身，不要去想外界的事情，而要关注自己的内在，将自己的精神拉回自身。

3. 将全身进一步放松，将大脑放松，体验全身和大脑放松的舒服感觉。

4. 全身和大脑放松的感觉逐渐延长，由开始的几秒钟、几分钟，逐渐延长到十几分钟，以至越来越长。

5. 如果杂念出现，应自动觉察到并让其自动消失。

6. 静坐的时间，可长可短，自行掌握。调理重病、大病者，当然保持较长时间较好。

7. 静坐时衣着宽松，不要紧束身体，衣服要厚薄适宜，精神愉悦，平静，全身放松，练习前先清理干净大小便，以免中途中断练功。

8. 练习过程中或在一定的阶段中，全身或肌肉皮肤有发痒、发热、发冷、蚂蚁爬行、风吹、打哈欠、嗳气、排气、肠鸣、肌肉酸痛等均属正常现象，不必理会，使其自然消失即可。

9. 剧烈运动后、精神紧张、生气发怒、饮酒、过饱、过饥、饭后，均不宜静坐。并注意选择空气清新，环境气温适宜之处，过冷、过热、大风、过于潮湿、空气污浊等处，均不宜静坐。

10. 静坐结束后可双手相对搓热，用双手指掌自下而上摩擦头面，搓双耳，搓后颈等处，用双手十指梳理头发，指尖摩擦头皮，然后拍打双肩、腰背、双腿，活动双膝、足踝、足趾，

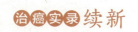

完成此次练习。并注意不要立即饮冷，冲洗冷水等。两手掌搓热熨双眼部，再慢慢睁开眼睛。

以上是根据实践经验，初步练习静坐的基本方法。只要认真练习，精神好转，疲乏减少至消失，食欲增加，睡眠改善，情绪好转，纠结减少，经络、气血运行通畅，无病强身，有病治病，定能取得良好的效果。

静坐是一门高深的学问和锻炼的功法，古往今来有许多大师和有大成就者练习此法。本文以基本的方法，全面展示静坐要点，希望对患者康复及有养生需要者提供帮助。欲进一步深入学习，可拜读历代大师及专家的专著。

养生站桩功

一、自然站式

练习开始时，先将全身架构调整妥当，要内清虚，外松稳，松和自然。内念不外游，外事不内侵，头直，目正，气息平和，扫除心虑，悠然清静。含胸拔背，下颌微内收。虚领顶颈，口眼轻闭。舌轻抵上腭，全身放松。

自然松静站立，手指相对，掌心互照，两脚分开与肩同宽，含胸拔背。

两膝微屈，五趾抓地，下沉涌泉，坐胯松腰。两脚分开，平行一致，两足或呈内八字，全脚掌着地，重心落在两脚心。

松腰胯，两手自然垂于腰侧。或叠放抱于丹田部，或呈圆形抱球状。距丹田部位 25～35cm。

松腕虚腋，上体端正。

自然腹式呼吸，以柔和，轻慢，细长为准。不要憋气，更不要突然中断呼吸。

站桩时间，开始以 5～10 分钟，以后逐渐增加至 20 分钟、30 分钟，以至更长时间。摆好架势之后，要站立不动，不要随意移动，精神集中，收回意念，全身放松，不要有意用力，感觉全身与周围空气混为一体，与天地融为一体。

二、站桩式

站桩式基本方法同上。

下肢可呈半马步或马步式站桩。

手可呈抱球状，亦可呈前拱式，即两手虎口交叉，两掌重叠或两手合掌，成立掌式。也可分别置于腹部，双手可抬至肚脐部或胸下的位置，呈抱树状，或向上抬至胸前，手指伸开自然放松，手心向内。肩部放松不要耸起，肌肉放松，使双肩向下沉堕。双肘之肘尖部下垂朝向下方。收腹、提肛、松腰松胯。

高位站桩，微屈膝，与自然站式相似，适宜于老年人，身体虚弱及病情较重者。

中位站桩屈膝较多，需一定体力支持，适宜于经过练习有一定基础，或身体健康者练习。

低位站桩臀部下坐，好似坐于椅上，需付出较多体能，适宜于身体强健，或更进一步的站桩练习者。

以上是初步练习站桩功的基本功法。可以根据练习者的年龄、性别、体质和健康状况选择使用。

摘抄著名武术学家前辈曾有《站桩歌》如下。

发系云天脚踩地，两臂松撑抱球圆。

十指茫茫放光线，气平心静体自安。

全身虚灵随风动，漫如游泳空气间。

向上托起千斤力，向下浮按水中船。

松紧自如得整劲，身体强壮似神仙。

站桩是一门高深的学问和锻炼功法。古往今来有许多大师或大成就者练习此法。本文以基本的方法全面展示站桩要点，只要认真练习，精神好转，疲乏减少至消失，食欲增加，睡眠改善，情绪好转，纠结减少，经络、气血运行通畅，无病强身，有病治病，希望对患者康复及养生者提供帮助。欲进一步深造者，可拜读历代大师及专家的专著。

食物的五行属性和辨证择食

《汉书·郦食其传》指出："王者以民为天，而民以食为天。"比喻食物是人们赖以生存的最重要的东西。无论是健康者，还是有疾病缠身者，都应该非常重视食物的选择和食用。许多食物都具有"药食同源"的特点，下面介绍有关五行生克制化，辨证择食的内容。以便能使食物养生保健，促进健康，而不是相反的作用。

《黄帝内经》是中医学最早的医学巨著，被称为"医家圣典"，分为《素问》和《灵枢》两部，也是最高深的养生宝典。

五味入五脏就是重要的食物养生内容之一。我们要在日常生活之中，谨慎调和饮食五味，对养生和治病甚有帮助。

一、五味归属五脏的规律

1. 五味所入

《素问·宣明五气》指出："五味所入：酸入肝，辛入肺，苦入心，咸入肾，甘入脾，是为五入。"这种饮食五味归属五脏的理论，是根据五行归类的原则制定的。五脏与五行的关系：肝属木，主疏泄，肝为将军之官，开窍于目。心属火，主血脉，心为君主之官，开窍于舌。脾属土，脾统血，主运化，主升清，开窍于口。肺属金，肺主气司呼吸，肺主宣发，肃降，开窍于鼻。肾主水，肾藏精，肾为先天之本，肾主生殖，开窍于耳。

2. 五脏宜食

《素问·脏气法时论》曰："肝色青，宜食甘，粳米、牛肉、枣、葵皆甘。心色赤，宜食酸，小豆、犬肉、李、韭皆酸。肺色白，宜食苦，麦、羊肉、杏、薤皆苦。脾色黄，宜食咸，大豆、豕肉、栗、藿皆咸。肾色黑，宜食辛，黄黍、鸡肉、桃、葱皆辛。辛散、酸收、甘缓、苦坚、咸软。毒药攻邪，五谷为养，五果为助，五畜为益，五菜为充，气味合而服之，以补精益气。此五者，有辛酸甘苦咸，各有所利，或散或收，或缓或急，或坚或软，四时五脏，病随五味所宜也。"五脏五味所宜，因时因机而宜，或取其属，或取其势，或取其味，或取其性，或取其生制，或取其承化，而非拘于一格。

3. 五脏之苦所宜

如"肝苦急，急食甘以缓之；心苦缓，急食酸以收之；脾苦湿，急食苦以燥；肺苦气上逆，急食苦以泄之；肾苦燥，急食辛以润之。"

4. 五脏之色所宜

肝对应的颜色是青色，适宜食用甘甜味的食物，如粳米、牛肉、枣、葵都是甘甜的。肝苦于急，急食甘以缓之。

心对应的颜色是红色，适宜食用酸味的食物，如李子、韭菜都是酸的。心苦于缓，宜酸物收之。

肺对应的颜色是白色，适宜食用苦味的食物，小麦、羊肉、杏、薤都是苦的。肺苦于气上逆，宜食苦物泄之。

脾对应的颜色是黄色，脾脏恶湿，湿邪容易困脾，使脾运化水湿功能受损。苦有燥湿作用，用苍术，白术等可以燥湿健脾。

肾对应的颜色是黑色，适宜食用辛味的食物，黄黍、鸡肉、桃、葱都是辛的。肾苦于燥，宜辛物润之。

二、五味食物的功效

生肝：酸味能滋养肝脏，酸能敛、能涩。有敛肝止泻，止喘，涩精，敛汗，缩尿等作用，可用于虚汗、泄泻、尿频、咳嗽等。酸味食物有增强消化功能和保护肝脏的作用。以酸味为主的有酸梅、石榴、西红柿、山楂、橙子等。

生心：苦味能滋养心气。古有良药苦口之说，苦味食物能泄、能燥、能坚阴，有清热泻火，清热燥湿作用，所以苦味药可治疗热证、火证、湿证，如胸中烦闷、口渴多痰、心悸烦躁等症状。具有除湿和利尿的作用。像陈皮、茶叶、苦杏仁、苦瓜、百合等，常吃能防止毒素的积累，防治各种疮症。

入脾：甘能补，能和，缓急。性甘的食物可以补养气血、调和药性、解药食之毒、消解疲劳，还具有缓痉止痛等作用。如红糖、桂圆肉、蜂蜜、米面食品等，都是补甘的食物。

入肺：辛能散、能行，有宣散发汗、理气行气、活血等作用。风寒湿邪，外感表证，气血积滞者宜服。常吃的葱、姜、蒜、辣椒、胡椒，均是以辛味为主的食物，这些食物有调理气血、疏通经络的作用。

入肾：咸能下、能软。有泄下、软坚、散结和补益阴血等作用。如盐、海带、紫菜、海藻、牡蛎、海蜇等都是咸味食品，有软坚散结，泻热通便等作用。

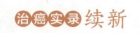

三、因人择食，因病制宜

古代医学家张仲景曾言：所食之味，有与病相宜，有与身为害。若得宜则益体，害则成疾。所以根据自己的体质或病患，辨证择食是非常重要的。

五味应适宜五脏。《素问·脏气法时论》亦有提到：肝病者宜食甘，心病者宜食酸，肺病者宜食苦，脾病者宜食咸，肾病者宜食辛。

在日常应用时要因病制宜，辨清虚实，才能准确运用。比如，肝病食甘，脾病食咸，肺病食苦是根据五行相克理论确定的。木克土，为肝克脾土，所克之脏。土克水，是脾克肾水，所克之脏。而肺病食苦是火克金，克己之脏，以上分别适用于肝病、脾病及肺病之实证，而不能用于肝、脾、肺之虚证。而心病者食酸，肾病者食辛，是根据五行相生理论确定的。虚则补其母，适用于心病，肾病的虚证。而如心病，肾病为实证则不适合运用，故在运用时要根据五行相生克乘侮的机制明辨虚实，才能调理好不同的五味。

四、五味不适宜有损健康

依据五行学说的生克乘侮理论分析，不适当地过度摄食五味，偏嗜饮食会损伤五脏、并造成相应的疾病。

1. 过食酸味肝气偏盛

《素问·生气通天论》说："味过于酸，肝气以津，脾气乃绝。"《灵枢·五味论》说："酸……多食之，令人癃。"酸味入肝脏，故味酸食物走肝以养肝。有疏肝行气，解郁通滞的作用。但过食酸味食物，使肝气偏盛。肝属"木"，脾属"土"，而肝木是克脾土的，肝脏功能偏亢，则脾土就会因肝强受乘而弱，造成木克土。因此如有消化不良，腹胀胃酸，腹泻肿满，胃溃疡，胃炎，肠炎，小便不畅者，不宜多食酸，否则会增多不适或加重病情。因酸有收敛作用，过食酸味食物，使气机运行阻滞，故有可能出现"癃"，即小便排泄不畅通的病症。

脾病不可食酸。酸走筋入肝，酸味食物有收敛、固涩、生津、开胃等功效，适当的食用适量的酸味食物，可促进消化功能、增强肝脏的解毒能力，调味的醋也有抑菌杀菌，舒畅气机的作用。

2. 过食咸味肾气偏旺

咸味食物有催吐、润下、软坚、补肾等功效，食之得当，对人体有益。味过于咸，大骨气劳，短肌，心气抑。《灵枢·五味论》说："咸……多食之，令人渴。""多食咸，令人血脉凝泣而变色。"咸味入肾，故味咸食物走肾以养肾。但过食咸味，致肾自伤，骨骼软弱。进一步影响到其他脏腑，如肾水侮脾土可见脾主肌肉之功能衰弱，肌肉瘦削、萎缩。肾属水而心厉火，如肾气偏旺，会克制心血的功能。肾水乘心火可见心脏之气凝结，使血脉瘀滞，运行不畅。有心脏虚弱、高血压、冠心病等心病、血病者，不要食咸。

3. 过食甘味土克水

甘味有补养气血，补充热量，益胃解毒等作用。味过于甘，心气喘满，色黑，肾气不衡。《灵枢·五味论》说："甘……多食之，令人悗心。"甘味指甜味和淡味的食物，其均入脾脏，故甘甜的食物走脾以养脾。甘有"缓"的特性，过食甘味食物会使上焦心肺气机运行不畅而有心悸喘满；甘入脾，脾属"土"，肾属"水"，土克水，肾病不可食甘。甘走肉入脾，多食甘令人恶心、骨痛而发落，所以肉病不可食甘。食甘过多可影响糖脂代谢，增加血管压力，致使发生肥胖、糖尿病、脂肪肝、痛风、高血压、心脏疾病和脑卒中的风险升高。食甜过多导致土克水，致肾气虚弱，引起记忆力下降，故有糖尿病、肥胖症、厌食症和肾病等患者少食甘。

4. 过食苦味损肺

味过于苦，脾气不濡，胃气乃厚。《灵枢·五味论》说："苦……多食之，令人变呕。"苦味入心，故味苦食物走心以养心。如苦瓜、茶叶味苦，入心脏，两者均有清心泻火、解毒疗疮的作用，适用于心烦尿赤、口舌生疮、疮痈肿毒等病症。由于苦入心，过食苦味食物，会使心脏受伤，而又因心属"火"，脾胃属"土"，心病而"火不生土"，因此脾胃虚衰，出现"脾气不濡，胃气乃厚"的病症。容易上火者宜食苦味，以泄心火，养心阴。苦入心，肺属金，火克金，故有肺病的患者要少食苦。

5. 过食辛味损伤肝

味过于辛，筋脉沮弛，精神乃央。《灵枢·五味论》说："辛……多食之，令人洞心。"辛味指辛香、辛辣食物，入肺脏，故味辛食物走肺以养肺。如葱、姜味辛，辛入肺，所以可以宣肺通鼻、调治肺气不利的鼻塞、流涕等病症。因辛入肺，肺属"金"，肝属"木"，肺金乘肝木，肝主筋，故过食辛致使肝所主之筋脉为病而生肝病。有肝病者不宜食辛，有气病者不可食辛。而金胜反侮火，又使心所主之精神受到损伤。辛走气入肺，多食辛令人愠心，筋急而爪枯。辛味食物有祛风、解表、行气、活血等功效。其多为调料、调味品，食之得当，有增进食欲、帮助消化的作用。过食辛味食物，伤津、耗液而导致大便秘结、口舌生疮、伤气、耗血、并损伤肝的气血。

五、日常生活中的常见五味

1. 酸味食物

醋、西红柿、木瓜、红小豆、马齿苋、柑橘、橄榄、柠檬、杏、枇杷、橙子、山楂、石榴、乌梅、柚、芒果、李子、葡萄、酸枣、酸梨、百香果、蓝莓、番石榴、草莓等。

2. 苦味食物

苦菜、苦瓜、芦笋、芥蓝、莲子芯、大头菜、香椿、蒲公英、槐花、淡豆豉、山慈菇、酒、荷叶、茶叶、香橼、佛手、薤白、杏仁、百合、白果、桃仁、茄子、人参果、青橄榄、油柑、柚子等。

3. 辛味食物

葱、生姜、香菜、芥菜、白萝卜、洋葱、白芥子、茴香、蒜苗、油菜籽、油菜、萝卜子、青蒿、大蒜、大头菜、芹菜、芋头、韭菜子、肉桂、胡椒、紫苏、薄荷、辣椒、韭菜、香橼、薤白、陈皮、佛手、酒等。

4. 甘味食物

莲子、红枣、红薯、红糖、山药、香蕉、萝卜、丝瓜、竹笋、土豆、藕节、菠菜、南瓜、圆白菜、扁豆、芋头、豌豆、胡萝卜、白菜、冬瓜、黄瓜、豆腐、黑大豆、红小豆、绿豆、黄豆、薏苡仁、荞麦、粳米、糯米、高粱、玉米、小麦、黑木耳、蜂蜜、银耳、甘蔗、柿子、苹果、柑、荸荠、梨、花生、白砂糖、甜瓜、西瓜、山楂、菱角、桃、樱桃、橘、柚、黑芝麻、栗子、芒果、无花果、葡萄、核桃、桂圆、松子、香菇、芡实、枸杞子、椰子、菠萝等。

5.咸味食物

盐、大酱、苋菜、大麦、小米、紫菜、海带、海藻、海蜇、海参、蟹、田螺、牡蛎、榴莲等。